Folks,
this ain't
normal

Other Books by Joel Salatin

Folks, this ain't normal

*A Farmer's Advice for
Happier Hens, Healthier People,
and a Better World*

Joel Salatin

CENTER
STREET

New York   Boston   Nashville

Center Street
Hachette Book Group
237 Park Avenue
New York, NY 10017
www.centerstreet.com

Center Street is a division of Hachette Book Group, Inc.
The Center Street name and logo are trademarks of Hachette Book Group, Inc.

The publisher is not responsible for websites (or their content) that are not owned by the publisher.

Printed in the United States of America

First Edition: October 2011

10 9 8 7 6 5

Library of Congress Control Number: 2011928347

ISBN: 978-0-892-96819-0

Contents

Foreword
by Allan Nation

For twenty-five years I have watched Joel Salatin and his family struggle to make a living from a hundred open acres in northern Virginia. In addition to the usual weather vagaries that afflict all agricultural enterprises, Joel and other small farmers like him has had to struggle with government dictates and regulations that, intentionally or unintentionally, have denied him direct access to the marketplace. Most of these regulations are advertised as insuring that the American consumer gets healthy food, but in reality they actually prevent it. A policy of one-size-fits-all regulation means that a regulation that is a minor nuisance to a large industrial processor is a farm killer for a farmer trying to sell directly to a consumer.

As Joel makes clear in this book, these regulations are primarily designed to prevent access to the marketplace, not to regulate food quality or healthfulness. There are no regulations on the food served at a private party or a church social where the food is given away. The regulations only come into play when the food is sold. As Joel asks, what is it about private enterprise that makes the government believe small-scale food production is suddenly so dangerous?

In an era when local foods are all the rage, federal, state, and local regulations greatly hamper the growth of this alternative to industrial foods. No doubt many urban consumers will be shocked to read of the hostile harassment and intimidation put upon small-scale food producers by government inspectors whom Joel Salatin terms "the Food Police." In what other field are you considered guilty until proven innocent? And, when proven innocent, there is never a word of apology or an exculpatory press release? After a few such instances of this, would you keep trying to sell food direct to the consumer?

Unfortunately, this taxpayer-financed war against local food production has operated under the media radar. Hopefully, this book will bring it to the attention of all alternative food consumers. However, there is more to this struggle than just fighting power-mad government bureaucrats. It extends to the menus of restaurants, fast food emporiums, the purchasing policies of alternative food vendors such as Whole Foods, and even to sympathetic consumers like yourself.

The big problem is that everything new has to start small and with a simple and cheap production prototype. Few self-financed farmers have the wherewithal to start at the scale most publicly held corporate customers require. Small farmers sell their labor through their products. Consequently, they seek high-labor, low-capital systems of production just as farmers did a century ago. However, the marketplace is not as flexible as it was a century ago. A restaurant that only wants one cut of meat is of little benefit to a small-scale producer who has to sell all the meat from an animal. Similarly, making a farmer with a husband-and-wife labor force fill out reams of paperwork and forms before they can deliver one bite of food to a franchised food store is a cruel and unusual punishment.

Also, asking a "natural" production system to function year round is an oxymoron. Low capital input requires that the farm's production model is kept in sync with the natural seasons of production. For example, you cannot raise chickens, a tropical animal, outside in foot-deep snow. Making a small farmer perform year round like an industrial factory is a sure formula for his burnout and bankruptcy, plus a recipe for a dull eating experience in the off season for you, the consumer. As the Swiss say, "Winter cheese is boring cheese." In animal products, all the unique flavor nuances in heritage meat and milk come from the animal having consumed green, living grass. These flavors are not there when fed a diet exclusively of hay or silage. The small farmer's competitive edge comes from producing a highly flavorful, high-skill input, seasonal product that can be marketed through a short, inexpensive, distribution chain. Local marketing not only fits this requirement but is usually essential for a profitable, self-sustaining, small-scale farm.

For local food production to continue to grow, the whole regulatory and marketing system is going to have to compromise a bit and meet the farmer halfway. Personally, I am not a "my way or the highway" kind of guy. Like Joel, I do not wish to see industrial agriculture regulated out of business. I just wish to see the consumer allowed to have more of a choice. None of us in alternative agriculture are opposed to government-enforced health standards. What we are opposed to are standards that dictate a high-capital solution when a lower-capital alternative is possible. Tell us what the standard is and then let us devise a way to meet it. Devising lower-capital alternatives is our stock-in-trade, and we are really good at it. Turn us loose.

Joel Salatin is an excellent example of this creativity in creating low-capital production prototypes. He singlehandedly created the North American pastured chicken industry with his low-cost, movable broiler shelters. From using pigs to aerate his compost in the spring to using truly free-ranging chickens to control flies in his pastures, Joel has figured ways to produce food with a minimum of capital inputs and no toxic chemicals. Writing a monthly column in our publication, the *Stockman Grass Farmer,* Joel has shared his ideas, his successes and his failures, with all who cared to read it for twenty-five years. He has absolutely no fear of people following his lead ruining his business with competition. An excellent public speaker, he has traveled the world with his message of the need for revival of a Jeffersonian, intellectual approach to agriculture. Shocking most of his audiences, he shows up to speak in a conservative business suit, white shirt and tie, to indicate that he is a college-educated entrepreneur and not the rural hayseed or neo-hippie they were expecting. Regardless of his audience, he pulls no punches when discussing his libertarian economic beliefs, his social conservatism, or his religious faith. Needless to say this completely discombobulates those who consider all alternative food producers as being from the political left.

Personally, I have long thought that Joel Salatin's Polyface Farm was an excellent example of how high-value, direct-marketed farms like his could be an engine for rural economic development. Joel currently has fourteen employees; he buys all of the supplemental feed his pastured chickens and pigs eat locally, and his animals are all processed locally. Using sweat equity, he has built a two-million-dollar-a-year food business without any government loans, assistance, or subsidies. To me that's a story that should be on the front page of the *Wall Street Journal.*

And his farm is truly beautiful, with extra-green pastures fertilized with the manure of thousands of pastured chickens. In his forested areas, time-control grazed pigs have removed the thick understory and created an open, park-like environment. Small ponds stairstep up the mountainside behind his house, providing water for wildlife plus gravity-fed stockwater and pasture irrigation. If you wanted to jump-start an agritourism economy, nothing would do it better than a hundred farms like Joel's. More jobs, a prettier landscape, and healthier food, all created without any government spending. Doesn't this sound like what America is looking for right now? Here's how to help bring it about.

This meeting the farmer halfway extends to you the consumer. Most of us have been so conditioned by the industrial food system that we don't realize the conflict between our belief system and our expectations. For example, don't expect fresh, unfrozen, grass-fed beef and chicken in the dead of winter at your local store or restaurant. Try to learn enough about farm production prototypes so that you aren't taken in by faux natural systems such as free-range chickens from a confinement house with one tiny door open. Realize that a "USDA Certified Organic" label does not insure that a production method that mimics nature was used. For example, most "Certified Organic" beef comes from industrial-type feedlots, and winter-produced organic milk utilizes the same confinement prototype as industrial milk. Anything labeled "USDA Natural" means absolutely nothing as far as the production method used. "Looks like" and "sounds like" products are a way the industrial food producers profit from the hard marketing work of small-scale producers who really do have something different. Don't get taken in by these charlatans and spend more money for the same old crap with a new label.

As a concerned alternative food consumer, you need to be willing to take personal responsibility for the food you eat. Don't rely on the USDA or the FDA to vet farmers for you; do it yourself. Try to buy as much of your animal protein and dairy products from a farmer whose farm you occasionally visit and try to personally grow as many of the vegetables and eggs you eat as possible. This can start as small as a single flowerpot with a tomato plant in it.

You have your own doctor and dentist. You need a farmer like Joel Salatin on your team as well. That's the true local food revolution that is spreading across America. Be a part of it.

Introduction: How I Became Normal

My family and our farm, Polyface Farm, in many ways seem like an anachronism. We still don't have a TV in our house. We grow practically all of our own food — I think if we could figure out how to grow toilet paper and facial tissues, we could just about pull the plug on society.

Teresa, my wonderful and beautiful bride of thirty-plus years, spends many days a year making and canning applesauce, freezing sweet corn, fermenting pickles, and filling quart jars by the hundreds in our basement larder. We drink raw milk, sometimes acquired legally and sometimes not. Although our farm produces hundreds of beeves, hundreds of hogs, many thousands of chickens and eggs, turkeys, rabbits, vegetables, and forestry products — and maybe other things by the time you read this — none of it enters industrial food channels to be extruded, amalgamated, prostituted, irradiated, and adulterated. We sell directly to families, restaurants, and a smattering of retail boutiques.

In half a century, we've never bought a pound of chemical fertilizer and don't apply pesticides, herbicides, insecticides, or any other -cide to our plants and animals. Our animals don't do drugs. Instead, we move them almost daily in a tightly choreographed ballet from pasture spot to pasture spot. They aren't confined in concentrated animal feeding operations. The herbivores receive no grain and the omnivores receive local, non–transgenic modified organism supplemental grains (GMO-free).

We don't participate in any government programs, period. No cost-share grants, no crop subsidies, no conservation easements, public or private. Our infrastructure is largely portable and nearly invisible.

In the winter, we house chickens, pigs, and rabbits in hoophouses, or tall tunnels, all together. This exquisite menagerie drives pathogens insane with confusion, rendering these disease agents impotent without any pharmaceuticals or toxic sanitizers.

My mom, Lucille, is a spry octogenarian who still tires plenty of women half her age if they try to follow her around. She lives fifty feet away from my house in a circa 1750 log home built of now-extinct American chestnut, glory of North American forests until about 1900. We heat both Mom's house and our old house with an ultra-modern outdoor wood furnace, or water stove, with fuel that we harvest from our own farm.

My dad, Bill, passed away in 1988 after serving in the Navy in World War II, receiving a degree in economics, and working for Texas Oil as a bilingual accountant in Venezuela for nearly a decade before buying a farm there. Mom was in a health and physical education master's program at Indiana University when she met my dad, who was getting his undergraduate degree on the GI Bill. They married and began their farming life in Venezuela, but it was not to be. Political unrest expropriated the farm in 1960 and they lost all their life savings and the dream of farming in a developing country. Returning to the United States, they looked at farms within a day's drive of Washington, D.C., hoping that the political winds would change and allow them to return to their beloved thousand-acre farm bounded by a wide river on the equator in the Venezuelan highlands.

It was not to be. They found this farm in Virginia's Shenandoah Valley, far and away the most eroded, gullied, decrepit — did I say cheap? — farm anywhere. They put a mortgage on it in the summer of 1961 and moved in with their two children, Art, seven, and Joel (me), four, and a very pregnant Mom carrying my unborn sister, Loretta.

When I finally arrived at the same middle age Dad and Mom were when they started over, their dogged determination and perseverance spoke to me more forcefully than any sermon. I couldn't imagine having the energy to start over. But start over they did. You will learn more about this farm and its healing as this book unfolds, but it is a story of carbon, soil building, ecological innovation, and a lifetime of swimming the wrong way.

I don't remember much about Venezuela except the final traumatic events as we fled from the rebellion and chaos that enveloped the countryside. I wish I had held on to my fluent Spanish, but alas, at that time in the Swoope, Virginia, community, speaking Spanish was considered either daft or insane, so Mom and Dad reluctantly decided not to fight that battle. Plenty of other battles existed due to community contempt toward outsiders, Yankees, and farmers who grew grass instead of corn and eschewed DDT and other lifesaving concoctions from the devil's pantry. Oh, did I mention that the Ku Klux Klan burned a cross and hay bale on our driveway so that we would know that the community knew we were communist spies? Welcome to Swoope.

Now, fifty years later, I don't think anyone in Swoope thinks we're communist spies, but in the era of McCarthyism, prejudice toward outsiders ran pretty deep. Today, we're good friends with some neighbors, and still shunned by others. But that's life when you swim upstream.

Throughout my childhood and into my teen years I was the child who truly loved the farm. My older brother would go on to a career of aviation mechanics, serving for fifteen years as a missionary pilot in Indonesia until one of his sons developed an illness that required returning stateside for better medical care. His family moved back to the farm in 1996 and he started his own small business as an airplane mechanic. My sister married an accountant and moved to Texas, near Dallas, where she and her husband have raised two children and she currently proudly works in the executive offices of the Boy Scouts of America. I was the one who chose a career as a farmer.

Did I say I wanted to farm? You need to understand, I just wanted to farm. I loved the farm. I loved chopping thistles — back when we used to have them. I loved gardening. I loved nursing baby lambs and calves. I loved hand milking the family cow. I started a flock of chickens at ten years old and peddled the eggs to neighbors and church members. Did I say I loved the farm? Teresa and I were high school sweethearts and married after college, she with a degree in home economics and I with a degree in English from the Christian liberal arts school Bob Jones University, but I really majored in debate. Would it surprise you if I told you I loved debate? I competed throughout high school and college.

Anything to do with communication, I was there — essay contests, forensics, drama, debate.

All my buddies have gone on to prestigious careers as attorneys, politicians, and motivational speakers. Me? I just wanted to farm. Never in my wildest dreams did I think I would write books and become one of the chief promoters for the integrity food tsunami sweeping America's landscape. People routinely ask Teresa, "Did you know what you were getting?" Ever my best friend, she laughs and says, "No, I thought I was marrying a farmer." Teresa grew up in a farm family, a sister with three brothers. She can hold her own, trust me.

My dad and mom worked off the farm in order to pay for it, she teaching high school health and physical education and he in accounting. But they experimented. Dad was a genius, I am now convinced. He developed a portable electric fence system in the early 1960s, understood soil development, composting, and nutrient density. He also understood debt and profitability, margins and value-added marketing. Although my parents never earned a living from the farm, they laid a foundation, an ethic, indeed a vision big enough to capture my wildest dreams.

Having worked part-time at the local daily newspaper during my junior and senior years in high school, I returned there to a full-time position after college. Teresa and I married and with parental support turned the farmhouse attic into a commodious penthouse apartment. We lived there for seven years until our daughter was born. My grandmother, who had moved into a mobile home in our yard when I was a teen, had passed away and my parents decided to exchange houses. They moved into a bigger and more stylish home and Teresa and I moved downstairs in the house where I grew up. I've never moved.

On September 24, 1982, over the advice of all my friends, both young and old, I returned to the farm full-time. Giving up a steady paycheck and work I enjoyed seemed insane. But I wanted to farm.

We homeschooled our two children, Daniel and Rachel, beginning at a time when homeschool parents were still being hauled off to jail for truancy violations and their children abducted by the education police and placed in foster care. Fortunately, those days are past, thanks to the Home School Legal Defense Association and certainly no thanks to the institutional education establishment. Both children had their own businesses and grew up butchering chickens, planting gardens, gathering eggs, canning vegetables, and selling to the hundreds of customers who bought our meat, poultry, and eggs.

In 1996 a family visited us from Texas, one of thousands who wanted to see the farm and learn how to process chickens. Their striking teenage daughter, Sheri, eventually married our son, Daniel, and they now have three children, Travis, Andrew, and Lauryn. They built their own house on the farm from lumber we milled at our sawmill from our own trees in our woods. As of this writing, Daniel handles day-to-day farm operations and tells me what I need to do. I wouldn't want it any other way.

Our daughter, Rachel, after a two-year degree in business and then another two-year degree in interior design, was working in the big city, but has wandered back to the farm, where she is using her creativity and design to help make this beautiful place more beautiful. She does all my PowerPoint photography, maintains a Polyface note card collection, creates maps, and — well — we're just all excited about her artsy-craftsy skills. We've been Plain Jane for too long. Rachel snazzies everything.

Our four generations living on the farm is perhaps my single greatest blessing. Surrounded by this emerald farm in God's creative crown, surrounded by abundance in the fields, the gardens, and the basement larder, feasting on compost-grown, pasture-raised food minimally prepared in our home kitchen, communing with family — this is normal. This is connection, foundation, heritage, tradition.

And yet most modern Americans can't conceive of living like this.

The United States now has too few farmers to merit counting on the national census form. As a culture, we don't cook at home. We don't have a larder. We're tuned in, plugged in, addicted to electronic gadgetry to the exclusion of a whippoorwill's midsummer song or a herd of cows lying down contentedly on the leeward side of a slope, indicating a thunderstorm in the offing. Most modern Americans can't conceive of a time without supermarkets, without refrigeration, stainless steel, plastic, bar codes, potato chips.

Urbanites routinely ask me, "What do you do out there on the farm? If you don't go to a movie, don't get takeout, don't bar hop, don't spend most evenings at soccer games — what on earth is there to do?" Oh, let me tell you. Each morning I step out into dew-speckled pastures, each drop a rainbow-studded diamond adorning orchardgrass, red clover, white clover, plantain, chickory — a whole salad bar bedazzled in morning's solar glory. I have thousands of expectant animals waiting for a fresh salad bar. They love me.

I love them. I love everything about this. The smell of new-mown hay. The magic of a calf sliding out in one final contractive heave from the cow, who immediately begins a gentle, throaty murmuring as she licks the calf and then pushes the wobbly baby to her engorged udder to nurse. What do you mean, "What is there to do?" What's there not to do? This circle of life has been ongoing for a long time. Longer than supermarkets. Longer than Tyson chicken houses. Longer than iPhones and video games.

Increasingly, I feel this cultural tension between my life and the life of modern Americans. To be sure, I don't want to go back to one bath per winter, fireplace heat, and pitchforks. In this book, I've chosen specific normalcies, well aware that we have had soil erosion since the beginning of time. We've had diseases since the beginning of time. Slavery has been normal in more cultures than not. Yes, I'm well aware of that. But a host of positive, wonderful cultural norms have existed that I submit provided a foundation for civilization's sustainability and regeneration.

Ours is certainly not an old culture. Yet in recent decades we've used more energy, destroyed more soil, created more pathogenicity (temporarily stopped some too, for sure), mutated more bacteria, and dumped more toxicity on the planet than all the cultures before us — combined. I love the United States, but I am not blind to the wrongs. I have no desire to live anywhere else, but that doesn't mean I think everything we're doing should be done or can be maintained.

On many levels, I am struck by the sheer abnormality of our situation. In this book, I'd like us to think broadly and deeply about how to restore normalcy, to reincorporate those foundations that sustain cultures — by using what we know and what we have in ways that honor and respect those upon whose shoulders we stand. By identifying and honoring historical normalcy, we present a loving legacy to those who have gone before. I think we owe such a gift to them. Let normalcy begin.

Folks, this ain't normal

Children, Chores, Humility, and Health

"We need something for our young people to do" is a common refrain in adult circles today. Daily news reports about roving teenagers getting into mischief during the wee hours of the morning don't make any sense to me. Every time I see that a group of young people has caused some fracas at 2 a.m. I wonder, "Who has time and energy to be out cavorting at 2 a.m.?"

Our children went to bed at 9 or 10 p.m. and were grateful for the opportunity. Our apprentices and interns normally dismiss themselves from our company and head off to bed as soon after dark as they can get there.

That young people today, at least when they are not in school, spend the day lounging around, hanging out, and then go into the wee hours burning off excess energy is aberrant in the first degree. Add to that the pastime of playing video games, exercising only thumb muscles and fingertips, and folks, we have a situation that just ain't normal.

When the biggest thrill in life is becoming competent enough on the video game to achieve level five performance, what kind of environment are we creating for our future leaders? When I sit in airports and watch these testosterone-exuding boys with their shriveled shoulders and E.T.-looking fingers passing the time on their laptops, I realize that this is normal for them. This isn't happening because they are sitting in an airport trying to while away the time. This is actually how many, if not most, of their hours are spent — recreation, entertainment, and playing around.

Contrast that with historical normalcy. Here is a list of chores for young people since time immemorial:

1. Chopping, cutting, and gathering firewood. In the days before petroleum and electricity, every able-bodied person contributed to keeping the household warm during the winter months. This wood accumulation required a knowledge of the forest and of what kind of wood burns well. Not all wood is created equal. Resinous woods like evergreens coat the inside of the chimney and unless mixed half and half with nonresinous will accumulate too much soot on the inside of the chimney or flue. This highly combustible residue can become a fire hazard. Whenever we cut down a pine tree, therefore, we want to look around for at least equal parts hardwoods to balance out the fuel for the fireplace or woodstove. Green wood cut from standing, living trees contains 30 percent or more water, and this moisture retards the fire because before the wood can burn it must evaporate the water.

A skilled wood gatherer knows to seek dead and dry wood for immediate burning but to stockpile the green wood for future burning. But all dead and downed wood is not equally dry. If the dead wood is up off the ground a little, it will be perfect. A standing snag is ideal most of the time. Sometimes it has already rotted and turned to powder — common in soft deciduous trees like poplar or red maple.

If the dead or downed wood is on the ground, it may be too rotten to burn. Burning wood is essentially an extremely fast rotting process: What soil microbes do over an extended period, a fire does in a short period. If the combustible carbon is already decomposed through the rotting process, nothing is left to burn.

All wood gives off about the same BTUs per pound, but different woods weigh different amounts per cubic foot. Heavy woods like white oak and hickory give off twice as much heat per cubic foot than light woods like poplar or white pine.

Gathering wood, then, requires a fair amount of knowledge to be done well. Beyond the knowledge is the skill to gather it efficiently. Obviously if we're going to the forest to bring in firewood, we will take our tools like a chainsaw (modern), crosscut or bucksaw (premodern), or ax (old). Or imagine the Native Americans who either used stone axes or built fires around big trees to fell them. That required yet another whole skill set — one that I don't possess.

But I do know how to run a chainsaw — a wonderful modern invention. I also know how to swing an ax, sharpen an ax, and replace the handle on an ax — all skills I developed as a youth. Once the wood is cut, it must be loaded into a vessel: trailer, pickup truck bed, hay wagon, whatever. It never ceases to amaze me when I go to the woods with our apprentices and interns how much I have to teach about efficiently gathering wood. First, we stack the branches with all the butts facing one way and uphill because the fluffy branch ends tend to build vertical height faster than the butts. If you stack the branches haphazardly, the pile gets too high too fast. By carefully placing the branches, we can get far more on the pile.

When we begin picking up the cut pieces of wood, we want to get the vessel as close to the wood as possible. No walking — pitch it into the vessel. If the piece is too big to throw, of course, then you may have to walk, but we want to keep backing the vessel into the cut wood to minimize walking. Obviously, if we pitch the wood to the vessel, we want to position our bodies between the vessel and the wood we're picking up. This way we can reduce the throw by the length of our bodies and our arms — usually a distance of nearly five feet.

By swiveling back and forth this way, we can load the wood twice as fast as if we're behind the pieces throwing them into the vessel. And three times faster than if we're picking them up in our arms and carrying them over to the trailer. I know some people are reading this thinking, "Wow, that sounds like a lot of work. I'm glad I just turn on the thermostat and the heat starts."

But now we get to the point of the story: Few activities can yield more satisfaction in the heart of a young person than riding in on a big load of firewood. This chore offers communing experiences with the forest, but not in a woo-woo cerebral academic kind of way. Rather, it's a visceral, healthy understanding of the forest's bounty, the diversity of its species, the different properties of each, the reality that some specimens died and some live until another day.

Some of my most satisfying experiences as a youth entailed gathering wood with Dad. Usually we would do this kind of work in the fall, the leaves turning brilliant colors, just enough nip in the air to invigorate the body. Perhaps my favorite work, still today, is working the woods. Few things are as satisfying as going into a jumbled-up mess, taking out the crooked trees, widow-makers (dead trees leaning up against their neighbors), dead trees fallen over, and walking out a couple of hours later with a beautiful order restored and excellent trees newly released (weeded) to grow better and healthier.

I consider it the ultimate multitasking. Not only have we reenergized the good trees and restored beauty and order, but we've accumulated our heating fuel at the same time. Whenever I throw that last piece of wood on the trailer, I like to take a few minutes, in the silence, and survey the site where I've worked. Branches neatly stacked will provide several years of housing for voles, chipmunks, and rabbits. Sometimes we chip them for livestock bedding. The good trees, standing straight and vigorous, reaching for the sky, will grow better now, unencumbered by the crooked, diseased, and scrub trees sapping soil and sun energy. What I could scarcely walk through two hours ago is now spacious, open, parklike, and organized.

The triumphant, exuberant spirit of our interns, riding in atop a trailer load of freshly gathered firewood, is testament to the deep personal satisfaction, the physical, emotional, and spiritual affirmation that such work engenders. This visceral, meaningful work makes the spirit soar with self-worth and accomplishment. This is the ultimate self-actualization. You won't find that at the end of a video game, no matter how many times you play.

I hope this examination helps illustrate the depth and breadth of historic youthful normalcy. Because generally gathering firewood is done with at least one other person. The social time, bonding, and camaraderie that is part of the process puts icing on the cake. Yes, it's work, but so is trying to figure out what to do with unruly youthful hormones at 2 a.m. Historically, normal youthful development entailed a meaningful contribution to the household. Work defines the individual. What is one of the first questions we ask when greeting new people? "What do you do?" That means, "What do you do for a living. What is your vocation? Your career? What defines you as a person?" Vocation clues us in to the person: engineer type, lawyer type, potter type, entrepreneur type, minister type, counselor type.

In the Jewish tradition, boys become men at thirteen years old. Any reading of colonial American biographies reveals unheard-of intrepidity among teenagers. In fact, the term "teenager" did not occur until the Industrial Revolution, when meaningful societal contributions by this age class began to wane. Until then, they were young adults. Many of the Pony Express riders were teens. These guys knew how to ride a horse, handle a gun, think on their feet, spot danger, be dependable.

Accumulating the wood, gathering it from the woods, was generally a communal chore. The daily task also entailed splitting and bringing the wood into the house.

2. Splitting wood was necessary to keep heat in the home. Normally accomplished with an ax, this chore has its own skill set. Reading the end of a piece of wood requires experience and careful observation. As wood dries, the moisture from the ends evaporates faster than what is stuck inside. This rapid drying on the end creates checks, or cracks. When setting up the block of wood to split, therefore, reading these checks reveals the natural inclination of the piece to split. Leveraging those small cracks makes the splitting much easier.

3. After splitting, the wood had to be brought into the house to keep the firebox full. By this time, the connection between gathering and necessity is clear. No wood, no heat. I remember well during my teen years taking my morning pee in the upstairs bathroom and seeing the stream splatter onto ice in the toilet bowl. That definitely motivates you to get the fire going, bring in wood, gather wood — the whole seamless chain of events to maintain house comfort.

This chore taught me both personal responsibility and dependability. If I got cold, it wasn't anybody's fault but my own. If I neglected to bring in enough wood to get through the night, I was victim of my own negligence. I had to think ahead, plan, be aware of outside temperature that determined how much wood we would burn for the night. I had to take note of the kind of wood. If it was a fast-burning wood, I needed more volume than if it was slower-burning wood. I needed a combination of big pieces to hold the fire and little pieces to make enough surface area to keep burning. This was all my responsibility.

But ultimately, this whole process painted a daily reminder of my dependency on nature to supply heat. It didn't come from a pipe. I participated in the effort of growing trees, then it was up to the rain and the sun. Participating in this great work steers us toward dependency on our ecological womb. Breaking this historical responsibility and dependency may seem like a good thing for a while, but if we use that freed-up time to become self-absorbed, or become Hollywood celebrity addicts, are we really better off? For all our extrication from these chores, are we better people? Are we more responsible people? Are we more aware of our ecological dependence? I'm not saying it's sinful to heat with natural gas or electricity. I do believe, however, that we must put more effort into remembering our responsibilities and dependency on the environment even if we don't participate in these traditional activities.

Here's a little-known chore: **4. Keeping animal protein in the chicken yard once a week during the winter.** One of the first man-sized chores for farm boys was providing some dead critter for the laying flock to eat in the winter when the grasshoppers and crickets were dormant. Since chickens are omnivores, they need animal protein, and that's hard to come by during the cold winter months.

Consequently, young boys had the chore of acquiring something for the chickens. Usually a squirrel, skunk, possum, raccoon, rabbit — something small. This required shooting or trapping, and is one reason why handbooks for boys written during the 1800s and early 1900s were dominated by homemade trapping devices. Often these boys were not yet old enough to carry guns, so they had to be ingenious at acquiring varmints some other way.

Matching wits against these animals that scurried around the home at night occupied many a youthful discussion and evening whittling, refining, tweaking by firelight. It occupied conversations at social gatherings and formed the warp and woof of meaningful collaboration. And it was the perfect job for young people seeking wise elderly counsel — from adults who had passed this way before and trapped or shot their fair share of the winter chicken yard protein.

Now, dear people, please close your eyes and meditate on this chore for a while, comparing it to the raucous nonsocial totally aberrant youthful passion pitting finger responses against a handheld video screen. Which do you think will really prepare young people to take their place in societal leadership? Which process actually lays a foundation of cleverness, persistence, and self-actualization to offer us world leaders who are not peer-dependent and who can think through the nuances of a problem?

For urban young people, building and launching model rockets, building and launching soapbox derby cars, and a host of other craft-type activities help develop these traditional skills. And they sure create great stories. How many times can you tell the story about hitting 100,000 in the Crazy Maniac Highway Destructo video game? But you can always tell the story about the crazy rocket that went sideways.

Here's a chore that predates me by about a decade: **5. Picking up cow dung from the barnyard.** When I was a youth, one of my old-timer neighbors told me about this chore that was one of the early rites of passage for young boys. Wheelbarrows have been around for a long time. Today they have pneumatic tires, but before that they had a simple metal wheel. Before the days of chemical fertilizer and agriculture experts telling farmers that manure wasn't even worth hauling to the field, farmers knew its benefits.

They didn't know all the scientific names for the various nutrients, the elements contained therein, or the enzymes saturated throughout, but they knew manure was magic. Always has been, always will be. For the record, although we know far more about manure than we did even a couple of decades ago, we still have much to learn. The more we know about nature, the more we know we don't know.

For centuries farmers tried to figure out how to be more resourceful with manure. In the days before electric fences and front-end loaders, manure spreaders and wood chippers, this required hand work. Gene Logsdon, in his wonderful book *Holy Shit*, explains the historic static barn manure pack. Created in the winter when the cows and sheep were not out on pastures as much, the barn manure and bedding pack was one of the only concentrations of nutrients on the typical farm. During the grazing season, the pastured animals spread their own manure but it was so widely distributed that its effects were not as noticeable. This bedding manure was so prized that farmers wanted to gather even the cow pats dropped outside during the night and place them inside the barn under the protection of the roof and into absorptive contact with straw: what I call a carbonaceous diaper.

Hence the chore of going around with the wheelbarrow and a fork, gingerly picking up these outside cow pies and wheeling them into the barn where they could be covered with straw and accumulated until spring. While this may not have been a favorite chore, it did indicate a rite of passage, because a boy who could run that wheelbarrow around the barnyard was just around the corner from becoming a man. I remember well coaching our own children to use the wheelbarrow, watching as they tried to balance it and urging them on with "Yes, you can do it! You can do it!" When finally the day came that they could operate it proficiently, I passed the baton.

I remember as if it were yesterday the first time my son, Daniel, drove the tractor by himself. He was about eight years old and we needed to pick up a wagon load of hay bales in a large flat field. The thirteen-acre field was expansive, and since I was picking up the bales by hand, he needed to drive as slowly as I could walk. The implement was a hay wagon, which is a fairly benign implement — not like a baler or mower.

Of course, Daniel had grown up around the tractor with me, so he knew where everything was: clutch, throttle, brake, gearshift, steering wheel. I put it in gear for him, let out the clutch, and then jumped off, leaving him standing in front of the seat holding on to the steering wheel. I began loading the hay bales and he drove expertly alongside, put-putting along in fine fashion. When we were finished, he stepped on the clutch to disengage the transmission and I jumped on the tractor to drive it to the barn. I'm sure insurance agents are flipping out right about now. Trust me, you don't know half of our stories.

That was a Saturday, and the next day at our church fellowship group Daniel beamed to everyone about what he had done. It was the only time he ever complained about homeschooling: "I wish I could go to a school tomorrow for show-and-tell." That was a rite of passage.

I remember when I was about the same age working with my dad. We were feeding a herd of cows in the winter and had the big dump truck full of hay bales. Dad needed to throw them off and I was his only crew. When you're feeding hay on a pasture, you want to put it out in a long line rather than a pile. This allows all the cows to get to the hay at once and it also reduces their tromping on it and wasting it. The easiest way to do this is to throw it off while the truck is moving.

So Dad put the truck in gear and let out the clutch, and I stood on the seat and steered. This 1951 International had a throttle on the dashboard, which meant you didn't have to push the gas pedal to make it go.

We were on a long, flat ridge. Dad put the truck in low first and then climbed into the back to throw off the hay. When we finished, he praised me for doing such a good job.

When our daughter Rachel was eight or nine years old, she began baking zucchini bread and pound cakes for our farm customers. Not only was she a truly gifted baker, but as a marketer, who could possibly refuse the cherubic face and expectant countenance of a child? "Yes, of course I'll buy one," the garden club ladies would say. And then the next week the patrons would come back and, crouching down to Rachel's height, gently pinch her cheek and gush, "Oh, my garden club ladies loved your pound cake at our luncheon. It was delicious."

What does that do for the personhood of a child? All of us crave affirmation, especially affirmation that genuinely recognizes our contribution to society. Being able to touch others in a meaningful way with our gifts and talents creates reciprocal affirmation. And while I may insult some people, I submit that this affirmation has a different quality, a different intensity, than simply being praised for winning a game. Perhaps acting in a dramatic production comes closer. But when we create something that we can sensually experience, and that represents our ingenuity, the gratitude on the part of the recipient speaks to deeper levels of our personhood.

In her early teen years, Rachel's baking business expanded. Then she added a housecleaning business, and by her midteens she was employing others. We homeschooled and never had a television in the house, which created time to pursue these entrepreneurial activities. Contrary to much popular opinion, I would suggest that this was the ultimate preparation for adulthood, rather than an adolescence of coddling and endless recreation.

Our son Daniel started a rabbit project when he was eight. Some friends moved to the city and their new lease restrictions excluded animals. Their three rabbits needed a new home and Daniel took them in. We built a portable rabbit shelter and he moved it around the yard, fertilizing and mowing. Knowing what rabbits are known for, we decided to add "RABBIT" to our farm offerings in the next season's product order blank. We assumed that not too many people ate rabbit, but hoped that enough would that Daniel would be able to sell some.

Within two weeks after the order blank went out, Daniel had orders for 150 rabbits. This was quite a tall order, even for rabbits. It launched his business and he gradually built it up to a sizable operation that recently has been commissioned to independent contractors on the farm.

I'm a big believer that children should have autonomous businesses. This teaches the value of a dollar, persistence, thrift, and good math skills. The earlier someone learns the difference between profit and loss, the better. I well remember Daniel going down to the farm store and purchasing half a ton of unmedicated rabbit pellets when he was about twelve years old. His nose just cleared the counter and the guys would josh with him: "Only half a ton? Why don't you get a whole ton?"

Daniel would matter-of-factly respond, "I don't have enough money for a ton." How many adults have not learned that lesson? Both of our children hit twenty years old with $20,000 in the bank. I don't believe in allowances — nobody should be paid to breathe. This was not pay for chores. It was self-earned, saved income from their businesses and provided a wonderful nest egg for future pursuits. That, my friends, is liberating and launching.

Our grandson Travis was only about five years old the first time he went with me to raise and lower the tractor front-end loader for something I was doing in the field. All he had to do was work the joystick that operates the hydraulics to move the loader up and down. He watched me closely for instructions and did what he'd seen his daddy and me do many times. His triumphant smile over helping me do something I couldn't have done by myself oozed affirmation. He barely touched the ground for the next day, making sure everyone knew he had helped Grandpa. We were a team, there in the field, old geezer and kindergartner, working together to solve a common problem, sharing in the triumph of a physical, seeable, measurable job well done.

Recently I was in Washington State conducting a seminar, and a middle-aged lady told me her grow-up story. She said when she was a girl, when school dismissed for the summer, the apple orchards in the area would lease the school buses and print a picking schedule in fliers in the newspaper. The school buses would come through the city on a schedule, just like the ice cream truck, and if you were older than ten years old, you could get on the bus and ride out to the orchards and pick apples for the day. This gave young people spending money, physical exercise, and affirmation as contributing members of society. At the end of the day, the buses would deliver them back home and they were richer than the money in their pockets.

Can you imagine such a reasonable activity occurring today? The insurance underwriter for the school district would go apoplectic that the buses were being used for something other than carting brains to school. Child labor laws would scream "Exploitation!" and criminalize even the notion of such an activity. I find it amazing that today our culture thinks it's sensible to put a sixteen-year-old behind the wheel of two thousand pounds of steel and send it hurtling down the expressway at seventy miles an hour, but if that same person pushes a lawnmower or operates a cordless drill, that power tool is too dangerous.

On our farm, we routinely have younger teens in the fifteen- to seventeen-year range wanting to come and work for the summer. Many are homeschooled and quite mature, eager to get on with their life's objectives, which in this case means starting a viable agriculture endeavor. But although we used to take them, we don't anymore due to overreaching occupational safety regulations that classify a cordless screwdriver as a power tool and therefore illegal for anyone under eighteen to operate.

The same teen who can't legally operate a four-wheeler, or all-terrain vehicle (ATV, commonly known in the vernacular as Japanese Cow Ponies), in a farm lane workplace environment can operate a jacked-up F-250 pickup on a crowded urban expressway. By denying these opportunities to bring value to their own lives and the community around them, we've relegated our young adults to teenage foolishness. Then as a culture we walk around shaking our heads in bewilderment at these young people with retarded maturity. Never in life do people have as much energy as in their teens, and to criminalize leveraging it is certainly one of our nation's greatest resource blunders.

Our culture now denies young people the very activities that build their self-worth and incorporate them as valuable members of society. Rather than seeing children as an asset, we now view them as a liability. If there is any expression of our society's aberrant behavior, it is certainly expressed in the "cost of children" analysis in the modern press. What happened to the day when they were considered a worthwhile asset?

Our societal paralysis to leverage youthful energy in a more mean-ingful way than soccer, ballet, and video games indicates profound imagination constipation. This protective timidity that denies our young people risk and self-actualization keeps them from attaining emotional, economic, and spiritual maturity.

Worse than being hurt on the job is growing up without a sense of self-worth. Gangs are a direct result of this societal abnormality. While I'm not naïve enough to believe that if we encouraged childhood work we wouldn't have gangs at all, I would argue that their proliferation has mirrored young people's eviction from visceral societal contribution.

Lest anyone think I'm proposing child labor, I also love to see chil-dren free to enjoy imaginative play. Our children grew up building dams in the creek, forts in the hay, forts in the firewood pile, forts in the woods. After reading *The Swiss Family Robinson*, Daniel and Rachel spent several days in the woods. Teresa and I weren't quite sure what they were doing, but we knew they were into a serious project. After three days, the children asked us to come and attack them — giving us clear directions on where to assault their stronghold first.

As Teresa and I approached along the designated path, Rachel and Daniel let loose with whooping and hollering, moving deftly from one booby trap to another, releasing a bag of sticks on us, then entangling us in string. When we finally made it through the hazards and arrived at their inner sanctum, we all had a wonderful laugh at their rendition of the classic book's story.

Compare that to spending all day in front of a video game trying to race a car around a track or decapitate the alien invaders. I am not a psychologist, but it seems to me that the video alternative is a far cry, as a personal development technique, from the forested fortress. The chil-dren tied, sawed, climbed, rolled, heaved, and built something with their own creativity. Video games confine creativity to someone else's software imagination. And we haven't even addressed the physical ben-efits of all that exercise — climbing up the trees to string twine and gathering armloads of sticks. Oh, and the site was half a mile from the house. They had to walk there and walk back. Precious memories.

My grandchildren's escapades are already epic. They have their flags and forts throughout the farm and barn, daily venturing forth to slay dragons and protect righteousness. Who needs amusement rides and

Disney when every day, with a little sweat and imagination, you can create your own castles and story lines? When I ask Travis and Andrew, sometimes with Lauryn tagging along, what they are up to, they regale me with fantastical stories, crisp descriptions of how the "bad guys" came over that "hill right there and we...we ambushed them right there and...and..." Trust me, folks, this narrative can go on through chores if you have the time to let it unfold.

Although childhood active playtime is wonderful, so is work. One particularly poignant illustration of this occurred when Daniel was about ten years old. A neighbor boy a year younger wanted to build a fort below his house, so he enlisted Daniel's support in the project. Since diaperhood, Daniel had been going with me to build fence, and I routinely paced myself by not stopping for a drink until I had achieved some specific point in the project. He would ask for a drink and I'd say, "No, we're not going to get a drink until I finish setting this post."

He went over to the neighbors' to build the fort the first morning of the project, and about two hours later the boy's mother called our house: "What's wrong with your son? He won't let my son have a drink of water until they've finished the first wall." We laughed ourselves silly over old ten-year-old slave driver Daniel. But folks, that is the stuff of life. That is the stuff of maturity. Persistence and faithfulness. Can these be learned equally from entertainment or recreational venues? If we relegate our young people to only find accomplishment from entertainment or winning the athletic trophy, have we not shortchanged their understanding of human value?

I like a great ball game as much as anybody, but all game and no meaningful work creates an unbelievably jaundiced view of life and our role in it. And that brings me to the sixth chore in this discussion:

6. Gardening. As recently as 1946, nearly 50 percent of all produce grown in America came out of backyard gardens. Hoeing, pulling weeds, planting vegetables, and then canning, freezing, dehydrating, and fermenting accounted for significant family time and energy. Laying by was not an option; it was a necessity. That someone would enter the nonproductive off-season with an empty larder was simply unthinkable. And foolhardy.

With the proliferation of just-in-time inventorying and supermarkets with long warehouse stays and a global inventory chain, this historically normal domestic activity has been relegated to unnecessary status. Such food production, preparation, and processing simply gets in the way of extracurricular outside-the-home activities.

When a child plays a video game, if the race car wrecks, in a few seconds the game gives him a new one and he goes right on playing. If he's fighting alien invaders and his character gets his head bashed in, the machine replaces the stricken victim in a few seconds and the game goes on. No one, at any other time in human history, has been able to replace their materials, their tools, even their playthings with such instant fabrication or resurrection.

Life is not like this at all. In real life, if you drive your car like a maniac and wrap it around a tree, you don't swagger away cavalierly from the catastrophe and receive a new car plopped down by the auto fairies in a few seconds. It's a real loss, with real consequences and real upheaval.

If your tomato plant dies because you failed to water it, you don't count to ten and watch a miraculous resurrection. Death is final. It's over. The hubris with which our young people enter life, living in this world of replacement and limitless instant gratification, engenders an arrogance toward life and ecology that is both scary and dangerous. No fear is the mantra of fools.

When we started our apprentice program at our farm I saw this illustrated daily. Though only thirteen at the time, Daniel had an awareness of danger, a situational awareness far superior to apprentices twice his age. He knew what happened if a tractor tire ran over something. He'd seen squashed buckets or bent metal. He knew what an errant tree falling could do. He was well aware that a random groundhog hole could dislodge a whole wagon load of hay and bury the stacker under a ton of bales. He knew how unpredictable — and violently strong — a cow kick could be in the corral, and where to position himself to not be the victim of such actions.

Apprentices twice his age were constantly putting themselves in dangerous positions. Not because they were foolhardy, but simply because they had not been in these situations and therefore had no clue about what could go wrong. Over the years, we've had only one apprentice we had to send home due to his inability to assess dangerous places. We actually feared for his life because he couldn't grasp the gravity of a given situation.

Knowing what to fear is the first step in knowing what to fix. I fear that we are bringing to our world a whole generation revved up on hubris, who think they have the world by the tail. Solomon, generally described as the wisest man who ever lived, said in the biblical book of Proverbs, "The fear of the Lord is the beginning of wisdom." If this doesn't denote appreciating the gravity of the situation, I don't know what does.

The gardener fears changes in the weather pattern, lack of water, soil loss, husbandry negligence. That so few in our generation have a visceral experience with any deprivation is why, in the face of mounting water shortages, soil erosion, atmospheric changes, and chemical toxicity most people can still drink their Coca-Cola, munch their nachos, and spend hours glued to sitcoms, oblivious to catastrophes building around them. The wise gardener studies his environment, watching for weeds, bugs, drought, flood, heat, cold, and soil changes.

Cultivating this habitat awareness and responding to its nuances allow the gardener to enter a world of mystery and grandeur. Ultimately all gardeners realize that their landscape depends on something much bigger than themselves. Seasonal cycles, frost dates, degree-days, day length, and even waxing and waning moon cycles all play a part in this majestic garden dance. It's a place of wonder and awe, ultimately impressing on the gardener a palpable humility toward this divine ecological umbilical.

The sheer joy expressed by schoolchildren in gardens when they first discover those plump potatoes, buried under green foliage all season, is the stuff of unbridled exuberance. No discovery could elicit a more enthusiastic response. No hidden treasure can excite more enthusiasm than those potatoes rolling out of the ground. One of my favorite interactions on our farm is when city children peek under laying hens and see eggs for the first time, the exhilaration as they catch their breath, open their mouth in a big smile of wonderment, and say to Mommy or Daddy, "Look! Eggs!" And if they happen to actually watch a chicken squat and lay an egg, you'd think they just discovered the moon.

I'm reminded of a study I read about when Teresa and I were contemplating homeschooling our children. The crux of the study was that the earlier a child learns specific spatial data, the less spiritual the child will be. Using the moon as an example, what these researchers found was that the sooner children learn that the moon is comprised of this and that elements and that it is so many miles away from the earth, the sooner they lose their awe and wonder toward the moon. It moves, in the human mind, from a majestic orb in the sky, a mystical object of wonderment, to simply a ho-hum rock.

Maintaining a sense of awe and mystery toward the universe, and cultivating a profound sense of dependency on something bigger than ourselves, seem to be a fundamental responsibility we adults should have toward our children. To abdicate this responsibility is to populate our culture with manipulators and dominion-thinkers on overdrive. For my religious right friends, remember that the first occupation of humanity was to be a gardener — with specific restrictions on hubris, known as the forbidden tree. Overreaching dominion resulted in paradise lost. That should instill fear in all of us to not take our dominion reach beyond our grasp of creation's rules.

Watching new life spring from last season's dead and decomposed relics instills hope. The garden's cycle helps young people understand that what is will not always be, that regeneration requires death and decomposition. Out of sacrifice springs life. To encounter that, to see it, touch it, taste it, smell it, gives old-fashioned common sense and reasoning abilities. It is the real world, not some artificial cyber-fantasy that titillates the mind with cerebral extravagance. The computer game cries for more, more, more. More violence, more drama, more excitement. More consumerism. It's like a cerebral drug trip, ever more demanding, less satisfying, dependency-enslaving.

The garden teaches balance. No gardener plants only one thing. Yes, industrial agriculture does that, but no gardener would think of such nonsense. Gardeners balance high plants with low plants, top growers with bottom growers, vegetables with flowers. The gardener learns about crowding plants, about earthworms, soil tilth, and a host of comparisons and contrasts that create a vibrant place. Carrying capacity expressed in seeds per square foot teaches discipline. If you want to grow ten corn plants per square foot, try it one time. You'll be sorely disappointed. Perhaps stacking people too close together has the same result.

Disciplining ourselves to respect and honor ecological limitations and patterns is part of wisdom. Failure to adhere to these principles should make us tremble with fear. It is this kind of humility, this kind of nurturing caregiving toward creation, that children who garden bring to their adult life. While I'm sure plenty of software designers have tried to duplicate this on a video screen, the difference between seeing something shrivel on a video display does not and cannot compare to watching the shriveling occur in real life.

In addition to attitudinal normalcy, I would suggest that gardens also strengthen children's immune systems. Autoimmune dysfunction is reaching unprecedented abnormal levels. Many researchers are working on this epidemic that is pointing more and more toward what is called the hygiene hypothesis.

Callaway, Harvey, and Nisbet, in a paper published in *Foodborne Pathogens and Illness*, discussed the hygiene hypothesis, which they say first began being bandied about in the mid-1990s and has increased in credibility among doctors and other experts. According to these researchers: "This hypothesis states that a lack of exposure of children (as well as adults) to dirt, commensal bacteria, and 'minor' pathogenic insults results in an immune system that does not function normally. This lack of antibodies to true pathogens in the immune system has resulted in the dramatic increase in allergies and asthma in developed countries over the past twenty years." The paper cites an American Academy of Allergy Asthma and Immunology estimate that from about 1990 to 2010, the number of people with allergies increased by 100 percent.

According to this hypothesis, the immune system becomes lethargic due to lack of true immunological exercise, a problem especially common in developed nations. My intuition, and probably yours, is that immune systems need exercise just like muscles.

Although this research is primarily aimed at sterile food, I would argue that it applies to any childhood devoid of soil contact. Most of us have heard our grandmothers say, "Every child should eat a pound of dirt before they're twelve," or some variation on that theme.

One of the central arguments in Jared Diamond's book *Guns, Germs and Steel* is that the cultures that ended up dominating the world were the ones that developed a greater array of immunities due to proximity to domestic livestock. For those of you who are already thinking along with me, yes indeed, a backyard rabbitry or chicken flock to complement the backyard garden would be a great addition to your child's immunological arsenal.

Splinters, blisters, and real dirt under the fingernails are all part of a normal childhood that builds immune systems. That, as a culture, we are reducing or even denying this immunological exercise is not only abnormal when viewed through the lens of history, but does not bode well for proper body and soul development. Indeed, it may prove devastating to children's health. Children's laboring in gardens is both attitudinally and physically positive. Weeding the beans and picking cucumbers should be seen as part of a healthy child development program. Certainly better than computer screens and television.

Where should these gardens be located? Any lawn, any flowerpot, and any windowsill offers a garden spot. Incorporating gardens into the family's domestic landscape is both normal and healthy. The notion that children actively engaged in food production exploit these little innocents just ain't normal. A normal childhood involves digging, planting, germinating, weeding, watering, and preparing. That nourishes both the immune system and the soul.

How about some things to do?

1. Grow things... anything. Indoor grow lights are still magic, and can bring sunlight indoors for remarkable discoveries.
2. Lobby for more lenient child labor opportunities so that once again teens can do historically normal work.
3. Instead of going on a cruise or Disney vacation, how about choosing a working ranch experience for the family, or an extremely rustic wilderness adventure where you make some traps and hunt for food?
4. Brainstorm entrepreneurial child-appropriate businesses — hand crafts, repair, tutoring, calligraphy, customized invitations, cleaning homes, mowing lawns, picking up rocks, hoeing weeds. The list of possibilities could fill many pages. Don't underestimate the creativity and resourcefulness of your sixteen-year-old unleashed on the community. Stay out of the way and let her run.

A Cat Is a Cow Is a Chicken Is My Aunt

No civilization has ever been in this state of environmental ignorance. In previous eras, people who lived in an area, whether they were newcomers or old-timers, had to be intimately aware of their surroundings and viscerally involved in rearing and preparing food for the table.

But in recent decades, in our culture, putting food on the table does not require any knowledge or involvement except how to scan a credit card, open a plastic bag, and nuke it in the microwave. No civilization in history has ever been able to be this disconnected from its ecological umbilical. And in more frequent dinnertime discussions, I'm finding more and more people wondering if a civilization this disconnected can actually survive.

Today we can live day to day to day, even a lifetime, without thinking about air, soil, water, lumber, and energy. If we do think about them, we think about them in the abstract. We don't have a visceral relationship with any of these essential resources.

For example, when I say "grass," most people associate that word, in its first sense, with lawns. And yet that is a paltry, uninformed notion of grass. Artificially planted and maintained two-inch turf grass is a far cry from the grass I'm talking about. I'm talking about native prairies, and *Little House on the Prairie*, where Ma and Pa Ingalls feared Laura would become lost if she went out of the house. The University of Nebraska still maintains an acre or two of this grass in Lincoln. It's twelve feet tall with stems more than half an inch thick. The first Europeans into Virginia's Shenandoah Valley wrote letters home describing grasses that could be tied in a knot above the horse's saddle.

When I say "pasture," do you think of it as a glorified lawn? Imagine grass as high as your head and so thick you can scarcely walk through it. That's grass. The point I'm making here is that as a culture, our references even to fundamental farming concepts stem from an urbanized mentality. Rather than viewing lawn as a downsized, unnatural, high-maintenance pasture, we view pasture as an upsized, high-maintenance lawn to be doted over, a money drain.

To have a discussion about normal living, normal ecology, all my readers need to understand how ignorant we've become as a culture. With our frame of reference skewed, our perceptions about farming, and our notions of what is environmentally enhancing or not, we approach farming with prejudicial brain damage. As a result, we have environmentalists spouting the ignorant notion that cows are belching methane and causing global warming. The scientific studies impugning the cow view her as taking, taking, taking, and not putting anything back.

That's like valuing children on the basis of diaper costs. Do they not have any redeeming value? I cringe when I read modern reports of how much children cost. A culture that creates a negative value on children has to be the least creative culture on earth. Children have always been valued as a treasure and a blessing. Throughout history, the cow has been considered an asset, and even worshipped in some cultures. She is the basis of dowries in nomadic societies, the ultimate currency. Ours must be the first culture in history that demonizes the cow.

The cow, perhaps more than anything else, represents civilization. Domesticating this multipurpose beast that can turn lowly grass into meat, milk, power, clothing, cordage, tools, lubricant, cleansers, and roofing materials arguably defined civilized living opportunities. Ecologically, the cow restarts the photosynethetic biomass accumulation process. Pretty important, I'd say.

Pruning is a universally accepted horticultural practice. On our shrubbery, our apple trees, our vineyards, pruning develops the foliage, strengthens the plant, and creates better fruit. An herbivore is a grass pruner. Without the herbivore, the forage would grow to senescence, fall over, and oxidize CO_2 into the atmosphere. The herbivorous pruning restarts the juvenile growth phase of the biomass engine — kind of like pushing a horticultural restart button. Without the herbivore, the photosynthetic activity — viewed like a solar collector — shuts down into dormancy. Throughout history and worldwide, the herbivore reawakens biomass, stimulating it to greater solar activity.

When farmers divorce the herbivore from fulfilling this ecological function, it cannot perform the positive function it is supposed to. In what will surely be a classic on this entire subject, Simon Fairlie's book *Meat: A Benign Extravagance* gives the math and apologetics for all the positives derived from herbivores. From antiscientific UN reports to religious broadsides, the antiherbivore campaign is both highly abnormal and incorrect.

Because some people use the cow abusively by denying this normal role is not reason to demonize the cow any more than it would be proper to eliminate automobiles because someone drives one recklessly. Not a single long-term tillage system on earth exists without an herbivorous component. You can't just substitute tofu (made from tillage — soybeans) for the herbivore. It doesn't work ecologically. Period. No matter how much you like tofu.

This is perhaps one of the biggest misunderstandings people have about farming ecology. In a desire to get rid of the cow, they want to substitute plants that require tillage. No long-term example exists in which tillage is sustainable. It always requires injection of biomass from outside the system or a soil-development pasture cycle. To think that plants which require tillage can build soil like perennial pasture indicates environmental absurdity.

Tillage, or stirring the soil, burns out organic matter due to the hyperoxygenation it creates. While this offers a tremendous amount of energy to a growing crop like squash, corn, or wheat, it comes at a price in soil degradation, and especially nitrogen retention. On our farm, we use the lawn around our house as a biomass importer for the vegetable garden. We mulch our vegetables with the grass clippings, which slowly decompose and build soil that the vegetables deplete. The lawn accumulates fertility and the garden depletes fertility. This is the nature of tilled versus perennial systems.

It doesn't matter whether the tillage is for cotton, corn, soybeans (tofu), peanuts, or tomatoes: Tillage always depletes soil organic matter and vital nutrients. This is why all traditional cropping systems demanded a multiyear pasturage component between cropping years. Newman Turner's ley farming system in Britain illustrated the soil-developing strength of pasturage. In this case, he would grow red clover and orchardgrass, for example, for three years and then grow one year of grain followed by a year of a root crop like turnips or beets before going back into forage.

The Argentina system of pasturage followed by two years of annuals like small grain, corn, or soybeans was developed because chemical fertilizer was too expensive or unavailable. Most sustainable farmers in America who grow annuals practice a multiyear rotation that includes pasturage. At the least, they grow a soil-developing cover crop between cycles. Cover crops are generally leafy annuals allowed to accumulate biomass and then tilled or mown ahead of another crop. The point is that the soil's biological economy requires putting something back. Historically, the herbivore-pasturage cycle put things back.

Some say, just because we use the cow to graze the soil-building pasture component, does that mean we have to eat her?

This is the kind of question that scares me. Rather than showing some new enlightenment, it illustrates a new state of absurdity. Who is going to handle these cows if they have no value other than as mowers? What happens when a cow gets old? Who is going to manage these cows to make sure they are on the field that needs them at the right time? Are you willing to pay a hundred dollars for a loaf of bread in order to finance the cow component necessary to rejuvenate the soil?

This brings me to one of the biggest abnormalities we're facing on the farm: anthropomorphism. This past summer, a group of well-meaning women near one of our rental farms turned us in to the animal control officers for abusing our cows. One of these ladies had driven by the paddock at 4 p.m. and saw the bunched-up 300-head herd, waiting patiently by the gate to the next paddock. We move the herd to their next paddock every day at about 4 p.m. and they get very used to the routine.

She called animal control, insisting that these cows looked like they were crowded, and since she didn't like crowds, the cows must be unhappy. Folks, this kind of ignorance just ain't normal. That our culture has the luxury to employ somebody to take this lady seriously is indeed abnormal in the history of civilization.

Realize that this herd had a couple of acres to spread out into had they wanted to do so. It wasn't as if they were corralled in a tight spot. They could have gone anywhere in the paddock. But cows are herding animals. Get it? Herding. Why do the wildebeests on the Serengeti bunch up when they could spread out over thousands of square miles? They bunch up for predator protection. This is instinctive herding behavior. Another advantage of bunching up is that bodies rubbing together disturbs the flies, keeping these irritants from landing. Swarming, disturbed flies are much easier for birds to catch in midair than when sitting on the backs of animals. From a nutrient standpoint, the crowding creates more aggressive hoof action to chip up their manure, treading it into the ground to stimulate fertility. It shades their urine so it seeps into the ground rather than evaporating.

A lot of cool things happen in that tightly grouped herd. It is all positive; not one negative thing. Animals are not people. Unfortunately, we've entered a time in our culture when the only interaction most people have with an animal is with a pet. Some people call their pets their children. In fact, many people are more concerned about the food nutrition for their pets than for their children. When Fido gets all-natural raw canine-primal pampering, the humans are glued to the TV munching nachos dipped in Velveeta. Are we missing something?

To put this subject in perspective, I receive letters from time to time pleading with me to quit raising livestock. The writers always include some metaphysical encounter or an epiphany that moved them into a higher spiritual dimension of oneness with cows and chickens. The result is a new understanding that animals are humans. They are just four-legged people, and if I would quit murdering them, then I would be a greater blessing to our world. The writers implore me to join them in this new level of understanding: A cow is a child is a fish is a fly is my daughter.

This does not indicate a new evolutionary heightened cosmic awareness, but a new devolutionary and unprecedented disconnectedness with our ecological umbilical. One writer provided me a list of quotations that she hoped would "inspire" me, beginning with the Bible's Job 12:7–8: "But ask now the beasts, and they shall teach you; and the fowls of the air, and they shall tell you: Or speak to the earth, and it shall teach you: and the fishes of the sea shall declare unto you." If this isn't consistent with my admonition to honor the pigness of the pig, I don't know what is. I learn from my animals every day. I learn from my carrots and tomatoes every day. I even learn from people — sometimes.

The writer of the letter, however, insisted that I take this biblically enjoined animal education and elevate the beasts to human equivalency. Not only does this misconstrue the biblical admonition, it also assumes that all teachers must be humans. Such insistence is nonsense. Practically everything can teach me something. Even inanimate objects, like a stubborn bolt on an engine or a water pump that won't prime — everything can teach. Just because I learn something from an entity does not make that entity human.

Included in this biblical passage is a broad "earth" concept. Who among us does not learn from the earth? But does that mean that a carrot must be worshipped? When I pluck that carrot from the ground, I mash it, rip the fibers apart, and pulp it in my mouth. It is absolutely and violently destroyed as a carrot. But that gives me the energy to plant another carrot; hence, carrothood is ensured through this sacrifice.

The fact that life requires sacrifice has profound spiritual ramifications. In order for something to live, something else must die. And that should provide us a lesson in how we serve one another and the creation and Creator around us. Everything is eating and being eaten. The perpetual sacrifice of one thing creates life for the next. To see this as regenerative is both mature and normal. To see it as violence that must be stopped is both abnormal and juvenile.

To take this one step further, I would even suggest that the sacrifice is elevated to sacredness based on the respect and honor bestowed on the sacrifice during its life. For example, if we string up a murderer, we don't call that a sacrifice; we call it just deserts. But if an honorable person is strung up, then he is immortalized as a sacrifice. The life well lived bestows upon the sacrifice its sacredness. And so how the chicken or carrot or cabbage lives defines the life's value consummated in the act of death — chomping, masticating, burying in our intestines to regenerate flesh of our flesh and bone of our bone. That no life can exist without sacrifice is a profound physical and spiritual truth. And the better the life, the greater the sacrifice.

I have no problem with vegetarians who choose to vote against industrial farming by eating that way. Teresa and I have always said that if we didn't know somebody like us, we'd practically be vegetarians too. And for the record, when Rush Limbaugh fires up his machine guns against the monkeys in the jungle, I don't think that's funny. Animals do indeed have rights, but that does not elevate them to humanhood. Where the animal rightists cross the line is when they call a cow or chicken a human. I do not try to argue with those folks. It's useless. And I won't spend time on that here. What I want to discuss is the level of ignorance about farming in general and animals specifically that makes even well-meaning people appear absurd.

For example, the following comes from a bulletin I picked up at a green living fair from United Poultry Concerns. A visitor who claimed to have toured Polyface Farm "on a sweltering day" questioned the animals' "freedom" and our "compassion" for the animals. "Chickens were in tiny cages with tin roofs in the beating sun, panting like mad. The cages were located over manure piles the birds were supposed to eat larvae from. Rabbits were kept in factory-farm conditions in suspended, barren wire cages." I won't quote the passages about other farms in the brochure, but I will take a look at these assertions since they deal with our farm.

First, realize that our farm has an open-door policy. The fact that anyone can come at any time, unannounced, to see anything, is certainly a transparency that is both vibrantly open but also risky. We don't screen people to be sure they comprehend what they see. First of all, we have to understand that these people violently oppose eating animals. On the front of the brochure, they quote author Joe Bob Briggs, writing online in *We Are the Weird*, "The waiter said, 'All of our chicken is free-range.' And I said, 'He doesn't look very free there on that plate.'" While this might elicit a smile, it's pure nonsense. A carrot doesn't seem very much like a carrot in my intestines, either. Give me a break.

The above visitor admits she toured Polyface on a sweltering day. It was a sweltering day, okay? I'll guarantee you that I was sweating way more than those chickens out there in the field. Animals have a dramatic ability to adapt to weather conditions. Have you ever watched ducks and geese swimming on a pond when it's freezing outside? Doesn't that look cold to you? And yet those ducks and geese are perfectly happy.

A friend told me his neighbor called animal control on him because his horses looked cold. It had snowed a couple of inches and the horses had some snow on their backs and were standing in the cold. The neighbor's ducks and geese were swimming contentedly on the pond. Not only were the horses not cold; they were as content as could be. In winter, these animals grow extra feathers, hair, and wool to give them more insulation against cold. Far more animals have been killed through respiratory trauma being locked in buildings than died being out in the cold.

A chicken is perfectly happy as long as she doesn't get wet and stays out of the wind. Although the quarters may be frigid, she'll be just fine. Haven't you ever seen a sparrow or chickadee sitting on a tree branch on a day so frigid you wouldn't want to be outside? And yet these tiny little creatures are chirping and swooping, seeming to have the time of their lives. Just because your cat would rather be inside doesn't mean it's abusive to have these animals in the cold.

Heat is the same way. Dogs pant. Cats even pant. And yes, on a sweltering day our chickens pant. I sweat. This is nature's way of dealing with heat, of the body getting rid of the heat. If every day were like this, we'd probably make some changes. In extremely hot areas like south Texas, pastured poultry producers take the summer off in their seasonal production just like here in Virginia we take the winter off. Not every single day is 70 degrees with blue skies and little puffy clouds.

These visitors probably didn't know that just before they arrived we were up there spraying water over the shelters to cool things off and give the birds some relief. This is life. We're all uncomfortable. That doesn't mean you're about to die. I wonder if these visitors returned home to air-conditioning that is destroying the planet through unsustainable energy use. It's so easy just to step onto someone's place and start finger-pointing, without any context, and with a jaundiced view toward animal welfare.

I wonder how many of the people who go apoplectic over alleged herbivore carbon footprints jet to Africa for photo-safaris. How many Nature Conservancy members burn copious amounts of fossil fuel toting their kiddos to soccer and ballet, then returning to air-conditioned comfort? Let's be big enough to recognize our inconsistencies. I'm inconsistent too, but it's a lot easier to spot it in others than myself.

The visitor says the birds were crammed into tiny cages. Interestingly, whenever one of these chickens inadvertently gets outside the shelter (or cage, as she calls them), the bird immediately begins circling, circling, circling, chirping an alarm, and trying to find a way back inside. Instinctively, the birds know they are vulnerable to predation outside. Besides, being social beings, they want to be inside with their mates. To think that these birds would rather be outside their "cages" indicates a profound lack of understanding regarding chickenness; a profound ignorance about predator and weather protection.

On that sweltering day, an afternoon thunderstorm would wreak havoc on those young broiler chickens. Their "cage" protected them from both the stifling sun and the violent rain that was boiling up, unseen, on the other side of the mountain to our west. Interestingly, the visitor says nothing about whether the chickens acted hot or uncomfortable. All she knew was that the shelter didn't look like a place she wanted to be, so she assumed it was a place the chickens didn't want to be. Until they are in their last two weeks of age, broilers can handle 100 degrees without any problem. When they get big, we put prop sticks under the shelters to create air convection sucking under the sheltered lid. If the author of the critical commentary was like most visitors, she wouldn't even have noticed these props, or felt their air current. Most visitors don't notice all these nuances of our care. But they know what they know what they know, and write about it in publications and spread their ignorance.

The comment about the birds being over manure piles they were supposed to eat larvae from is interesting to me. I have no clue what was going through the visitor's mind. Actually, cow manure contains seven essential enzymes necessary for bird digestion. Birds following herbivores is symbiotic, and one of the most elemental patterns in nature. Here again, I'm assuming the author of this report thought this was despicable. Actually, these lethargic broilers don't scratch the cow pie like the mature nonhybrid and aggressive, fully mature layers in our Eggmobiles do. But the cow manure still aids in the digestion. Just because a manure pile seems yucky to the visitor certainly does not mean it's yucky to the chicken. To the chicken, those manure piles are like Grandma's cookies. Yum. I've never known a chicken to show aversion to a cow pie, except for the one time when we brought some ivermectin-treated cows to our farm. The sterile cow pies had nothing to offer the chickens.

That we move these shelters every day to a fresh spot isn't even mentioned by this prejudiced visitor. The truth is that our birds at Polyface receive far more square footage per chicken in their lifetime than free-range flocks; they just don't receive it all at once. Instead, they receive a fresh piece of pasture every day so they can't soil the whole. That keeps things sanitary, keeps pathogens down, and keeps the pasture salad bar fresh to stimulate the appetite. Animals all eat dessert first. They notice staleness much sooner than a human.

In the final analysis, I assume a child's playpen would be considered abusive to this visitor. What's the point of a playpen? It's a protected environment to allow the child limited freedom at an age when unlimited freedom would invite harm. That is exactly what our field shelters are all about. These birds go out to the field before they are three weeks old. That's scarcely bigger than a sparrow. And it's a mighty tasty morsel for a crow or starling. And mighty vulnerable to weather shifts. What the visitor needed to say, to be honest, was that she considers domestic livestock inherently sinful. Come on, just be open about it.

Now let's go to the rabbits, suspended in factory farm–style cages. I wonder if this visitor has ever visited a factory rabbit operation? In multiple tiers, the cages reek of urine and feces. Ours has roomy cages, one level only, with chickens scratching through the droppings underneath. It's interesting that nowhere did this visitor indicate any noxious odors. That is a powerful omission, and shows she couldn't enjoy something different even when it hit her on the head.

Our rabbits receive forage routinely, another nonfactory reality. They receive high-quality hay in the winter and green chop in the summer.

I wonder if she saw the bunnies in portable field shelters nearby? She would have thought them too confined as well. But they receive a new spot every day and eat up to 75 percent of their diet off the pasture. In truth, on our farm the rabbits do push the "rabbitness" envelope harder than any other animal we raise.

The reason rabbits in the world are not in groups is because they are extremely susceptible to coccidiosis, a disease caused by a soil-borne protozoan parasite. Most commercial rabbitries feed a coccidiostat routinely and subtherapeutically to combat this problem. Whether it is technically an antibiotic is subject to debate. On our farm, we do not feed coccidiostats. By our suspending the rabbits above chickens on deep bedding, the manure and urine feed nitrogen to the carbonaceous bedding and eliminate odors. The composting bedding also grows bugs and worms that entice the chickens to scratch deeper and aerate the material, further encouraging bug and worm proliferation.

One other critical factor: Does (mother rabbits) eat their bunnies when disturbed or frightened. Who knows why, but stressed does will eat their bunnies. Having the does out where dogs, urban visitors, and machinery frightens them encourages this cannibalistic behavior. Our Raken (Rabbit-Chicken) house creates a soothing ambient chicken chatter that ameliorates fright from visitors. I suppose you could argue that rabbits should not be raised domestically because of these instinctive constraints.

I would argue that people eat rabbits. They are going to eat them whether we raise them or not. We may as well supplant factory rabbits with our kind rather than giving it all up to the industrial mindset. Furthermore, rabbitries have been part of domestic livestock for centuries. My son Daniel wanted to raise them as an independent business when he was eight years old, and his rabbit enterprise provided him an early farming endeavor that helped entice him into farming. I do not for a second apologize for this enterprise that helped shape his character and business acumen. Go point your finger somewhere else. The rabbit enterprise has been foundational to express the Danielness of Daniel.

The final statement in this visitor's report says there was no sign of compassion or freedom for the animals. What is freedom? What is compassion? Do you know what the animal considers freedom? Remember, I admit that the rabbit enterprise pushes the envelope as hard as anything we do here at Polyface. We certainly have our rough spots. But the trade-off of providing a stress-free life, with a natural forage-based diet, certainly offers some positives. And the fact that these rabbits are healthy without antibiotics and other props indicates their happiness in this environment. With that said, we are always looking for ways to do better.

And no compassion? Wow. Ouch. That's a pretty broad brush there, dear visitor. Perhaps she has not seen the sleepless nights, the days in sweltering heat providing additional care, running extra water lines. Which brings us back to the herd waiting to be moved, the herd that looked like a crowd. Another abuse charge was that we were not feeding them any hay. Since every other farmer in the county was feeding hay, she assumed we were starving them. And finally, she said they went four days without water.

The reason we were not feeding any hay was because with our grazing management, we had a nice forage stockpile ahead of them that we were systematically marching through one day, one paddock at a time. When we explained this to her, she responded, "Well, if you've already grazed it, what is there to eat?" We explained that we rested these paddocks. "How long?" she queried. "A hundred days." She had no clue about controlled grazing management, and did not even have the understanding to notice the cattle being moved every day into tall, rested forage.

The water, of course, was available to the herd in a portable trough that we also moved along with them every day. But the water trough could not be seen from the public road, so she assumed they had no water. We explained that the cattle drank out of a water trough that was always with them. Incredulous, she asked, "How does the water get there?" Trying to hold back our laughter, we explained, "We pump it through a pipe." Folks, this lady is a college-educated, upper-crust garden club type, well-intentioned as can be, but ignorant as a post. But the animal control officers, regardless of whether or not the charges are outrageous, must follow up each allegation as if it has merit.

After several days of our time squiring these officials around the farm, the top veterinarian said, "You don't have an animal problem. You have a people problem." The informant accused us of not being neighborly. We responded that neighborliness would have meant that she called us before the animal control people. That's what neighbors do. Cows want to be in a herd. They don't eat potatoes and pheasant; they eat grass. They like being outside in the winter just like deer and elk and moose and bison. They find places to shelter themselves; even the lee of a little ridge can make all the difference in the world.

And finally, sometimes everything isn't perfect. I'm sure these folks that demand that everything every day at Polyface be perfect never have a day when their house is a mess or their marriage takes an awkward turn. Judgmentalism combined with ignorance is a dangerous combination.

A perfect example is the crusade many animal rightists are waging against shipping chicks in the mail. Chicks are not human babies. When a bird lays a clutch of eggs to incubate, she can't lay all the eggs in one day. She lays them over the course of a week or more and then goes into a semihibernation state called setting. The first egg laid, exposed to ambient temperature, does not grow very fast. That embryo in effect waits on the others to be laid. Once the hen quits laying the clutch and begins setting on them, she has to stay on them and not let them be exposed to ambient temperature for more than a few minutes. Just enough time for her to get off the nest and grab some water. She eats very little during these roughly three weeks.

Finally, the eggs begin hatching. The first one to hatch is probably the first egg laid. The eggs will hatch over the course of twenty-four to seventy-two hours. If the hen gets off the nest to care for the early-hatched chicks, she will expose the not-yet-hatched embryos to the cold at their most vulnerable time. So she has to wait for the last one. God designed chicks, therefore, with a unique ability to survive just fine without feed and water for three days so that all their siblings can hatch before the mother hen takes them on their first meal outing. In case you're wondering, chicks don't nurse their mothers. The mothers take them to food, and from day one, chicks feed themselves. How about that, moms? Pretty cool, huh? Chicks are not human.

This unique quality allows chicks to be shipped through the mail without hurting them. People who want to close down this practice are actually hurting the alternative to chicken factories. Anybody up on these issues is well aware of the stench and other problems associated with concentrated animal feeding operations. David Imhoff's blockbuster book *The CAFO Reader* can dispel any ignorance about these industrial operations that view life mechanically rather than biologically. Factory farms don't need to send their chicks through the mail because due to their volume they have dedicated hatcheries and delivery vehicles to transport thousands of chicks to one factory house at a time.

Too often, factory farming detractors — of which I am one — fail to differentiate between animals raised well and those that are not. Their abhorrence of the industrial abuses swings their pendulum all the way over to a prejudicial view toward all animal consumption. At that point, the charges become disingenuous. To refuse to admit that systems exist that honor and respect the animals shows the true agenda — no livestock whatsoever. That is not only highly abnormal historically; it is both unrealistic and ecologically devastating.

The function that herbivores play, for example, in stimulating biomass accumulation is both powerful and real. Chickens have historically converted kitchen scraps into eggs. Pigs have historically scavenged domestic waste products as varied as whey, offal, forest mast, and spoiled grain. That a large percentage of landfilled material is animal-edible food waste should strike us as criminal. Rather than showering landfill administrators with greenie awards for injecting pipes into the anaerobic swill to collect biogas, we should be cycling all that edible waste through chickens and pigs so that it never goes to the landfill in the first place.

Instead, we send armies around the world to ensure cheap petroleum to energize chemical fertilizer factories to inject acidulated elemental Nitrogen, Potassium and Phosporus (N,P and K) into tilled soils to grow grain to be harvested, gas-dried, then transported to animal factories. And now that the landfills are filling too fast, we routinely incinerate these wet, edible wastes in energy-intensive systems that run at a net energy loss. It's insane. Nature's systems do not generate waste. When will we learn that there is no away? We say we'll throw it away, but away doesn't exist. That's why nature is full of loops and cycles.

People who think it's better to incinerate kitchen scraps, or biogas them at the landfill, than it is to feed these materials to pigs or chickens are out of touch with normalcy. Traditional recycling like this was foundational to the economy of a farmstead or village prior to this blip that we now know as cheap energy.

Another argument often touted by the anti–farm animal crowd (notice, they usually aren't opposed to pets) is that it generates too much manure. And they cite experts who finger manure as one of the top ten pollutants in America. Its two billion tons is seen as a liability rather than an asset.

Ecologically astute farmers realize that this manure is the answer to maintaining soil fertility and development. The problem is not the manure generation. The grains people are supposed to eat, presumably grown in places like the Midwest, are still mining the mountains of manure and biomass accumulated there during the millennia of grazing bison. What has become a curse through modern abnormal factory farming is supposed to be one of nature's greatest blessings. This carte blanche demonizing of a historical blessing indicates a profound disconnect to our ecological umbilical.

The antimeat crowd routinely argues that more people could be fed with grain directly than from the meat created by animals eating grain. In a world of starving people, how can we afford land-wasting models like animal production? Indeed, the most vehement of them charge that animal production increases famine.

Most articles promoting this notion greatly inflate the grain-meat conversion ratio, using outlandish figures like fifteen pounds of grain to one pound of meat. I don't know where these scientists get these figures, but it sure isn't from a farm. It's probably from some prejudicial software. The real numbers are about seven pounds for beef, three pounds for pork, and two pounds for poultry. But again, herbivores would not need any grain, and hogs could run with electric fencing on the nation's forests. If all kitchens had enough chickens attached to consume the table scraps, egg commerce would not exist. Perennial pasture completely changes these animals from liability into asset. And pasture is land-healing rather than land-debilitating like grains.

Furthermore, nobody in the world goes hungry due to lack of food production. It is distribution and other problems that create starvation. Because they can eat perennials that do not require tillage, herbivores are always preferred in impoverished societies. This is why the most efficacious famine-relief agencies I've been privileged to work with, like Heifer Project International, are founded on livestock. If you really want to help impoverished people, get them started in animal husbandry.

I find it strangely abnormal that people accuse meat eaters of elitism. "Why do you want people to starve?" they ask. The truth is that if someone had magical powers and could click their fingers, doubling the world's food production tomorrow, it would not find its way into one needy stomach. The ugly truth is that nobody goes hungry due to a lack of food. They go hungry due to a lack of distribution.

I know a lady in North Carolina who lives next to a yogurt factory. She raises pigs — that was the occasion of my acquaintance — on rotten milk. She said the factory throws away tractor-trailer loads of milk all the time — she can get as much of it as she wants, for free. Anyone who has worked in industrial food processing facilities knows that this is the case. If all the whey generated from cheesemaking went through hogs, like it did historically, we could produce the pork as a salvage and still get all the meat and manure. As it is, most of it is just thrown away or energy-intensively processed into organic fertilizer for potted geraniums in the homes of middle-class Americans.

These homes, by the way, could fertilize their geraniums with manure generated from a couple of chickens fed on kitchen scraps. Why are chickens dirtier than parakeets? I say get rid of the parakeets and put a couple of chickens in there. They'll make far less noise and give you beautiful eggs to boot. Talk about win-win.

The nutrient density of meat is far superior to grains, and far easier to come by. A no-livestock agenda actually starves people and impoverishes developing societies.

Much if not most of the land in perennial pasture, worldwide, is not suitable for tillage. Were it ripped up in tillage, the assault on the earth's precious soil resources would bring far more cruelty even than factory farming. The amount of nutrition per resource expenditure is more on perennial pasture than it is on tilled ground. The anti-animal prejudice here is quite apparent. So is the naiveté that tillage is ecologically neutral. It never has been and never will be.

Another argument advanced by the anti–farm animal crowd is that it uses too much water. Again, I've seen the numbers, and many of them are ridiculous. I don't know if they pull these numbers out of a hat.

All across the world, where historically normal (natural) herbivore-perennial patterns are being practiced, hydrology cycles show marked improvement. Springs run again; creeks remain viable longer into dry periods. Protective ground cover increases. The fact that anti-animal folks refuse to learn about these success stories does not dismiss their reality. Only a simpleton assumes that all beef is feedlot beef and creates numbers from that model as if it's the only one that exists. Why don't they qualify all their charges with the words "grain-fed" or "feedlot," rather than just saying "beef"? This broad-brush approach is neither fair nor scientifically accurate. And for the record, if they really want to save water, how about attacking flush toilets that use potable water?

The same dichotomy exists on the vegetable side. Too often these grain-only advocates do not differentiate between ecologically friendly plants and those that aren't. Failure to qualify the terms is a failure to appreciate the devastating effect grain production has had on the world's ecology.

Depending on which historian you read, our Shenandoah Valley lost three to eight feet of topsoil during its first two hundred years of European settlement. When our family moved to our farm in 1961, shale bedrock exposures on the hillsides provided a natural monument to years of soil loss under grain production. And now, after fifty years on these soilless barrens, using perennials and animals, lots of compost, and patience, the soil has rebounded and those wounds are covered with several inches of fertile soil. Except, of course, where we fenced out cattle. Those areas are still barren and soilless just like they were in 1961, even though we fenced them out and let trees begin growing.

In the last century, Iowa, breadbasket of America, has lost half of its topsoil. Wouldn't it have been better to return our omnivorous livestock to food salvage operations and utilize our techno-glitzy electric fence systems to mimic undulating bison herds on the Iowa fields? Until the advent of the electric fence, we couldn't really duplicate the kind of management on a private-property scale that nature accomplished in the wild. But now we can, so we have no excuse not to return to historically accurate land management normalcy with herbivores. This is the land management, by the way, that created the deep soils we've been mining for the last century growing grains since vacating our Shenandoah Valley's eroded soils.

Remember, people, you always need to compare what somebody says against historical and philosophical authenticity. The dearth of

farming-ecology understanding is ubiquitous in our culture. I appreciate that I'm ignorant about things. Having grown up deprived of TV
and in turn depriving my own children of TV, I'm extremely ignorant
about Hollywood, movies, and celebrities. I've heard of *Bonanza* and
The Beverly Hillbillies, but I really prefer cowboy shows or comedies if
I'm going to watch something. Okay, okay, I'm not that bad...but I'm
pretty bad.

I really like those old shows. I've decided the way to know you're
becoming an old fogey is when the only shows you like are sponsored
by Depends, the Scooter Store, and Viagra. Ha!

Back to our discussion about ignorance: Seriously, what is important
to know? What we spend our time discovering and learning is a direct
reflection or result of what we believe to be important. When I look at a
bookstore shelf during layovers at airports, one of my favorite pastimes,
much to Teresa's alarm —"Another book? Where do you expect me to
put it?" — I'm attracted to the subjects I deem important. This is a fact
of life, and for the record, I do buy things from every side of the argument and political spectrum. I like to know what the other side thinks —
and often I learn things I didn't know.

One of my messages in this book is to try to awaken a thirst and hunger for some basic food and farming knowledge before our appetite for
cerebral and academic techno-subjects crowds out all of this historically normal knowledge. This is why it's more important, in my humble
opinion, to acquaint your children with your local farmers than with
Bambi. Wouldn't you agree that it's just as important to attend a forest
walk-through with a logger as with a birdwatching club?

Wouldn't it be as valuable to go process your Thanksgiving turkey, or
at least spend some time with it in the field, as it is to face-paint your
five-year-old and stick colored feather-shaped construction paper in her
hair? Farms and food production should be, I submit, at least as important as who pierced their navel in Hollywood this week. Please tell me
I'm not the only one who believes this. Please. As a culture, we think
we're well educated, but I'm not sure that what we've learned necessarily helps us survive.

I'm talking about the skills and knowledge contained, for example,
in the Foxfire books. The back-to-the-land books of the hippie era are
still some of the best living manuals out there. Country craft and

farmsteading enjoy an interest revival every time things look bleak. To me, it seems prudent to acquaint ourselves with some of this information before a meltdown occurs. A rudimentary, basic understanding of things won't crowd out our celebrity information or keep us from knowing how to use a cell phone. Trust me, it won't. I love people, and I love learning. And it seems to me that an educated person should know a few basic things about farm ecology. Not much, just a little. Just a little. I offer the next examples in the spirit of explanation.

"You don't have roosters with your laying hens. How do they lay eggs?" Dear folks, chickens don't need roosters to lay eggs. They need roosters to hatch eggs, but not to lay them. Just like women don't need men to lay eggs; they just need a man to hatch one. A mere century ago, not one in a hundred would have been ignorant of this common agrarian knowledge.

The next common one: "Oh, there's the bull, 'cause he has horns." Dear hearts, horns do not make a bull. It ain't what's on top of the head that counts. It's what's between the legs. I don't know if horns have anything to do with horniness, but they sure don't have anything to do with masculinity.

A farmer friend of mine told me recently about a busload of middle school children who came to his farm for a tour. The first two boys off the bus asked, "Where is the salsa tree?" They thought they could go pick salsa, like apples and peaches. Oh my. What do they put on SAT tests to measure this? Does anybody care? How little can a person know about food and still make educated decisions about it? Is this knowledge going to change before they enter the voting booth? Now that's a scary thought.

Do you know the difference between hay and straw? Straw is the stalk and leaves of a small grain plant. Stover is the leftovers of a corn plant. Hay is solar-dried forage. When forage gets tall, you cut it and let it lie in the sun. The sun dehydrates it so it can be packed together without molding. Hay is edible for the animals and straw is generally used for bedding because the edible part came off in the grain, which is really a big fat seed. If forage is packed together before it dehydrates, and you exclude the air with airtight packaging (silo, plastic) it ferments, making silage.

In order to get hay equally dried, it is windrowed to let the air blow through it and get the underneath leaves turned up to the drying sun. A windrow is a long tube of hay. A baler picks up the windrow and forms the hay into packages: round bales, little square bales, little round bales, or large square bales. Each of these has a different machine and different reason for use.

How do you herd cows? Cows have a flight zone. Since their eyes are on the sides of their head, they have far more peripheral vision than people. They can see about 300 degrees around themselves. If we could do that, it would be equivalent to having eyes in the back of our heads. Depending on our approach toward the cow, she either wants to go past us, turn around and stand off at us, or turn tail and run away. All these responses are a result of how we approach her flight zone.

Trees grow out, not up. They only grow up right at their buds. That is why you can put a rope on a tree and it stays at the same height. Once bark forms, that height does not change. The cambium grows the tree horizontally, in diameter, but not vertically. Otherwise that hammock we stretched between those two trees this year would be a foot higher next year and a foot higher the year after that. Wouldn't that be funny?

Farmers speak in precise language. A cow is a female who has had two calves. A first-calf heifer is a female who has had only one calf. A heifer is a female who has not calved. A bred heifer is a female who is pregnant but has not yet calved. A bull calf is a young uncastrated male. A bull is an uncastrated male old enough to breed — and that is far from full-grown, believe me. A calf is an unweaned bovine of either sex. A heifer calf is a female calf; a bull calf is a male calf. A stocker is a weaned calf prior to finishing. A finisher is a calf almost big enough to slaughter — it's being finished. An open cow is one that is not pregnant. A dry cow is nonlactating. A fresh cow is one that has very recently calved, and a freshening cow is one that is just about to calve. A bull can cover (breed) about thirty to fifty cows.

Folks, that's just cows. And believe it or not, virtually every American knew all this lingo a scant century ago. Every species has this same level of nomenclature. Not long ago, common knowledge included the difference between a wether (castrated male sheep) and a ram (breeding-age male sheep). A ram lamb and ewe lamb. A shoat (castrated male pig) and a gilt (unbred female pig). Sow and boar. And then you have the whole grouping thing: herd, flock, gaggle (geese). And as if that's not enough, the birthing takes on distinctives: cows calve, sheep lamb, rabbits kindle, hogs farrow, horses foal.

Can you name four vegetables that grow underground? Potatoes, carrots, onions, beets, salsify, parsnips, turnips. How about four that grow above ground? Corn, peppers, broccoli, cauliflower, Brussels sprouts, kohlrabi, green beans, lettuce, peas, melons, squash, cucumber. Tomatoes are a fruit. Which vegetables can handle a frost? Which ones have to be planted after frost? Which ones are legumes? Which ones grow tall? Which ones need trellises? Which ones are perennials? Asparagus, rhubarb.

Everywhere children and gardening mix, the enthusiasm for learning this heritage agrarian wisdom is insatiable. To interact with nature and food in this visceral functional way is foundational to developing common sense. When people lose touch with these cornerstones of existence, their thinking gets all screwy. Staying grounded, very literally, and staying anchored in sensibleness require relationships with food production. This is one reason we encourage people to come and visit our farm. We want people to interact with the animals, the gardens, the earthworms.

I just recently watched a French-produced video called *Micro-Cosmos*. It's been out since 1996 — so I'm behind the times — but it uses high-magnification photography to show, as its subtitle declares, "It's *Jurassic Park* in Your Own Backyard!" Everything we see, the air we breathe, the food we eat, is all dependent on a vast microscopic and insect-sized community. It is more grand, more beautiful than anything we can imagine.

When we as people view this vastly complex, diverse universe as some sort of cerebral science experiment, we lose our functional moorings. This magical, marvelous food on our plate, this sustenance we absorb, has a story to tell. It has a journey. It leaves a footprint. It leaves a legacy. To eat with reckless abandon, without conscience, without knowledge; folks, this ain't normal.

What should we do about this? Obviously, everyone can't move to a farm. But if this matters to you, here are some doable things to reconnect and reeducate.

1. Spend some serious time on a farm. Many farms now have work days, or work-share opportunities. Ask your farmer — you do know your farmer, don't you? — about labor opportunities. And when you go, assume that you don't know anything and you've never really worked a day in your life. This spirit will prepare you to absorb the information and the sore muscles awaiting you.

2. Involve your family in gardening. Community gardens, school gardens, your own backyard. Opportunities exist everywhere to grow something. A simple plastic solarium on the southern exposure of your house can provide both winter warmth and horticultural delight. If you make it big enough, you could put in a dining table.

3. I'm serious about the parakeets replaced with chickens.

4. All sanitation departments and solid waste administrators should campaign immediately to feed all edibles to on-site animals. Period and amen.

5. Forgo the Bambi vacation and visit a local farm in your area. Just spend time there. Spread a picnic in the field with the cows. I'm suggesting cows rather than chickens or pigs for a reason, by the way. A huddle of cows surrounding your picnic is certainly as exciting as watching squirrels in a city park. Don't get in the farmer's way. Make it clear that you simply want to learn, to connect, to observe.

6. Realize that agendas drive data, not the other way around.

7. Eat more grass-fed beef and less chicken or pork.

8. Read things you're sure will disagree with your current thinking. If you're a die-hard anti-animal person, read *Meat*. If you're a die-hard global warming advocate, read Glenn Beck. If you're a Rush Limbaugh fan, read James W. Loewen's *Lies My Teachers Told Me*. It'll do your mind good and get your heart rate up.

9. Raise some animals and prepare them for dinner. Small animals are best in urban settings. A cow might be a bit large for a backyard. But chickens and rabbits are extremely compatible with urban settings. At our farm, we welcome children to help dress chickens — the parents are squeamish. Children younger than ten don't have a problem with it. Once they hit twelve, it's not cool anymore. Timing is everything.

10. Take your children hunting, or send them with a friend who does. Learn how to dress game and prepare it. This is as ancient an education as humanity, and connecting to it may offer some of the best lessons for our future. People unable to connect with their predator persona may be missing something that helps complete their humanity. Injecting ourselves into our ecology is part of our mission, and truly a connection to our human birthright.

Hog Killin's and Laying
in the Larder

Where is all the food in your neighborhood? Think about it. Where is it? Down at the supermarket. At the Costco warehouse. Standard figures say that the average town has only three days' supply of food within its borders. A simple three-day interruption is enough to starve out a town.

From blizzards to floods, hurricanes to earthquakes, and even to longshoremen's strikes and Teamsters' interruptions, not to mention fuel anomalies, a three-day inventory of food is not very long. Certainly not when compared to historical normalcy.

I've been to the Powhatan village near the Jameston/Williamsburg living museum complex more than once, and it always captivates me even more than the European villages. These are the Native Americans who made squatty homes by bending over saplings, then covering them with skins and leaves. A circle of stones in the center contained a small fire, but the smoke did not draw well due to the shape of the house. Although the hole in the quasi-dome's center was over the fire, no chimney created a draft to suck up the smoke.

As a result, the upper reaches of these shelters always filled with smoke. For sure, the lower reaches had more smoke than would be healthy too, and that no doubt accounted for some physical ailments.

But I'm fascinated, when I go into one, to see the larder hanging up there in that smoke. The entire upper third of the shelter is a network of poles lashed together and holding smoked meat, berries, and vegetables.

Smoking is perhaps one of the oldest methods of food preservation, and certainly one of the most low-tech. When our son Daniel was about twelve years old with an avid appetite for Tom Brown survival books, he built a crude hot smoker in the backyard out of a barrel and ditch covered in corrugated roofing scraps. Smoking works, and these clever Native Americans incorporated it into their crude homes, laying by in a pantry literally over their heads.

Can you imagine lying down with your beloved every night and staring up into the murky ceiling of your home, looking at a multimonth supply of preserved food? Compare that to lying down with your beloved in a home with half a dozen blinking LCD lights — one for the cell phone base, one on the computer, one on the coffee maker — are you with me here? A humming refrigerator dependent on uninterrupted electricity no doubt generated by fuel dependent on a global transportation grid. The only nonperishable food in the house is sealed condiment bottles — salsa, ketchup, mustard, pickles — in the pantry and a few cans of processed commercial soup or dehydrated soup concentrate.

Talk about vulnerable. At best, real sustenance wouldn't last more than a couple of days, or perhaps a week. I suppose Homeland Security would consider those Powhatan villagers diabolically subversive, labeling them hoarders, to think about laying by.

Think about that iconic living history museum, Williamsburg, Virginia, during its bustling colonial vibrancy. Where was the food? Not down at the supermarket. Not at Costco. It was in those cellars, both wine and root, the larder. Goodness, today most young people have never heard the word "larder." And even the smaller version, "pantry," is going out of vogue. Now we're building living quarters with a nook — we don't even have kitchens.

How about during the time of Laura Ingalls and *Little House on the Prairie*? Where was the food? Not at the supermarket. Not at Costco warehouses.

The first supermarket supposedly appeared on the American landscape in 1946. That is not very long ago. Until then, where was all the food? Dear folks, the food was in homes, gardens, local fields, and forests. It was near kitchens, near tables, near bedsides. It was in the pantry, the cellar, the backyard.

I am well aware that people starved to death in earlier days. Of course, people are starving to death today — probably more than at any time in human history. At the same time, roughly half of all the human-edible food produced on the planet never gets eaten. It spoils in warehouses and shipping containers. It bruises during transportation. It exceeds sell-by status in logistical distribution snafus. It doesn't get to the refugee camp because a group of thugs holds a Red Cross truck at gunpoint.

If anyone could snap their fingers tomorrow and double the world's food production, not one single child would get a better meal than she got today. The world is throwing away mountains of food every day. Nobody goes hungry because of lack of food; they go hungry due to a lack of distribution. The underlying cause for that logistical transportation breakdown can be poverty, poor infrastructure like roads, sociopolitical upheaval, or something else. Food academics and advocates who have coined the term "urban food deserts" to describe inner-city situations where tobacco and soda are readily available but not meat and fresh tomatoes do not help the cause by saying this is a racial issue. The fact that most of these areas' demographics are predominantly African American has nothing to do with why farmers' markets, supermarkets, and real food stores don't want to locate there. These gang-infested, drug-heavy areas are simply not conducive to business — any kind of business. Legitimate business interests tend to shy away from poor inner-city areas, regardless of color, ethnicity, or religion.

Every time community gardens and embedded food production/processing enterprises get a toehold in these rough areas, it has a civilizing effect. I can't praise Will Allen's Growing Power, centered in Milwaukee, enough for bringing hope and opportunity to these areas. He is indeed the quintessential entrepreneur-prophet. The intensive production models he develops through biomimicry using high-tech hoophouses and synergistic multispeciated stacking, from fish to vegetables to vermicomposting, is remarkable and absolutely knocks the socks off of anything being bandied about by the industrial food fraternity.

When I went to Terra Madre, the international Slow Food

convivium founded by Carlo Petrini and held in Turin, Italy, a few years ago, I made a point to attend every African delegation presentation I could. Simultaneous translation was marvelous. Every single one of the African presenters I heard said something like this: "What is killing our local food system is cheap Western dumping. We have plenty of resources. We have plenty of knowledge. We have plenty of workers. If you westerners (primarily America, often via the United Nations and other relief organizations) would just stay out and quit displacing our indigenous economy and food systems with poor-quality commodities, we can feed ourselves, thank you."

In fact, our American delegation spent most of our time apologizing for our nation's actions and assuring delegates from other countries that we did not agree with America's food and agriculture policies. It was quite an eye-opening experience that I'll never forget. Whenever I think of it, the earnest, pleading passion of those African delegates rings in my ears.

This reminds me of an exchange I had in Canada a couple of years ago when I was in Ontario giving a speech. At the banquet meal, we were seated at round tables, about six people per table. I picked a seat at random, waited for the other five spots to fill, then we all sat down as the banquet hall filled up. I sat down and the guy next to me blurted out to the table, "I hate Christians."

"Well, this might be different," I thought, especially since I am one. Normally in these kinds of situations, everyone introduces themselves around the table amid magnanimous handshaking, smiles, and the deafening noise coming from all the other shuffling feet, scooting chairs, and introductions. Not at this table.

"I hate Christians." Everyone kind of looked quizzically at the guy, not quite sure whether he wanted a response or had more to say on the subject. I waited long enough to figure he wanted a response, and asked, "Why?" I don't know, it just seemed like the right next thing to say at the time. Wouldn't you?

"Their charity destroys developing countries," he answered. Turns out, he had just returned from a six-month video stint in a couple of African countries. He said several times he watched shipping containers of clothes, sent primarily by well-meaning conservative Christian missionary groups, completely destroy village economies. He explained

that people are people, and all cultures have deadbeats as well as entrepreneurial go-getters. The go-getters in these cultures are the village
shopkeepers and merchants.

When a container of foreign goodies arrives in the village, everyone
mobs the freebies and takes the Western handouts. This collapses the
local business and these displaced go-getters become the famous war-
lords we in the West have all learned are the nexus of all those people's
problems. This same story has been corroborated since and makes me
careful about how I help. Help is not always a handout. Help can also
be a butt-out. And help is not always about material possessions. Sometimes it requires faith in people to go through their societal evolution,
that they can indeed learn from their mistakes.

Interesting that the man identified Christian charity as the problem
and did not indicate that meddling and dumping by the UN or other
governmental-type groups creates the same problems. I think they do. I
don't know why, but my intuition suggests that voluntary private charity
probably wreaks less havoc than government charity, extracted by violence from an otherwise more charitable citizenry. And if you don't
think it's violent, just refuse to pay your taxes this year. Charity achieved
by force can never work.

Food security involves both quantity and quality. A new security
issue in recent years is the threat of bioterrorism, which would probably
fit under both categories. I'd like to talk about it a bit because it is such
a hot issue.

This is especially important because I'm considered a bioterrorist by
the defenders of the industrial food system. I am not, of course, but the
label is very real and very disturbing. The reason for the outrageous
label, of course, is because on our Polyface Farm we don't vaccinate,
medicate, acidulate, eradicate, irradiate, adulterate, or confiscate. Our
animals, therefore, threaten all our neighbors' livestock with diseases
and, by extension, the entire planet's food supply. All because our pastured chickens commiserate with red-winged blackbirds and indigo
buntings, which in turn take all our viruses to science-based environmentally controlled factory chicken houses and threaten to destroy the
planet's food supply. I am not making this up. More about this later.

At any rate, let's suppose I were a bioterrorist and I wanted to taint the
food supply. I think I'd want to make a big splash, get to as much food as

possible. Would I go to a small farm? I don't think so. I'd go to the larg-est farm I could find, especially one of those with a "No Trespassing" sign in front. Most of them don't have any people around. Nobody wants to work there because they stink to high heaven. If you drive up to them at 2 p.m., all you hear are feed augers, electric fans, and clank-ing feeders. Usually nobody is around.

And if I wanted to taint some food, would I go to someone's home pantry? I don't think so. I'd go to a huge warehouse with lots of employ-ees receiving low wages and just putting in their time. The mountains of food there would be an enticing target indeed. Is everyone with me on this? Bioterrorists aren't going to attack your pastured livestock farmer or your Community Supported Agriculture garden. Especially since most of these operations are more labor-intensive and have people running around — who actually like being there and care about what happens.

At the beginning of this chapter, I asked, "Where is all the food in your neighborhood?" A century ago the answer would have been that it was in the home or very near the home. Storing food in huge ware-houses, in a few distribution centers around the country, or in the silos of a few processors is vulnerable to bioterrorism precisely because it ain't normal.

Now let's go to the quantity issue. At our house, we have mountains of food. Teresa cans and freezes summer produce and fills our larder with hundreds of quarts of home-processed food. I can walk down to the basement anytime and count the jars. I can physically see those jars. Do you know how comforting that is? I can open the freezer and see bags of corn, packages of steak and sausage.

Routinely, Teresa hands me her shopping list: green beans, apple-sauce, sweet pickles, relish, squash, pickled beets. I dutifully — like all good husbands should — go to the basement and bring back the various seasonally produced, laid-by items. No money exchanges hands in this transaction. This is true home economics.

We didn't start this as a result of the Y2K scare. We do it because it's normal. I find it fascinating that greenies think they've really arrived in their journey to restore food security when they go down to the farmers' market and shop for a couple of apples to munch on and some artisanal homemade chutney. Don't get me wrong: I'm all in favor of patronizing farmers' markets. But be honest, now, when was the last time you saw someone — especially an upper-class environmentalist — walk up to a vegetable vendor at a farmers' market and ask, "Could I buy three bushels of green beans next week? I want to can about sixty quarts for our winter supply, and I'd like to do them next week if you have them."

The first thing that would happen in such an instance would be a panicked scream: "Is there a doctor here? A paramedic? We need help here right now! We've got a farmer in full cardiac arrest!"

The ugly truth is that if people actually went to farmers' markets to buy serious food, they'd wipe out the whole place in about twenty minutes. The average person is still under the aberrant delusion that food should be somebody else's responsibility until I'm ready to eat it. Most farmers' market buyers can only buy enough to fill one hand because the other is holding the leash for Fifi, the upscale, perfectly manicured poodle, or other canine of equal pampering. I like little ribboned bottles of condiments and cute bow-tied mini-breads. But I want to see people really buying their food, displacing their supermarket patronage, period.

I was on a radio talk show in Vermont one January and the host was giving me a hard time about organic food prices. "I had a party at my house last week and wanted to serve corn on the cob, so I went down to the supermarket and the regular corn was $2.49 for a dozen ears and the organic was $4.89. How can you justify that?"

Wrong question. The question is, "Why do you need fresh sweet corn in Vermont in January? You should be eating canned, frozen, or parched corn that you made late in the summer when farmers could scarcely give their corn away because people were over that and going for the fall squash and potatoes." He should have been feeding these guests from his own larder, amassed months earlier when farmers' market vendors were feeding half their late-season success to the compost pile. It happens everywhere and all the time. Restoring normalcy is our problem — you and me — not somebody else's problem.

How many of us lobby for green energy or protected lands, but don't engage with the local bounty to lay by for tomorrow's unseasonal reality? That we tend to not even think about this as a foundation for solutions in our food systems shows how quickly we want other people to solve these issues. Our ecology and our food systems are simply a visible manifestation of all the value systems, or thought processes, of every individual in the culture. One person, or one organization, or one group cannot fundamentally change things. It's the collective understanding of many that moves things from peripheral lunacy to cultural shift.

I don't know how tomato plants do it, but somehow they know when the first frost is coming. They will produce at a nice steady pace all summer long, a nice flow that you can handle. But all of a sudden, one week before frost, they shift into overdrive and dump buckets in your lap. It happens every year. And every year, vegetable growers at farmers' markets dump wheelbarrow loads of excess tomatoes right at the end of the season.

Where are the people lining up to buy them at half price, blemished along with the rest, to go home and make fruit leather, juice through the food mill, diced tomatoes, or canned whole tomatoes? Or ketchup or salsa? Throughout human history, before supermarkets, this end-of-season flurry of activity was normal in every household. Children cranked the food mill. Mom oversaw her expanding larder. Dad snitzed apples for applesauce and apple butter.

Have you ever been to a hog killin'? Virginia pork is legendary, of course. Let me describe a hog killin'. You have to wait until fall when the nights are just frosty a bit and the days are well above freezing but not enough to take off your jacket. I'm purposely being unscientific here, trying to explain it the way an old-timer would have known. After the first frost kills the flies and the weather is nippy enough to enjoy sitting around the fire of an evenin', you set up two large kettles and ready the scalding tub.

The scalding tub is like a sheet metal bathtub, sunken in the ground, sitting on some heavy steel grates. You go to the shed and get the tripod, a three-pole contraption that sets up like a teepee but has two wooden pegs on it near the top. The poles are about ten feet long. You sharpen knives and get out the big half-round log that acts as a cutting table. It's scarred with thousands of knife slashes accumulated during its long history.

Early the next morning, with all in readiness, you go to the hog lot and load anywhere from three to ten hogs in a trailer. You want to make sure you load all you're going to kill the first time. Once you shoot that first one and some blood gets in the trailer, you'll never load another hog in that trailer that day. This is wisdom. The number depends on how many you have to do and how much help you have. The menfolk load the hogs, get the fire going under the scald tub, and wash down the half-log table with lye soap and start the other fires under the two kettles partly full of water.

The womenfolk are putting together lunch, and that's no mean task. They're peeling potatoes for mashed potatoes — enough to feed twenty people. The turkey or two went in early, along with the ham. A big pot of green beans with pork fat is simmering on the stove, along with stewed tomatoes, baked apples with cinnamon on top, and homemade noodles with chicken broth. Three varieties of homemade pickles from earlier in the summer need to be put on a pickle tray. Boiled eggs need to be peeled for deviled eggs, and sweet potato casserole needs fixin'. You get the picture. Sourdough is rising in the warm spot above the stove in preparation for sourdough rolls.

Crack! The first .22 caliber rifle shot indicates the start of the day. The oldest and wisest man sticks the hog in the carotid artery to commence bleeding, and then steps over to whisk his finger through the scald water. It needs to be just hot enough that he can't keep his finger in more than an eight-inch swish through. Just right. All the men grab the hog and slide it out of the trailer and over to the scald trough. Using ropes wrapped around the hog, they lower it in and pull it back and forth, sloshing the water up and over the skin.

The oldest and wisest man kneels down to jerk a few hairs. Not quite ready yet. Another minute in the water. Still. Check. Ahh, just right. Between his thumb and forefinger, he pinches some hair and it comes out easily. Crack! Another hog goes down. The first hog, hauled out of the water onto a wide board, gets attacked by all the young boys wielding small metal saucer-shaped hog scrapers. A wooden handle attaches to the scraper, and with this tool they scrape the hair off the skin.

In about ten minutes they all hoist the hog onto the first tripod, sticking the wooden pegs through the leader ligament on the hind legs of the hog. They heave the poles upright until the hog's head is dangling just above the ground. One man dips a bucket of hot water from one of the kettles and sloshes it on the hanging carcass to rinse and cleanse the skin. An experienced man steps over and begins cutting down the belly to let the entrails roll out. Grandma stands to the side, because now we're getting into the women's business. She directs where the pancreas, lungs (lights), liver, heart, and kidneys go. The goal is to get all the hogs killed and hung on poles before lunch so they have time to chill. The chilling firms the meat and fat, making it easier to cut and process.

The men feast first, and then the women. Lots of joking, joshing, storytelling. "Remember when . . ." is a common refrain. After lunch, all but the oldest women go back to the hanging hogs. The men gather round and lug the first one killed over to the cutting table. There, it's cut into ham, shoulder, bacon, tenderloin or pork chops (that's the same cut — one with bone, one without), and ribs. Meanwhile, most of the organs have gone into one of the kettles and are seething nicely.

Back fat above the loin is cut off and then diced into pieces that go into the other kettle (copper) for lard and cracklin's. The men heave the hams, shoulders, and bellies onto their shoulders and carry them to the curing house, where they are rubbed with salt, brown sugar, and pepper, then completely immersed in those ingredients. Young women cut up the skin pieces into cubes and then prepare pans to receive the ponhoss (a decidedly and distinctly Shenandoah Valley heritage specialty).

The seething organ broth is about ready for its next step. With a slotted spoon, the pieces are carefully pulled out and cornmeal is added, along with some salt and pepper, until the whole kettle turns into a porridge consistency — kind of like cream of wheat or oatmeal. One person stirs it constantly so it won't burn or stick on the bottom of the kettle. At just the right moment, everyone forms a long line with the bread pans and a dishrag or hot mitten, and someone ladles the ponhoss into the pans. Each is carried to a table to chill.

Meanwhile, the sausage grinder is whirring away with the trim pieces and the last of the carcasses meet dissection. In the fading sunset, the hot oil from the skin and fat gets pressed out in the lard press. The leftover skin pieces are delightful cracklin's and add the final delectable taste to a very historically normal and secure food day. As the old folks say, "A good time was had by all."

My last hog killin' was on my father-in-law's farm in about 1985, and I still miss it terribly. It finally got too hard to get enough people together, what with Little League and soccer games, movies and night shift at the plant. The old folks gradually died off and the young people were too glued to the television to care. Now when they want tenderloin they go to Wal-Mart or Kroger. Instead of all that food going home at the end of the day to people's houses, where it waited for a dinner to call it by name, those hogs aren't raised anymore. They are confined in factory houses, far away from our Shenandoah Valley, trucked many miles, and processed in huge factories by nameless, faceless people who are themselves employee numbers in an industrial system.

Folks, this ain't normal. The defining characteristic of normal food, of secure food, is that it waits, in state, for us to call from our kitchens. Sadly, today our rural communities are as dependent on the supermarket and its concomitant chain of factory farms, truckers, processors, and warehouse forklift operators as any urban area.

I was in New York recently, in the Delaware Highlands, where in the past two decades 350 family dairy farms have turned into a scant fifty struggling dairies. In this place of breathtaking beauty and resource bounty, most residents eat the same food as the much-decried food deserts of inner cities. The Spam sold at the corner general store comes from the same supply chain, the same grinder, the same factory, as the Spam sold in the corner store in the impoverished inner city. And it's all wrapped in plastic, kept for months in a distant warehouse, inaccessible to the community. Unknown and unseen.

Remember, in the mid-1940s, nearly half of all vegetables in the United States were grown in home vegetable gardens. The Victory Garden effort was our country's last curtain call in the food security theater. That stage is now practically vacant. Witness the panic that sets in when weather forecasters warn of impending snow or other weather disturbances. Without being cocky, I'm confident that our family could eat for months from what we have stored in our larder. It's right under our noses, in our own castle.

This is not only normal, it's secure. When food is spread out among the households of a community, it's less vulnerable to anything, be it weather, politics, economics, or bioterrorism. Part of ecology is preparing for tough times. Plants store energy in their roots. Squirrels bury nuts against winter's snows. Bees busily make honey all season in order to survive the winter. Trees shed their leaves to conserve carbohydrates that will renew their growth in the spring. The whole world pulses with this preparation and awareness toward security.

We're acting like a mama bear facing hibernation who, rather than eating extra to put on fat for the long sleep, lies around watching the leaves fall hoping someone will come and feed her in January. Indeed, it begs the question of whether a civilization this irresponsible toward the primal requisites for survival can or even should survive. Food security is not in the supermarket. It's not in the government. It's not at the emergency services division.

True food security is the historical normalcy of packing it in during the abundant times, building that in-house larder, and resting easy knowing that our little ones are not dependent on next week's farmers' market or the electronic cashiers at the supermarket.

One more nuance before we close this chapter. Historically, normal food could be seen by the community. Since it was grown in proximity to its use, people could measure how much was out there. They could prepare. The farther food production moves away, the less we can really know what's out there. Do you think it's wise to depend on government statisticians to know whether enough food exists for you and your family? Who would you rather trust with your food interests — your local farmers or a bureaucrat from Washington, D.C.? When the government comes out with numbers like "lowest stockpiles of wheat in twenty years," what does that mean? Is this for people or animals? Where is it?

The old adage "figures lie and liars figure" may be appropriate here. Are you ready to depend on the same folks who created the latest government boondoggle or debacle for your family's sustenance? Or for that matter, are you ready to put your faith in Monsanto to take care of you?

We have neighbors — I'll call them Cleve and Matilda — who would be the bane of liberal environmentalists. Stay with me here — this may be a teachable moment. Members of the National Rifle Association, they hunt avidly and procure all their meat that way. They scavenge firewood from neighbors' woods to fill their home-built outdoor wood furnace that supplies all their domestic heat. Their huge garden, filled with blackberries, strawberries, and vegetables, offers a cornucopia of bounty, which they freely share with neighbors, including us. They can, freeze, and dry their bounty.

They don't go out much. Their entertainment is puttering in the garden, processing their homegrown bounty, or doing woodworking projects for neighbors. They don't buy new vehicles, seldom or never eat out, do fix-it jobs in the community to earn their living. They don't earn huge amounts of money but they don't spend much. They don't buy things or shop — their clothes are common working threads, worn out and eventually discarded for rags. They listen to Rush Limbaugh and plant fruit trees around their homestead, located off the road and secluded amid gardens, fruits, and woodpile.

Now let's meet another family, living in suburbia, utterly dependent on industrial food, helter-skeltering daily between charitable and recreational activities. Shopping and getting take-out food routinely, amassing twenty pairs of shoes and a dozen trousers. Jetting to Disney World for vacation, and popping pharmaceuticals for mental and physical survival. Big paychecks, lots of paper wrappers, big lawn to mow, and nice annual donation to an environmental organization. Goodness, maybe they even sit on the board of a prestigious greenie.org.

Let me ask you a question: Of these two scenarios, who is the true environmentalist? Who is really connecting to a normal relationship to an earth womb? In the final analysis, which of these two families really gets it? I won't answer: It's a rhetorical question. As a culture, we are quick to stereotype and marginalize, but in my experience, some of the most normal-living people are the ones who make the least noise about it. Cleve and Matilda are living it, not talking about it. Surrounded by the fruits of their domestic normalcy, their bounty is transparent, visible, measurable, knowable.

Our Polyface customers can visit our farm. They can see the cows in the field, the chickens on the pasture, and the pigs in the woods. Stockpiling during abundance is sensible. Whistling nonchalantly and cavalierly through the day, assuming that Monsanto and Tyson will somehow always come through for us, is putting your faith in some pretty dubious people. Try to go visit their farms and see how far you get. Ask them for their data and see if they'll show it to you. Do you really trust them?

When the food for a community is transparent, measurable, and nearby, the sense of abundance is palpable. Indeed, this sense is still one of my most powerful childhood memories: my grandfather's garden. Some of my most poignant and precious childhood memories are the late-summer visits to Indiana, to visit my grandfather — a true master gardener — and grandmother. His large meticulously kept garden burst with abundance. Lining three sides of it, a T-topped Concord grape trellis literally dripped with fruity sweetness. The heavy grape clusters hung by the hundreds at my eight-year-old eye level, filling my senses with ecstasy.

Why would we rather surround our homes with lawn instead of grape arbors? The first business of the household is security, and surely food is at the top of that list. To be sure, I don't think Tyson will collapse tomorrow. But wouldn't a thinking person realize that those chickens are more vulnerable to disease, pathogens, Teamster strikes, and global policy shifts than the chickens grown by our pastured farmer? And especially than the chickens we bought in bulk and stashed in our freezer for the year? Those chickens are in our house. They are within our grasp. We can measure them. We can glance at them anytime to make sure they haven't gotten away or been diverted by some global elitist's agenda. They're home.

That's secure and normal. So what can we do? Here are some ideas.

1. Find and patronize local farmers, in whatever venue you desire, and then ask them if you can help solve their salvage or abundance problem. What is extra that you can acquire, perhaps at a discount in volume, to reduce throwaways?
2. Preserve food yourself: dehydrating, canning, lacto-fermenting, parching, freezing, processing. A host of books exist to get you started. Ask your grandmother how she did it. Commit to preserve one thing so it's not daunting.
3. Take a fast food sabbatical — just one week, for starters. Fix a meal but make plenty so you have leftovers for lunches.
4. Turn off the TV and read to the kids for two hours one night. I'll bet they'll want more and you might turn it into a couple nights a week. You might actually be more lovable than when you're harried and hurried, bustling them off to some extraneous entertainment event. And reading together doesn't take any energy.

5. Postpone the vacation trip and discover your local farm treasures.

6. Buy a big freezer so you can buy meat in bulk and lay by. Get the money by selling your big flat-screen TV and canceling your Netflix account.

7. Start a domestic hobby: woodworking, candle making, quilting, knitting, carving, repairing anything (furniture, appliances, electronics). These are the skills and crafts that have undergirded civilizations for centuries.

8. Begin limiting your video game use. I saw a news report recently that measured average video game use by American men between the ages of twenty-five and thirty-five: twenty hours per week. Do you mean the flower of America's masculinity can't think of anything more important to do with twenty hours a week than sit in front of a video screen? Folks, this ain't normal. Can't we unplug already?

9. If you have any land at all, grow something. Anything edible.

Wrappings, Trappings, and Foil

I'm writing this chapter on my laptop 34,000 feet above the Pacific Ocean on my way home after spending a month giving speeches in New Zealand and Australia — a long time to be away from home. We left Sydney an hour ago and I've just finished the Virgin Australia–provided lunch and decided this is a good way to launch into the topic of food packaging. Lest any VA executives decide to wreak vengeance on me for the following diatribe, this would apply to any airline in the world, flying anywhere. I might as well incur the wrath of all of them. No sense being picky.

Anyway, this meal has grown. Normally when you eat, the stuff on your plate diminishes, but in a commercial airplane, it grows. It comes in a nice orderly tray with each food item encased in tight plastic packaging. Throughout the meal, and then until the flight attendants come to pick up the pieces, it grows and grows into an unruly pile of plastic, aluminum foil, and paper.

Let's see. First I had to poke a hole through the utensil plastic bag. This contained a plastic fork, spoon, and knife, plus a coffee and tea stirrer (after all, this is Virgin Australia), and pouches for sugar, salt, and pepper. As soon as you poke a hole in the utensil bag, it expands and bounces around the tray among the yet-unopened delicacies. I take the aluminum foil (doesn't aluminum have something to do with Alzheimer's?) off the hot lamb, vegetable, and white rice tray. I fold it neatly and try to find a corner to place it. As I reach for the plastic-encased roll, the cuff of my blazer catches the aluminum foil I just folded and sends it fluttering to the floor under my feet. No room to pick it up until all of us in the aisle fold up our trays. It will have to stay for a while.

I go ahead and open the roll. Now I have another fluttery piece of plastic. The butter is in a tray with aluminum foil on top. I rip the aluminum foil back and that doubles the size of the little bite-sized package. I dump the salt and pepper on the lamb/rice/vegetables, which gives me two small corners of paper to discard. The plastic-topped square dish holding the salad needs some dressing. Time to open the plastic canister of balsamic vinegar — which of course makes it double in size too. Fortunately, some clever, clever engineer figured out how to make the plastic top for the salad so it would nest under the little square dish. Very neat.

About this time, another flight attendant comes by offering drinks. They've given me a wineglass (after all, this is Virgin Australia), but I've never cottoned to wine, so I ask for orange juice. Of course, they don't put the orange juice in my wineglass — how gauche would that be — and hand me over a — you guessed it — plastic cup of orange juice. I begin eating the salad, roll, and lamb. And as I begin eating the lamb, I wonder where it came from.

Yesterday, I was outside of Mudgee in New South Wales and went past an unusually deplorable-looking flock of sheep. True, they were the exception and not the rule (in fact, my host said that farm routinely had dozens of dead sheep lying out in the fields), because I certainly have enjoyed Australian lamb for these couple of weeks — but I've been dining with the farmers who grew the lamb. This is the first I've eaten from unknown sources. Does anyone at Virgin Australia visit farms to see where their lamb comes from? In fact, this probably isn't even Australian lamb — it's probably from New Zealand. Does anybody know? Does anybody care?

Having finished my lamb/rice/vegetable hot dish, my eyes spy a packet of crackers and sharp cheddar cheese in the teacup. I open the crackers and try to stuff the plastic baggie back into the teacup. It has expanded to twice the size of the teacup. And I haven't even tackled the plastic shrink wrap on the slice of cheese. I rip it off the cheese and try to stuff both into the teacup. Impossible — they just keep jumping out. I wedge them between my legs discreetly, under the tray table.

After polishing them off, I go for the square plastic bowl containing banana cake. Like the salad, the plastic top can be put underneath for nesting. Very clever. Only one more thing to go: the after-dinner bite-sized chocolate bar, double wrapped in paper and aluminum foil. The outer paper begs all eaters to save the koala bear, and has the cute and typically sad-faced likeness of a koala in need. The aluminum foil inner, made from basalt mines destroying Australian farmland, comes off easily and I savor the little chocolate. Finishing off the last of my orange juice, I now have a tray heaped with fluttering paper, plastic, and aluminum foil, which I retrieve from the floor under my feet and mash into the lamb dish, hoping its weight will keep the lightweight plastic from showering down on my clothes and laptop as the flight attendant takes it all away.

Oh, I didn't open the little milk creamer because I'm tired of drinking tea. I never used the plastic spoon or the stirrer, or the wineglass. Or the teacup. But I sure grew a tray of plastic, paper, and aluminum foil. Very productive waste stream. Folks, this ain't normal.

Could I dare to ask a couple of questions? First of all, why can't all beverages be served in paper cups? Paper comes from trees. Paper sequesters carbon. It decomposes. Trees grow from sunlight. I've gotten to where I won't even take drinks on the airplane because of the plastic cup — and on a long flight, each passenger uses two or three of them. Multiply that by all the passengers on the plane, then all the planes in the sky, and suddenly you have tractor-trailer loads of plastic every day. When we may be heading into peak oil and the landfills are overloaded, why in the world are we using plastic? It's crazy.

Now for the meal. Why couldn't they have two big pots of soup up in the galley, with tight lids in case of turbulence, one with vegetarian cheese soup or broccoli soup — there are lots of great-tasting and filling vegetarian soups. And the other would be a rich lamb stew with vegetables. The flight attendants would come down the aisles with a stack of paper bowls and serving pots, ladling it into passengers' bowls. You don't need all this variety. Goodness, if you wanted to serve cheese and crackers with it, bring the tray down and let passengers reach over and grab the cheese slices and crackers of their choice. No wrap, no aluminum, no nothing.

The fruit could be an apple or plum or banana — something without a lot of mess and juice. Dessert could be cookies from a local bakery, using local flour, served out of a tray: Take one, take one, take one. I'm sure someone could figure out a dispenser that would keep takers from touching other cookies. After all, we can't have commingling fingers. That would be nasty. That's why at dinner parties, church potlucks, and Christmas shindigs nobody would think of making a cookie tray in which a person could touch more than one item.

There you have it. Lunch is finished and the paper cups nest together during pickup. The paper bowls nest together during pickup. The only utensil required is a spoon and it can be made of wood. I'm hearing more and more that the alleged greenie supposedly compostable cornstarch utensils in fact do not break down. But wood sure will. No plastic. The paper and fruit rinds can decompose and certainly do not need to go into a landfill. Of course, nonbleached paper would be best. The point is, I've just described a very nutritious but simple in-flight meal without this mountain of toxic packaging material.

I realize plastic and airplanes hatched and grew simultaneously, but what did they do before this sudden blip of human history known as the petroleum era? When people traveled they still had to eat. Travel in those days often required days on horseback, or in a carriage without refrigeration, plastic, or aluminum foil. They took dehydrated fruit, jerky, heavy bread, various nuts, and water. Why is that so bad? Unfortunately, many Americans have never encountered heavy European breads — the kind that can satisfy and fill you with a good handful. Chewed slowly — you don't have a choice — these heavy black and brown breads are nutrient-dense and incredibly tasty.

My favorite food item to take when I travel is a bag of mixed nuts. It's not messy, goes through security extremely well, is shelf stable at ambient temperature, and doesn't go stale. A little goes a long way. Ditto for dried fruits from raisins to apricots to apple slices. And jerky. Oh, baby! That's the cat's meow. When we harvest deer on our farm, Daniel and Sheri make a wonderful jerky out of the loins. You have to be careful eating it because it's so nutrient-dense. A small handful swells to the size of a basketball in your stomach. It's extremely filling, lightweight, tasty, and long-lasting. This, in fact, was the food of choice before modern days. If I had an airline, I'd offer jerky, yes indeed.

I've concentrated so far on airline food because it probably epitomizes modern society's fixation with encasing every morsel of food in plastic. Even bite-sized morsels. Not only was this not done a mere century ago, it was impossible. Mass production of customized wrapping material had not progressed to allow economical individual wrapping. Add to that our fixation on individual choice and noncommunal dipping, and we have a veritable daily mountain of waste exhausting from our food system.

Imagine every morsel of food leaving a trail of waste. Compare that to old-fashioned canning, meat curing, dehydrating (both vegetables and meats), and daily preparation from raw ingredients. Prior to preservative packaging, most food simply waited in its stable raw state until it was prepared right before eating. Root cellars and kitchen pantries held root crops, onions, garlic, apples, pears, and squash nearby without packaging or refrigeration.

In our family, the old basement under the house doubles as a root cellar. We've stored potatoes dug in early September all the way until little new potatoes are available the following May. Yes, the eyes might sprout a bit and they might look a little wizened, but they eat just fine and never go into a plastic bag of any kind. Ditto for onions, butternut squash, and sweet potatoes. We keep carrots in the garden under a deep layer of mulch all winter. When we want them, we pull aside the mulch and spade up another couple feet of row. The mulch blanket protects them from freezing. They get sweeter and sweeter as the winter goes along.

Cold-weather crops like cabbage will hold for a long time in the root cellar. Not as long as potatoes, but certainly well into the winter — until you're ready to give up cabbage, anyway. Cold frames and kitchen gardens were and should still be used extensively as season extenders to keep cool-hardy vegetables and leafy greens available throughout the winter. As long as plants grow near their point of consumption, they don't need a lot of packaging to get them to the table. Plants grown near a kitchen can be transported in reusable caddies or boxes.

The longer and farther something ships, the more packaging it requires. If the same effort at extending transport and shelf life through packaging had gone into extending production seasons, we'd be much farther down the road toward sustainability and normalcy. Instead, the food preparation assumption is that we must ship ungodly truckloads of off-season produce to northern tiers and hold it in warehouses until consumption.

Perhaps no one has ever achieved season extension success like Eliot Coleman, author of *Four-Season Harvest* and gardener extraordinaire, whose January baby carrots in Maine have become the schoolchild's most luxurious lunchbox trading item. That many if not most people in Maine (and everywhere else for that matter, but particularly in Maine where Eliot's innovations and expertise are easily accessible to all) who want fresh leafy greens in January buy them at the supermarket after they've been bleached and plastic-bag shipped from California or beyond is not a tribute to modern technology; it's an unprecedented abdication of personal responsibility and a ubiquitous benchmark of abnormality.

Any heirloom-type gardening book has plenty of diagrams about season extension techniques. The French made individual glass bulbs. I'll talk more about season extension in the next chapter, but it's as much a component of packaging as it is about localizing a food system. Season extension, though very important, is only one part of the packaging issue. Another is preservation.

The art of canning, whether by pressure or warm-water bath, allowed homes to preserve seasonal bounty in reusable glass jars for years. When Teresa sends me shopping in the winter, I go to the basement and choose from hundreds of quarts of food, from canned venison and chicken to relish, pickles, and sauerkraut. I will discuss this later as a part of normal food security, but in this chapter I want to promote home preservation as a normal way to package food prior to this totally abnormal blip in human history called the industrial or petrochemical age.

A century ago households did not generate the mountains of plastic, aluminum, and steel wastes that our food system generates today. These wasteful packaging options simply did not exist. I would argue that it is worth rediscovering the home economics of domestic food preservation simply to reduce the waste stream. That alone begs a return to normalcy. Nutrition, taste, and security add to the need for normalcy, but waste alone is justification enough.

Think about highly processed foods. Packaging around potato chips and snacks. A century ago, all those potatoes were in root cellars or cool warehouses. They were not sitting in millions of plastic bags on super-market shelves, in delivery trucks, and on top of people's refrigerators. For months. Maybe years. And they certainly weren't sitting in crinkly airtight four-color bags, already slivered and fried into chips.

In our own farm business, we've fought these battles, sometimes win-ning and sometimes losing. A century ago, virtually all chicken was sold fresh and local. When my dad and mom farmed in Venezuela dur-ing the late 1950s, we sold all chickens live at the village market. Street vendors would come and choose the chickens they thought they could sell on their route through the city, and affix those birds to a pole they would sling over their shoulder. Walking from house to house, they would hawk (no pun intended) the live chickens.

If the señora wanted to cook chicken for supper, she would dicker with the chicken vendor, buy one, and dress it out on the back stoop. Then she'd cook it for supper. In many places in third world countries today, if you walk into a country restaurant and order chicken, they will go out and pull one out of a crate, dress it, and cook it. When the num-ber in the crate gets low, they'll dispatch a boy on a bicycle to scoot over to the chicken farmer and bring another batch of birds to the restau-rant. I personally think this is very cool.

Today, however, the logistics of chicken commerce make package-free difficult. Most of our patrons do not want to dress a chicken on the back stoop. They want it plucked and gutted and looking completely dead and clean in a plastic bag. When I began selling chickens at Poly-face Farm thirty years ago, customers had to bring their own cooler so we could put the birds in something. We did not put them in bags at all. People would take them home, sometimes cut them up, but certainly bag and freeze the birds themselves. Some people used compostable butcher paper instead of plastic. Today, most supermarkets hardly even carry butcher paper. Most people don't even know what it is.

Even with our wonderful and with-it customers today, we have found selling unbagged birds to be no longer acceptable. So we succumbed to the plastic bag. Then more recently, our customers asked, and then demanded, that we offer cut-ups. We resisted. We dug in our heels, but the unrelenting requests finally convinced us to offer this service. In marketing, you can be nostalgically behind the times until you become so archaic you're obsolete. There's a fine line between nostalgic and archaic.

As soon as Polyface began offering this service, we had the problem of packaging. How many pieces do you put in a package, and what kind of packaging do you use? Supermarkets use Styrofoam — another petroleum product. Here again, our whole perception of normal is delineated by an invention only a few decades old. Can you imagine a day before Styrofoam? What did they do? They all sat around and starved to death because no petroleum-derived conveyance existed yet. Give me a break.

Anyway, we looked at paper trays. Because so few are used, they are extremely expensive. And they do get soggy easily. So we opted for Styrofoam, but we didn't like it. After a year of disquietedness, Daniel suggested we forget the trays and just use a simple little plastic bag. I was dubious — this seemed too nonstandard to me. After all, your customers will only tolerate so much weirdness. You can be a nudist, and you can be a Buddhist, but a nudist Buddhist — that's just too weird. But I gave in and we tried it. He argued that our customers didn't need to see the chicken; they knew it was good. All we needed was a way to hand it to them.

Sure enough, Daniel was right. On this one, our customers stepped right up to the plate and never batted an eye. Suddenly, what had been pallet loads of Styrofoam trays dried up to a few boxes of baggies. Hallelujah! I heard one of our longtime customers talking us up to another lady a few weeks ago and she said buying straight from the farm was imperative if for no other reason than to reduce food's collateral damage — oops, I mean waste stream.

As I sit here winding down this chapter, they've just brought me water in a plastic bottle. Why couldn't they give everyone a paper cup and tell them to hold on to it for the duration of the flight? Then they could come by with a big thermos of water on a cart and fill your cup. Goodness, even the flights that give you a plastic glass and fill it with water are still pouring water from plastic water bottles. It's insane. On many of these long flights, one passenger will use and throw away several plastic cups. Is anybody thinking about this? Hello, airline executives? Who will be the first one to really step out and commit to a compostable waste stream?

From my window seat I was finally able to convey my food tray over to the attendant — after plastic wrappings fluttered off of it twice and I contorted my body around this laptop and did a forward dive to the floor to retrieve the errant petroleum pieces. Can you imagine how we would have fed ourselves on planes a hundred years ago had we not discovered plastic? Goodness, we might have been relegated to eating jerky, nuts, dried apricots, and heavy German bread. Consigned to such unsophisticated fare, we might have gotten to our destination without indigestion.

Why is this so hard? This is the question that haunts me. This is the point of this book — or at least one of them. To me, the answer seems so simple. As I sit here on this jumbo jet carrying 350 people, am I the only one thinking about these things? The guy next to me is multitasking — watching an in-seat video while playing a game on his microcomputer. Everyone has headsets on and most are watching some form of entertainment. All wonderful, thoughtful, honorable people, I'm sure. But I'll bet not one of them realizes, or meditates on, the fact that we've just participated in a completely abnormal food experience. As if the flying were not abnormal enough, encasing every morsel of our meal in petroleum, and filling cubic meters of precious cabin space with plastic and aluminum — folks, this ain't normal.

To reduce packaging debris, here are some things we can do.

1. Preserve your own food in season. Buy extra in season and spend a day preserving it yourself. Even if that means freezing it in plastic baggies, it will be less material than from a grocery store.
2. Airlines should offer compostable containers and water from reusable vessels. The heavy stew would be nice too, but I'll not wander too far from the ranch on these suggestions.
3. If you have a garden, put some real emphasis on extending its productive season with cool-season crops like brassicas, carrots, beets, and greens.
4. Take containers to the farmers' market — boxes or cloth bags.
5. Reduce your purchasing of all processed foods. That's where the packaging is. If you must buy at the supermarket, buy unprocessed. The fresh, raw produce is usually not enshrouded in plastic.

6. Keep a healthy arsenal of resealable containers to stow leftovers from mealtimes. These handy-dandy baggie sealers — forget them. Stackable Tupperware works just fine and lasts a lifetime. And it burps.

7. For lunches at work or school, send leftovers in resealable containers. Send an apple and some cheese slices. Unprocessed and home-packaged in washable containers works just fine. When you start cooking meals, you'll have leftovers to put in these nifty reusable containers. This includes sandwiches — Teresa has sandwich-sized reusable containers. No need to wrap the sandwich in a plastic bag.

8. The thermos still works. Squatty ones to keep potato salad cold or stews hot, a thermos is perhaps the ultimate reusable packaging. And they look cool too.

Lawn Farms and Kitchen Chickens

The average morsel of food sees more of America than the farmer who grows it, traveling fifteen hundred miles from field to fork. Folks, this ain't normal. Numerous people have tried to express the magnitude of this irregularity with different statistics. For example, it takes fifteen calories of energy to put one calorie on the table, and four of those are in transportation.

Long-distance distribution now defines the modern food system, and yet as recently as 1946 the average food-miles in America was less than one hundred. The refrigerated rail car, which probably revolution-ized food shipping more than anything else, was not invented until the late 1920s. The first supermarket developed in the mid-1940s. Today, in Canada and the United States, only 5 percent of the food consumed in a bioregion is actually grown there.

In other words, when you go to the supermarket, 95 percent of what's for sale came from some other state. And yet imagine what is on the shelves in the supermarket. Imagine walking down the aisles, and then ask yourself, "What could be grown within a hundred miles of this location?" Go ahead, close your eyes and imagine. When I'm giving a local foods presentation, I often ask for people to close their eyes and then yell out what could be grown locally.

In most areas of the country, the list is huge:

dairy	oats
beef	barley
potatoes	honey
tomatoes	pigs
cherries	carrots
grapes	beets
apples	cabbage
chicken	cucumbers
wheat	coffee
corn	

Okay, I was just seeing if you were on your toes with that last one. This is not a definitive list by any means, but you get the picture. Most of what we eat can indeed be grown nearby. But it can't often be grown year-round, and therein lies the conundrum. You cannot have a viable local food system without a seasonal eating commitment. That includes preserving seasonal production for nonseasonal consumption.

For this discussion, let's assume we're on the same page about eating seasonally, including storing for the off-season. Is this realistic? Most people today, even the ones who embrace local food systems, really don't think it's possible. After all, local food would limit our options. Local food can't be grown in the same abundance as industrial food in far-off, more productive areas. After all, the reason potatoes come from Idaho is because they grow well there. To grow them elsewhere would reduce efficiency. The reason Washington State grows apples is because they grow best there. Efficiency is when each area of the country grows what it is best suited for and imports everything else. And then by growing more of that one thing in one place, we achieve economies of scale. That is all part of modern scientific agriculture. So goes today's thinking.

It would be nice if it were true. Such thinking takes a mechanistic view toward nature rather than a biological view. We'll talk more about that in the chapter devoted to monospeciation. Right now, let's just deal with the question, "Is a local food system realistic?" If it's not realistic, then we'd all better jump on the Monsanto bandwagon. If the food system I espouse actually creates starvation, then I don't have a very acceptable model.

This issue seems most acute and misunderstood in populous, irrigated, agriculturally rich California. "You don't really think California could feed itself, do you?" The query comes from right and left, greenie and industrialist. Indeed, California provides perhaps the ultimate litmus test for the viability of bioregional food systems. I'm not a scientist or a statistician; I'm just a country boy who spends a lot of time communing with cows and pigs out in the woods and fields, so take this for what it's worth.

When Californians ask how they can feed themselves, they generally assume continued exports at today's levels. After all, California grows most of the nation's mesclun mix, strawberries, almonds, and a host of other products. California supplies the lion's share of off-season fresh produce to the northern tier and East Coast. Here's my intuition: If all the petroleum in diesel fuel currently expended sending trucks across the continent to supply out-of-season produce to cold areas were turned into plastic film to cover season-extension greenhouses and tall tunnels (unheated greenhouses) in the East and North, California could feed itself on the newly freed-up land.

You see, dear folks, we can't just place a Band-Aid here and there and return to normalcy. Everything relates to everything. You can't deal with a problem in one sector without dealing with problems in many sectors. Things are too abnormal to be able to isolate sectors and touch one without affecting any others. It doesn't work that way.

I wish it could be easier. But unless and until the East and North step up to their bioregional responsibilities, California will be unable to feed itself. Of course, if Californians decided to feed themselves anyway, hang the rest of the country, then the rest of us would need a crash course in season extension. That probably won't happen. In fact, many would argue that turning diesel fuel into laminated hoop-house covers is also tilting at windmills, what with our country's fascination with building roads and extracting petroleum. You might be right, but I'm still going to advocate for an answer, regardless of how unlikely it may be.

Why do easterners have to eat herring from Monterey Bay? Why? Don't they have cod and swordfish? I like variety as much as anyone, but are we thinking about these things? Sometimes I think we're like the mountain climber who when asked why he climbs, responds, "Because it's there." Do we just eat these things because they are there? Because they are available? Heaven help us to be more conscious than that. The question of California's food localization can only be answered in the broader context of food localization everywhere. The East and North should have acres, acres, and acres of season-extending plastic covers. It would just take a reallocation of resources.

In my opinion, if there is one extremely legitimate use for petroleum besides running wood chippers and front-end loaders to handle compost, it's making plastic for season extension. That one thing has broad ramifications. It parks many of the trucks. That reduces road-building and repair costs and exhaust. It reduces all the energy needed to smelt the steel to build the engines and chassis. It reduces packaging. It increases transparency because the food is grown closer to the point of consumption. This is major. It's simple, yet profound.

With the trucks parked, greenhouses, tall tunnels, and more seasonal, localized eating, can we feed ourselves? We still have to answer that burning question. Here are several thoughts.

First, half of all food fit for human consumption never gets eaten. We know that. Much of that loss is attributable to long-distance transportation and warehousing. Go Dumpster diving if you don't believe me. Whole books have been written about this issue, and the statistics are unbelievable. Look at what comes out the back door of a restaurant, a supermarket, any industrial food processing facility. Second, plenty of wasted land exists. Land is moving out of production at an extremely rapid rate, both as a result of the aging farmer and due to land being purchased by nonfarmers. The average age of America's farmers is now approaching sixty, but thirty-five years of age is considered by business analysts to be the median age of the practitioners in a vibrant economic sector. Farming has not seen that age in a long, long time.

As we age, we become less innovative and less aggressive. We don't have the energy to keep up the pace like we did in our younger days. Older farmers become less productive, regardless of what they grow. That means many farmers are hanging on, just doing enough to get by. As these farmers die, the land often passes to children who are not farmers. Often, too, one spouse, usually the widow, hangs on for a few years before a final dissolution of the farm.

After one of our apprentices completed his term here at Polyface, he went back to his family's twelve acres in upstate New York. Planning to start with that small acreage and see what developed, he was stunned to receive requests from three different landowners in the area, a total of a thousand acres, to take over their land. "Just do something with it," they begged.

I've been in that area several times recently, and it is comprised of mile after mile after mile of neglected prime farmland. This is not rocky or sandy or highly eroded soil. It is rich land, ready for someone to steward. I spoke at a conference in New York this winter where another presenter was a Cornell professor, and he said they had just completed an assay of recently abandoned farmland in New York. This was land that had been actively farmed just ten or fifteen years ago and was now reverting to saplings and brush in the early stages of forestal succession. The total acreage — 3.2 million. That's not land lost to development, highways, or parks. That's just abandoned prime farmland, still privately owned by old defunct farmers or their children. Or, as is often the case, a new owner whose e-commerce money found its way into land investment. While New York may have more of this phenomenon than normal — property taxes drove out many of these farmers — this abandonment is not unusual. The same is true in most areas of the country.

I correspond with inmates, partly because I'm opposed to prisons. That doesn't mean I'm soft on crime; quite the contrary. But throwing someone in prison at a cost of $40,000 per year just so he can pour Coca-Cola on the TV set in an argument with another inmate over which show to watch doesn't do anybody any good. I'm for swift punishment and then a second chance. Whipping posts seem like a great idea to me. Prisons don't reform. That's like a one-month time out for a child. Forget it. Administer the board of education to the seat of knowledge, give the child a hug, and go on with life.

For years I've sent my books free to any inmate who wrote me wondering about the possibility of farming upon release from prison. I want these folks to have a chance at something worthwhile, and I'm happy to hear from someone who wants to make something of himself, but in recent years I haven't been able to get my books into prisons due to new rules about what inmates can receive. Very frustrating.

Anyway, I still correspond with them, and I got a letter recently from an inmate in Pennsylvania who wanted to farm. He wrote three farmers in the neighborhood where he grew up, explained his situation, and asked each if he could rent a few acres to get started. He reported to me that not only did all three write back to him, but all offered him their entire farm "because my kids aren't going to do anything with it."

I routinely receive letters from elderly farmers wanting to rent or give away their land to some young person who will love it and care for it. These aging farmers say their children will just sell it for development.

One of the most interesting daylong workshops I have been involved in recently occurred here in Virginia a couple of years ago when one of our state's top environmental organizations, the Piedmont Environmental Council (PEC), hosted a matchmaking session, pairing up landowners with wannabe farmers. Environmental organizations historically have not necessarily been friendly to working farmers. In many ways, I am not friendly toward most working farmers. Unfortunately, though, too often the environmentalists do not differentiate strongly enough between good farmers and destructive farmers. Most of us are prone to paint with a broader brush than necessary. I'll admit that I do it too, especially toward the USDA. I'll go on record right here that there are some wonderful, wonderful people at the USDA. You just have to look hard to find them, and they don't justify the organization. Wonderful people are wonderful wherever they are, government, NGO, corporate, whatever.

From my vantage point, the PEC's constituency, primarily financially well-heeled landowners who acquired farms with urban wealth, too often viewed farmers as the enemy. After all, farmers raised cows that melted the polar caps with burps. Farmers killed eagles with chemicals. You get the picture. I can assure you that in my conservative farming neighborhood, "environmentalist" is a four-letter word. To these new environmental landowners, the landscape use of choice, therefore, did not involve seeking friendship and counsel from the local farming community. It involved mowing. Essentially, these farms were turned into glorified lawns. To keep them pretty, these environmental farmers would mow a couple times a year to keep the brush and saplings back. And that was the extent of their landscape plan.

Gradually, the PEC staff realized that this was certainly not an ecological use of the land. Simply driving over the land with a mower a couple of times a year was neither productive nor environmentally enhancing. It was energy consumptive and biomass wasteful. To ameliorate the situation, they conceived a plan to act as matchmaker between their landed gentrified constituency and environmentally minded active farmers — the differentiated good guys in commercial farming. Farmers like me. It was the first workshop I've seen in America where the term "tenure" was used as a positive possibility. This European idea, whereby land is rented for ninety-nine years, offers non-landed stewards a stable base for operations. It also allows the landed gentry freedom from management for a long time.

With the spike in land prices in the last two decades, we may be entering a new era of land management whereby landownership becomes a defensive economic plan for people who have wealth to hang on to it. Land management, on the other hand, may become an offensive economic plan for those who want to acquire wealth. Actually, landownership as practiced in America is uniquely American. No other culture has this same property worship in their psyche. Canada and Australia come close, but the mystique is still not as great as it is in the United States. Historically, normal land control involved a tribe. If not tribal, then it was through royalty, which concentrated land control in the hands of a few. Peasants rarely let themselves dream of controlling land.

At the risk of sounding soft on property rights, I don't think I should be able to do things on my land that adversely affect my neighbors. That notion elevates community to a point of tribal arbitration. If every corporation or individual that polluted waterways or poisoned adjacent land were personally punished for the people they poisoned, we'd have a different environmental ethic in this country. The challenge ahead is to put loving stewards on the land who can massage it into soil building and biomass recycling. Right now too many environmentalists and open space advocates want to preserve farmland, without any regard to farmers. You can't preserve farmland without preserving farmers. What makes farmland aesthetic is the nurturing and massaging that farmers do to the landscape. Without the farmer, the landscape reverts to wasteland. Stewardship demands that people bring their innovation and sweat to the landscape to make it harness more solar energy and build soil faster than nature would if left to its own devices. Carefully orchestrated disturbance is the key to innovation — ecologically, emotionally, and economically. Albert Einstein said you cannot have construction without first having destruction.

If you're going to plant a garden in a lawn, you don't throw some carrot seeds over your shoulder and proclaim, "I have a garden." No, you have to get a shovel and spade and do some disturbance. Innovative succession ecologically takes disturbance, just like everything else in life. The Egyptian metaphor of the phoenix rising from the ashes speaks to the contrast between the two. Everybody loves to focus on the phoenix without appreciating the ashes that allowed the new to rise.

Having a baby is disturbing. But who wants to live in a world without babies? They are the key to new ideas and innovation. So to lock up land is to turn it into an ecological couch potato — unexercised and underutilized. Unless and until the people who want to preserve farmland can sit around a table and figure out how to preserve farmers, we're not solving the need of the hour, which is land stewardship.

I was in St. Louis giving a seminar recently and had a wonderful time touring inner-city farms. I saw a two-acre site sandwiched between an expressway and a parking garage that was not only extremely productive, but a focus for composting and community revitalization. Next, I toured a restaurant garden at Schlafly Bottleworks carved out of an old asphalt supermarket parking lot. The garden enabled the restaurant to grow most of its high-end salad and vegetables on the compost it generated from kitchen scraps.

Then the highlight — a twelfth of an acre farm presided over by several twenty-somethings dedicated to biomass recycling and local food, built on the lot formerly occupied by a condominium. The building had fallen into disrepair and turned into a haven for crack addicts. The city demolished it and these young people transformed the spot into a productive farm. When they dug a hole to insert a post to hold a trellis, the hole went through discarded electrical wires, blue jeans, and teacups. With a chicken recycling yard, vermicompost, and intensive raised beds, this tiny farm was producing all the produce to feed twenty people year-round.

Kitchen scraps went into the chicken yard. The chickens ate just about everything, scratching, eating, and pooping. This residue buildup then went to the earthworms, housed in bins. The alimentary canal in the worms sterilizes the manure and scrap residue and ratchets the fertility potency up a few more notches. Excess worms are fed to the chickens for animal protein and the whole system runs in a self-contained cycle except for the injection of kitchen scraps. The earthworm castings, or vermicompost, provides the ultimate base for fertility, both in the garden soil and potting mixtures for starting sets.

A simple makeshift kitchen under a hoophouse provided a hangout haven for neighborhood youth, who were jazzed about food production and preparation. Rather than build an expensive and heavy-footprinted conventional building to house the kitchen, they erected hoops and covered them in plastic. The whole structure cost very little, was erected in a day, and does not qualify as a building. Because it isn't a building, it didn't need a permit with footers, inspections, and the associated bureaucratic wrangling. The whole structure could be torn down and reerected somewhere else easily enough, which offered flexibility to the whole enterprise.

By installing some cabinets, an oven, and hanging utensils from a discarded bicycle rim suspended from the hoops, these young people have a fully functional kitchen for food preparation and preservation. The whole light footprint was ingenious. Located in an impoverished neighborhood, the little farm showcased every kind of biologically enhancing technique, from tier gardening to fertility management. At the time, the neighborhood was bringing too many kitchen scraps for the allowable half dozen chickens to recycle. The young visionary farmers were negotiating with the city council for freedom to expand their token flock in order to convert more community kitchen scraps into high-quality compost.

I asked these young people, "How much of the produce eaten in St. Louis could be produced like this in the city limits?" Their response was quick and firm: "Every single pound of produce could be grown within the city." Indeed, the same could be said for many cities, particularly the ones that are undergoing rapid depopulation as a result of manufacturing job losses, like Detroit. On the East Coast, Baltimore has 40,000 acres of vacant land.

These young visionaries had been mentored by America's urban farm guru, Will Allen, who founded Growing Power in Milwaukee. Mixing fish, simulated rivers, pots, hoophouses, and vermicompost, Allen's inner-city farms are off-the-scale more productive than any industrial single-species farm. His model proves the viability of urban farming as a real answer to feeding food deserts and urban populations. His model simulates natural ecosystems, recreating what nature does extensively in an extremely intensive way. The foundation is food waste. Hundreds of tons. "And we haven't even scratched the surface," he says.

He builds compost piles with the food waste, eventually running everything through worms. He calls them "my babies," and loves to reach down into the rich black vermicompost and bring up handfuls of wriggling, healthy worms. The vermicompost provides the foundation for pots growing a copious variety of lettuce and produce watered from fish tanks. The nutrient-dense fish tank water is purified just like a natural stream by running through a labyrinth of hydrologic (water-loving) plants.

An offshoot model, called SPIN (Small Plot Intensive) Farming, is gaining traction around the world. I met a young farmer in British Columbia recently who radiated farming entrepreneurial success. He owns no land, but has access to half an acre, and makes $50,000 off of it — a full-time income. For most people who have never visited these highly productive, intensive, integrated, multidimensional, stacked models, the sheer productive capacity per cubic foot (they use cubic, not linear, due to the vertical stacking of symbiotic plants and animals) is simply mind-boggling.

Too many of us are wowed by combines driving in formation across expanses of grain fields, or fifty-foot vegetable-picking rigs moving slowly through California produce fields. But big-machinery, single-species, extensive industrial systems don't hold a candle to the square foot yield of these intricately designed systems. The industrial systems are awesome because of how extensive they are. The embedded urban farming systems are awesome because of how intensive they are. The same is true on our pasture-based livestock farm. The symbiosis of multispeciation works the same way in animals as it does in plants.

Combining plants and animals gets the best of all worlds. That's the way nature does it.

The fact is that surrounding cities and towns around this nation, in hamlets both rural and urban, millions of acres of wasteland are begging for productive exercise. These acres can be pressed into service to grow food for their locales. We have the land and the know-how. When the culture wants it to happen, these lands will be stewarded anew by ecological farmers. No inherent barrier exists to keep this from happening. The only reason it is not happening yet is because most Americans still think it's normal and fine for the average morsel of food to travel fifteen hundred miles from field to fork. The day when that becomes energy expensive or ecologically repugnant, these lands will again produce food.

America has thirty-five million acres of lawn and thirty-six million acres devoted to housing and feeding recreational horses, and that doesn't even count golf courses. I spoke at a Fortune 500 consortium on the topic "Scaling Up Without Selling Your Soul" and stayed overnight in accommodations more expansive than 90 percent of the world's homes. I needed a GPS to navigate from the bed to the toilet. I never saw any other people in my room, but there was plenty of room for half a dozen without my noticing. It was obscene. Why does anyone need that luxury — in a desert, yet?

When I got up in the morning, sprinklers were running all over the place. Hedges, lawns, trees. Nothing edible, of course. I don't have anything against flowers and beauty, but I think vegetables, grapes, and apple trees are pretty too. Apparently all institutional landscapers have signed some sort of code that views edible landscaping as if it's a scourge upon the earth. Why?

Recently I facilitated a daylong discussion at a prestigious rural boarding school in the South that was wrestling with what to do about the surrounding farmland. Like many schools started in the 1800s, this one historically fed itself from its farm. Students worked in the dairy as part of their whole-person development. Old pictures in the administration building showed sheep grazing the front lawn. Fruit trees dotted the landscape around the dormitories and classroom buildings. Now this farm was a liability. I've been involved with numerous situations like this, and I've got one thing to say about a boarding school that views its farm as a liability: Folks, this ain't normal. How could producing all the food for the entire campus become a bone of contention on the board of trustees, the proverbial albatross around the neck of the institution? The trustees see the farm hemorrhaging cash every year and want to dump it on the bloated real estate market.

Others desperately want to reincorporate the farm into the curriculum. The environmental sciences teachers have a loyal following of students ready to plant gardens and feed earthworm beds. During this particular day at this particular school, I was amazed at how every time half the group wanted to move forward with edible landscaping and portable livestock operations to feed the school, the admissions department would give voice to the elephant in the room: "But the parents who want to send their kids to a college-prep boarding school don't want them working with compost piles. They don't want to come on parents' day and see sheep on the lawn."

How sad that we've become so sophisticated as a culture that food production has become yucky. According to the March 12, 2010, *Washington Post*, in Maryland, Montgomery County schools superintendent Jerry Weast sent out a memo on February 26 stating, "Because vegetable gardens are a food source for pests, create liabilities for children with food allergies and have other associated concerns, the Department of Facilities Management staff has not approved gardens designed to produce food." Amazing! Folks, this ain't normal. Demonizing gardens should be right up there with swearing at the pope, or at least as sacrilegious as burning the flag. What does this guy eat? Good grief, Charlie Brown.

A few months earlier, according to the report, Donna Marchick, a program administrator at the Department of Facilities Management, wrote to teachers at Maryvale Elementary School, "As you know, food-bearing plants attract pests. Maryland law restricts the use of pesticides on school grounds. Therefore, planting of food-bearing plants is prohibited by MCPS [Montgomery County Public Schools]." According to *Washington Post* correspondent Jane Black, the prohibition did not include butterfly gardens and rain gardens. Can you imagine the prejudice toward food and gardens with which these young people will enter life?

Local food systems must be integrated. In her great book *City Chicks*,

Pat Foreman tells about a town in Belgium that offered three chickens to any household that wanted them. Two thousand families signed up for the birds. Those six thousand hens, in the first month of the program, dropped compostable biomass to the landfill by one hundred tons. This was the ultimate recycling program.

If every kitchen in America had enough chickens attached to it to eat all of the scraps coming out of that kitchen, no egg industry or commerce would be necessary in the whole country. Imagine shutting down the entire egg industry. Greenies and animal welfarists decry battery cages and industrial chicken conditions, and I agree they are deplorable. But let's go all the way and link the chickens to their historical jobs, as salvagers of scraps and food waste.

Anybody can keep a couple of chickens in their home. They are certainly no dirtier than parakeets, much less noisy, and far more productive and useful. What's not to love? Institutional dining service directors receive awards from environmental groups for instituting a composting program that carts food service wastes ten miles away to some composting site. Well whoop-de-doo. How about putting a small chicken house adjacent to the kitchen so the garbage doesn't have to be trucked anywhere? Just feed it to the chickens and bring the eggs inside. Now we've got multiple benefits with one simple action.

That would eliminate all the grain that needs to be produced to feed the chickens. Reducing the grain production would reduce the amount of tilled land, which would reduce erosion, which would free up more land to be covered in perennials, which would build soil and ultimately stimulate springs to flow again. I know this sounds like the nursery rhyme about The House that Jack Built, but it's true. When you start really going to the heart of the problem, all sorts of ancillary benefits accrue. When you tiptoe around the edges with distant compost piles and nonintegrated solutions, you create another problem, such as how to transport the waste and pay for the fuel to transport it. Let's grab the low-hanging fruit, the obvious stuff. The rest will work itself out.

When I was in Italy several years ago at Terra Madre in Turin, I was impressed by the small lawns and the highway gardens. Spaces around houses in the city were filled with vegetables, not turfgrass. At the intersections of the expressways the land between exit and entrance ramps wasn't mowed with big batwing mowers like here in America. These expansive acreages were divided into quarter-acre plots, each with its toolshed and sleeping shack. Urbanites would come out to the garden plots on the weekend and cart the week's produce back into town to eat and share with friends.

What a great idea. When I was in Mexico, I saw that the expressways are mowed by family milk cows, tethered each day to mow a new circle. Late in the afternoon, as you drive along, you can see the owners gathering their cows to milk them, and then bringing them back for the evening. The city parks are mowed with cows. Grazing the commons has been part of culture for a long time. This notion that food production is dirty and people need to be protected from its sights and smells has taken hold in our culture only because of the atrocities within the industrial food system.

Can you imagine mowing interstates with cows and gardening in the cloverleafs in the United States? Animal rightists would pitch a fit over abusing animals by having them graze when we all know the charitable thing to do is run mowing machines over the grass. Insurance companies would go apoplectic over the possibility of an errant vehicle running through someone's garden or their weekend shack. Zero tolerance. Here's my question: How about zero tolerance for anti-ecological food production? If someone would like to garden by the highway and they're happy to take the risk, why not let them garden?

My daughter-in-law Sheri thinks that all the interstate medians should be planted with orchards tended by inmates. The inmates go out there to spray weeds anyway. Why not let them prune trees and pick fruit, selling it back to the community in prison farmers' markets? They'd get out in the fresh air, earn some money, and do something meaningful. I'd buy from them. How about you?

Innovation always requires risk. That's the nature of the game. Would we have gone into space without risk? Would we have an automobile without risk? Would the Wright brothers have flown today? No, they would have abandoned the very notion of flight. Their insurance company would have said their exposure was too high. I think we'd better quit administering tests in school. The risk of emotional trauma is too high. Where does this kind of timidity stop? A society ruled by fear is stagnant. The level of fear exhibited by our culture today just ain't normal.

Would Lewis and Clark have set off today on their journey? Of course not. It would have been too scary. It would have taken Congress ten years to decide if the expedition should be launched or not. But when it comes to killing, a simple executive order and we're ready to go, Mr. President. Yessirreee. Bring on the big guns. Shoot 'em up. Can you imagine today's Homeland Security bunch checking out the dudes who signed up for the Lewis and Clark expedition? They wouldn't have gotten approval for decades.

The truth is that if we poked edible landscaping everywhere it could be poked, we'd grow so much food we couldn't eat it all. With the advent of the supermarket and the abdication of personal food responsibility, the entire fabric of local food systems has been lost. From abattoirs to canneries to home gardens, the infrastructure that supported community-embedded butchers, bakers, and candlestick makers has given way to megamarkets and global trafficking.

The only reason this kind of food mileage and disconnection can occur is because cheap energy masks the costs. If the true cost of fuel, including the cost of maintaining Middle Eastern stability, were actually added to transportation costs, food-miles would not look efficient. If energy were as dear as it was before the petroleum age, refrigerated warehouses, climate control, and shipping mesclun mix from California to Boston would be prohibitively expensive. Historically, energy required significantly more effort. Cutting firewood without a chainsaw, toting it on an animal-powered wagon, growing the feed for those beasts — this took roughly a third of American farmland.

Petroleum and cheap fuel freed that third of the farmland to grow crops, which turned into surpluses, which dropped prices, which screamed for governmental remedy. Price support structures and subsidies are only a scant several decades old. Imagine an agriculture that had to make decisions on real-time economics.

Today's market-manipulative government intervention masks the true costs of supermarket food. Meanwhile, it prejudices local food viability. People have traded historically strong local food systems for fragile and detrimental industrial food systems. As a culture, we've traded our backyard gardens and neighborhood farms for Chinese imports and chemicalized, fumigated megafields susceptible to every disease known to plants and animals.

If we take the production results normalized by John Jeavons, bio-intensive garden guru, we could grow all the produce for America in just the lawns and horse paddocks without needing any farmland. Farms could then concentrate on more nutrient-dense things like cheese, meat, and poultry that aren't mostly water and therefore can be shipped more efficiently. Heavy, water-dense produce and fruit are extremely inefficient to ship because they contain so much water. One of the strongest arguments for local food systems is to quit shipping all that water in the vegetables. Local food systems are the backbone of any sensible food model. They have stood the test of time because they make sense when measured for energy, motion, and logistics. This blip known as the petroleum age, or the cheap energy age, does not change the essential rules that have made local food production the backbone of all secure villages.

No culture has ever survived when it couldn't feed itself. The strongest communities are the ones that can feed themselves. That is historical normalcy. Yesterday, today, and tomorrow. Let's rebuild it.

What can we do?

1. Edible landscaping. I cannot stress this enough. College campuses, lawns, anywhere plants can grow, move them toward edible rather than ornamental. It doesn't take any longer to prune an apple tree than an ornamental pear.
2. Use the margins. Road rights-of-way, parks, underneath power lines. Public spaces and unused places — fill them in with food plants.
3. Eat bioregionally. Save the distance stuff for extremely special events; does Boston need fresh strawberries in January?
4. Build a solarium on the south side of your house in which to grow plants.
5. Replace the parakeets with two chickens. They won't make as much noise, and they'll lay eggs.

Dino-the-Dinosaur–Shaped Nuggets Don't Grow on Chickens

"How do you make a hamburger?" The patron whispered it into my ear at a buying club delivery. Incredulous that I heard her correctly, I asked her to repeat the question.

"How do you make a hamburger?" Indeed, I had heard it correctly. I asked her the only question I could muster: "Are you for real?"

"Yes," she pleaded. "My husband and I have been vegetarians for about ten years, and now that we know pasture-based livestock is the best way to heal the planet, he wants a hamburger and I don't know how to make one." I am not making this up.

Not long ago we had a glitch in our bank statement that required getting some help on the bank computer. Our wonderful banker and loan officer set Teresa up in her office and helped her through the issues. In gratitude, we prepared a little gift package of pork chops, eggs, steaks, and a chicken and dropped it off to her. The next day we received a gracious phone call: "Thanks for the goodies. I'm okay with everything except the chicken. What do you do with a whole chicken?" Sharp, college-educated mom with grown children. What do you do with a whole chicken? Really? Are you kidding?

Back when I started selling chicken more than forty years ago, every woman in America knew how to cut up a chicken. I'm being sexist on purpose here, because I enjoy being sexist. Most of our customers are women. Men only grunt and stand in front of the refrigerator, staring inside, mumbling, "I can't find it." Only males who are chefs can stare into the cavernous depths of the refrigerator and actually retrieve something.

So forty years ago, every woman knew how to cut up a chicken. It was part of general knowledge. It was like learning to ride a bike, or read, or tie your shoes. It was part of domestic skills, like hammering a nail, running a washing machine, turning on the vacuum cleaner, or running a lawnmower. Today, more than half of our patrons don't even know that a chicken has bones.

I've got news for you, ladies. Chicken nuggets in the shape of Dino the dinosaur are not part of a chicken's anatomy. You won't find any muscle groups titled "Nuggets." Boneless, skinless breast wasn't even available in the supermarket before 1970. If your recipe called for bone-less skinless breast, you did the carving yourself. And when it was done, you also had neck, backbone, wings, thighs, and legs. And you cooked those, and ate them.

I was recently speaking in Toronto to an annual gathering of rural and small-city politicians. One councilman from a town of 50,000 told me about a farmer just outside his city who grows vegetables on a fairly large scale — like fifty acres of squash. The year previously, he had a massive crop failure and was penalized on his contract for not produc-ing up to the agreement. Desperate to ensure that didn't happen again, the next year he planted half again as much acreage as he thought he might need. Yes, you already guessed the outcome: perfect season and bumper crop.

He'd planted fifty acres of butternut squash and made his contract in just fifteen. The buyer didn't want any more so he had thirty-five acres of butternut squash in the field with no market. I don't know about you, but I love butternut squash about as much as sweet potatoes. And it's extremely versatile, from simple baking to luxury pies. This council-man, who was heavily involved in local food issues, including the food bank, found out about the situation and tried to marshal forces to go harvest and salvage what would have amounted to a couple tractor-trailer loads of squash.

In the end, however, his pleas fell on deaf ears because nobody knew what to do with it. He finished this narrative: "We can't even begin talking about local food until we get enough culinary expertise to know what to do with things when they are available. Nobody even knows how to cook anymore." Sadly, he is right. Cultivating the domestic culinary arts may be a bigger issue in restoring food normalcy than distribution, production, or anything.

Chef Anne Cooper of Farm to School fame says one of the hurdles they have in getting real food into cafeterias is teaching the children how to eat chicken containing bones. "What do you do with these?" they ask, completely bamboozled by this strange substance they've found embedded in the meat. Reminds me of the group of kids staring into an aquarium looking for the fish stick.

At a large university in Kentucky that hosted a food conference where I spoke, my hosts told me this story. I'll abbreviate and paraphrase. The previous year, in a "go local, go green" initiative, the school contracted with a fairly large grass-fed beef operation to supply the ground beef. Without the typical fillers and slurry salvage — remember the movie *Food, Inc.* where that ammoniated slurry comes down the chute pouring into boxes on a conveyor bound for America's burgers? — these burgers must be chewed. When they began serving them, the students rebelled, complaining, "We're not used to chewing our hamburgers." Folks, I am not making this up — I'm telling it to you just like it was told to me. Finally, the school backed off from the campaign, and by the time I spoke there, the next year, they had hired a public relations firm to sell chewable hamburgers to the student body. That was ongoing at the time and appearing successful. It might be too early to chalk up a win, but it seems headed that way. Gracious.

A Washington, D.C., art teacher came up to me after I'd done a presentation and said she was retiring at the end of the year. Being an astute male, I quickly responded, "Oh, you couldn't be old enough to retire."

She said, "Well, not really, but I'm frustrated."

"Why?" I asked.

"Last week I assigned my normal early-in-the-year art project to my tenth graders. I always have them bring in a cooking pot to draw. Cooking pots come in all shapes and sizes, but their lines are fairly simple. They all looked at me like I was from Pluto, so I asked them,

'What's the problem?' And they said, 'We don't have a cooking pot at home.'"

She continued, "In shock, I asked them, 'What do you cook in?' They replied, 'Oh, we just open the box and put it in the microwave.'" And that, dear people, had gotten this high school art teacher worked up into such a tizzy that she was headed for high grass at the exit door.

A friend was buying staples at the supermarket recently. He had flour, salt, sugar, bags of potatoes, boxes of butter, and the lady behind him in the checkout line asked, "What do you eat?"

He replied, "What do you mean?"

"You don't have anything in there to eat. How do you eat?" she persisted.

After some give-and-take like this, he finally realized that she had never seen staples. To her, this cart of staples was completely foreign. He looked in her cart, and everything was ready-to-eat, whether it was frozen pizza, canned ravioli, or canned soup. It was all completely processed and just needed to be heated in a microwave. To her, my friend had nothing to eat. Amazing. No civilization has ever spent more money remodeling and gadgetizing its kitchens, but been more lost as to where they are. It's like getting a jet airplane to go ten miles away. We put all this techno-glitz into our kitchens to impress people, and then don't spend any time there. Folks, this ain't normal.

Historically, kitchens have always been the centerpiece of the household. Something was always simmering, baking, roasting, rising, or something. The entertainment center has replaced the kitchen as the hub of the house. That is unfortunate, because you cannot have a normal ecology without a normal domestic culinary expertise and involvement.

I hear that many young people today think scratch cooking means you have to use a can opener. No, my dears, scratch cooking is when you use unprocessed ingredients and put them together to create something to eat. Amazingly, you can make a lot of stuff in your kitchen.

Sheri, our daughter-in-law, developed a quick and easy recipe for making lard in a slow cooker or crock pot. All it takes is pork fat. Our Weston A. Price Foundation (WAPF) member customers were pleading for lard because it's so much better nutritionally than vegetable oils and trans fats, but we couldn't make it for them legally due to food regulations and the dutiful food police who enforce them. Pie crust made with lard, french fries cooked in lard, even hush puppies cooked in lard. I'm sounding like Bubba's shrimp dishes in *Forrest Gump*. If you've never cooked in lard, you're missing something.

You can make jam, jelly, gelatin. Our farm sells chicken feet for gelatin and Jewish mother's soup. Sally Fallon, founder of WAPF, has done the world a great favor with her *Nourishing Traditions* book to bring alive the culinary arts. To list all the permutations of this work would be too laborious, but certainly the tsunami of interest in scratch cooking and whole foods preparation is a wonderful cultural shift. Promising to extricate women from kitchen drudgery, the processed food industry has done a masterful job of impugning the do-it-yourselfer. In her fabulous book *Radical Homemakers*, Shannon Hayes describes this backlash against modern culture's marginalization of the domestic culinary arts. If anyone needs a push to reenter this historically normal world, she will get you over the hump.

Contrary to popular opinion, scratch cooking from real local food does not require 24/7 duty. This is not about being barefoot, pregnant, and in the kitchen. I agree with Shannon, who says that Grandma would have given her right arm to have the timesaving gadgetry enjoyed by today's homemakers. What can be simpler than popping a roast, some potatoes, carrots, and onions in a slow cooker at 7 a.m. and setting it on the table at 6 p.m.? No cans to throw away; no boxes to throw away. And if you have a cute slow cooker, you don't even need a separate serving dish.

That meal just sits there and slowly percolates all day, using only 40 watts of power, and it's low-risk. Because it cooks slowly, it won't dry out if supper is late. It will be done long before necessary. Forgiving, low-energy, and it took all of ten minutes to cobble together. Home cooking is like any skill — the more you do it, the better you get. What may seem daunting right now will eventually become routine. And lest anyone is afraid to wade out into your kitchen, let me encourage you with a little truism. Everyone has heard the saying, "If it's worth doing, it's worth doing right." I have news for you — that's wrong.

The truth is this: "If it's worth doing, it's worth doing poorly first." Who ever does anything right the first time? And yet we've had that "worth doing right" drummed into our heads for so long, we're afraid of doing something new lest we make a fool of ourselves or have a flop.

Imagine watching a diaper-clad infant pulling herself up on a chair for the first time. She toddles, pulls, toddles, pulls, and finally stands, unsteady and unsure, kind of looking around, not knowing whether to be pleased with herself or terrified. Adults watching exclaim, "Oh, look at Roxanne! She's standing! Look at her, everybody. Roxanne, what a big girl. We're so proud of you."

About that time, Roxanne completely loses her balance and plops down on her diaper, grinning and bobble-heading around at all the sudden acclaim. Can you imagine adults then shouting at her, "Roxanne, for crying out loud. If you can't stand any better than that, just quit. If it's worth doing, it's worth doing right." No, of course you can't imagine that, and neither can I. So why is it that when we become adults, we're scared to death of plopping back down? It's not just because we don't have on diapers anymore. It's because we're paralyzed by the fear of failure. Something happens in our psyche to intimidate us, to cripple us with fear of the unknown. Look, folks, I know that kitchen looks foreboding, enigmatic. I know that whole beef roast thawing in the kitchen sink looks primal. But take your first step, dive in, do it poorly first. Who cares if the cake falls the first time? Who cares if the ice cream sticks to the sides of the churn? Who cares if the cookies are crunchy instead of soft and moist? Just get in there and do it. As you cultivate the skill, you'll do more with less, more in less time, and better than you ever thought possible.

We had an intern one summer who had just finished four years of dietetic school in a prestigious eastern university and she had never cooked anything in her life. Not one thing. The summer interning with us, she ventured into this great unknown and supplemented her dietetic degree with something real: culinary experience. If this isn't an example of disassociated learning, I don't know what is.

Lest anyone think I'm some sort of foodie, I'm not. Not by a long shot. I can shred cheese, make a great omelet, fry sausage. I've only cooked two times in my life, each time for nine months (we have two children — hint, hint), and that was enough for me, but Teresa, my bride of thirty-plus years, is a wonderful culinary expert from the old school. She's not a foodie either, but the oohs and ahs that her meals elicit are legendary. It's good food, simply prepared, and served with hospitality.

She bakes cakes from scratch, makes custard from raw cow's milk, makes pudding from scratch, ice cream, and heavy soups. I happen to be a soup lover. Her homemade tomato soup, from our homegrown tomatoes, fresh butter, and raw milk — let me tell you, it's to die for. Split pea soup, lentil soup, beef stew, potato soup. Believe me, you never had anything like this out of a can or a bag, and the ingredient list is pronounceable and short. Nothing strange, and almost no packaging to throw away.

What are kitchens for? In modern developed countries, they are the unpackaging center. They are a repository of grazable nuggets, whereby family members may come by on a whim and munch on something prepared by an entity that seldom has wellness as a goal. The goal for this preparation entity usually has something to do with increasing sales or market share. Nutritional integrity might be buried in a corporate value statement somewhere, but what do the words mean? Nutritional according to Monsanto? Heaven help us.

Kitchens are the vital link between the field and the plate. Field food products need to be diced, sliced, pureed, sautéed, marinated, and a host of other things. Why do people readily deny themselves the satisfaction of preparation integrity? Indeed, time spent mashing, stirring, and measuring offers meditation time to bond with the farmer. I think farmers who sell into the industrial food system deny themselves the satisfaction of knowing that their food will be touched by hands lovingly preparing it for those dearest to themselves.

One of our interns recently came from a commodity dairy farm. When the dairy tanker left the farm gate, she had no idea where it was going, who would eat it, and what would be done to it. But when she came to Polyface and interacted with patrons who took the chickens she'd raised and dressed, she looked in the eyes of the people for whom she'd been growing. Suddenly those early mornings moving shelters, feeding chickens, plucking, gutting, and bagging became relationally special. For her, it closed the emotional loop.

Every Thanksgiving, when our family sits down to our celebratory meal, we know that several thousand others are sitting down to a meal enjoying the work of our hands. It's not just some cerebral, academic awareness. It is visceral. We have talked with them, laughed with them. They have walked our fields. Indeed, we have courted each other. This intimate relationship with food has been preceded by a courtship, if you will. The dinner dance partner is here, properly courted, properly romanced, properly relationed. That's what kitchens are for.

That we need to address this emotional tie in these terms today indicates how far away from normalcy our culture has come. Prior to very recent days, the preparer had to be aware of seasons — of what is available when. Menus changed on what was available nearby. Those twinges of wistful dreaming in January for the first spears of spring asparagus, the first rhubarb stems, simply help anchor us to reality and make us appreciate life more deeply.

Delayed gratification is a powerful emotional reality, and tempers many things. Perhaps even things like road rage would lessen if we all tuned in to seasonal cycles. Perhaps even Wall Street, with its insatiable growth mentality, would see value in a rest cycle. Oh, sorry, we call that a depression, don't we? Why must we be disappointed at anything except red hot? Hockey stick charts don't last. The kitchen is where the normal person becomes grounded, joins the food team, and passes ultimate landscape connections to the next generation. Abdicating that responsibility creates a self-centered, myopic generation. I've heard the little ditty about the family that prays together stays together. I would suggest that it is equally valid to say that the family that cooks together stays together. That Jesus commanded the Last Supper to commemorate his death, until His return, is not just cutesy storytelling. The togetherness enjoyed and enjoined in that traditional sacrament stands as a monument to purposeful existence.

Favorite meals and favorite dishes form many of a family's deepest memories. One of my aunts never bought a dishwasher. When people asked her why, she said, "Because that's something I can do with my children." Isn't that great? Making the kitchen the focal point of domestic camaraderie exceeds anything else. When families begin placing importance on food, they make a political, societal statement. To actually care about food, to think about it, to see it as a conscious act is indeed a revolutionary thought in today's world.

That America was born out of the Boston Tea Party illustrates that how we view food and what we're willing to do about it fundamentally defines our cultural view. How tragic that so many families today completely abdicate this opportunity to vote with their food dollar. With every bite, we are either healing or hurting our neighbors, the soil, and ultimately the world. That's why at Polyface our little cooler bags have a phrase etched on their side: "Healing the Planet One Bite at a Time."

Culinary expertise is the fulcrum between farms and health. I would even go so far as to say that our nation can only be as physically healthy as the vibrancy of its household kitchens. The less emphasis we put on that critical component of the food system, the less we obviously care about everything else in the food system: the farm, the soil, and ultimately our own health. No health system in the world, public or private, can ultimately work if a culture exits its kitchens and essentially subcontracts that important work to others. Nobody is as interested in your health as you should be. Nobody is as interested in what will become flesh of your flesh and bone of your bones as you should be.

The notion that we can extricate ourselves en masse from our kitchens and preserve food integrity is foolish. It goes right along with saying good farming doesn't require more farmers. We can't have farming integrity without more farmers. As a culture, we pat ourselves on the back for extricating our populace from farming. I submit that better farming requires a more intimate acquaintance with the land, which in turn requires more eyes and ears and brains on that land. Can you imagine saying, "Let's get rid of half the teachers in order to get economies of scale and efficiencies in education?" Just like most of us would argue that more teachers generally create a better educational experience, I argue that more farmers make better food and more people actively cooking make better dining.

It never ceases to amaze me how jazzed people are about celebrities. The average person is far more interested in the latest Hollywood buzz than what's for dinner. Folks, that ain't normal. At four o'clock on Monday, more than half of all Americans have no clue what's for dinner. I'm not suggesting that we obsess about food, but there's a long way between where we are and obsession. Wouldn't it be neat if as a culture we were as interested in our kitchens as we are about the latest celebrity hookup or breakup? What if nobody watched TV one night because everyone was in the kitchen cooking dinner from ingredients they'd sourced from local farmers? The kids wouldn't be bombarded with advertisements for chicken nuggets. The family could actually talk and smell wonderful odors together. They could enjoy the craftsmanship from their own hands, instead of the goop at the hands of industrial factories fabricating artificial meals out of pseudo-food.

Our food system, as a culture, will only be as good as our commitment to and knowledge of the domestic culinary arts. Indeed, we could calibrate the health of our bodies and our soils — perhaps even our souls — based on the time spent in our kitchens. With modern devices, we can leverage minutes into hours; with practice, we become more skillful. With dedication, we can return to culinary normalcy.

Here are some doable suggestions.

1. Pick a meal, any meal, and fix it completely from unprocessed food. Breakfast is easy: eggs, sausage or bacon, whole fruit, raw milk. Then move on to lunch and dinner.
2. Process something simple, like applesauce. Buy some apples and cook them down, run them through a food mill. Don't have one? Go out and splurge. Your family will go crazy.
3. Bake a cake, from scratch. No mixes, no boxes. From scratch: like add flour, butter (not margarine — yuck), eggs. From scratch. Use honey instead of sugar. Watch the faces glow. This is good stuff.
4. Allow the person who cooks to *not* clean up the kitchen. Taking turns this way reduces the chores. Try to corral the whole family in the kitchen for half an hour after the meal just to talk — no electronic devices.
5. Make a little batch of mayonnaise from scratch. It's possible. This condiment is ubiquitous and enigmatic; doing that will empower you to take over the world.

We Only Serve White Meat Here

Fast food now defines America's food landscape. As Prince Charles so eloquently articulates, a culture is defined by religion, architecture, and food. Viewed this way, America's food culture would certainly be considered fast.

Eric Schlosser certainly did all of us a favor with his blockbuster best seller *Fast Food Nation*, describing the development and penetration of this oddity. So pervasive is fast food that most Americans cannot imagine a foodscape sans golden arches. That a quarter of all food is now consumed in automobiles is certainly abnormal.

I remember family trips when we traveled all day in the car. Mom would fix sandwiches and goodies to keep us occupied because stopping was too time-consuming, too expensive, and just unhandy. Besides, like most men, my dad viewed traveling on a vacation as a hunt: The prey was the destination. The sooner we arrived at the destination, the sooner the hunt could be successful.

But eating in the car in any other circumstances was unheard of. Today, cars practically have built-in kitchens, with tray holders, coffee warmers, cup holders. In those days, we didn't even have seat belts in the backseat. Imagine no Starbucks, no McDonald's, no Subway. Imagine having to go in, sit down at a table, and order from a note-taking waitress just to get a cup of coffee. Can you imagine? This was normal until after World War II.

It may shock you that I don't have a major problem with fast food per se. A convenient quick meal is actually quite a great invention. In our home, Teresa keeps frozen hamburger patties on hand so if we want a quick burger we can peel off a patty and cook it. The burger patties are next to the pork chops, beefsteaks, and chuck roasts.

The stash in our home freezer represents all the parts of the animal. I want to explore the abnormality of fast food not on the basis of quick meals, but rather on how difficult it is for this model to patronize local food. After all, what can be quicker food than dropping by the Brunswick stew pot, ladling out a bowl, and slurping it down? People have been doing that for centuries at ye olde corner tavern and ye olde kitchen table.

The abnormality is not so much that people want a quick bite to eat. The abnormality is in the percentage of quick meals, the narrow variety in content, and the consistency demanded by today's fast food chains and how these protocols deny local supply. My example of dipping stew out of a pot on the way through the kitchen, or even cooking up a burger patty for a quick lunch, does not inherently preclude local food sourcing. The problem develops when my sourcing is too narrow and too common to create a balance with the rest of the animal. A chicken is not all breast, nor a cow all ground, nor a hog all loin. In the final analysis, we must use the whole animal, all the potatoes, both long ones and short round ones, all the tomatoes, including the not perfect round. Are you with me? Plate variety is foundational to making sure everything gets used.

As a small farmer, I need to sell the whole animal. So does the food industry, and it's invented ingenious ways to do that by locating a steak house on one corner and a burger joint on the other. Between the two, the whole animal gets used. But fast food, because of its volume and narrow-spectrum use, inherently creates a conundrum for local supply.

Our experience with the wonderful fast food restaurant chain Chipotle Mexican Grill has really brought this home to me. This is one fast food outfit whose heart is definitely in the right place. They keep pushing the envelope on local sourcing and ecologically friendly food. Using traditional long- and slow-cooking techniques, open kitchens, and integrity sourcing, their innovations have created quite a stir in the fast food industry.

In full disclosure, our farm has been the pork supplier for their Charlottesville restaurant since 2008 and for their Harrisonburg location since it opened in 2010. I think explaining a bit of this story might help put things in perspective. By the time Chipotle approached us about being a supplier, our farm was servicing some thirty restaurants — mostly white tablecloth — in western and central Virginia. In short, we are a large player in the local food sourcing scene.

When Steve Ells, founder of Chipotle, first visited our farm, he really wanted the pastured chicken. But when we figured up how many chickens it would take to supply just one restaurant, it totaled some two thousand per week because they only use dark meat. It's juicier than the white. We would have had to find another outlet for the breasts. And of course they wanted a steady supply year-round. Pastured poultry on a foot of snow when the temperature is zero is not a good combination. And the chicken for Chipotle would need to be deboned, and processed under federal inspection. This kind of service is not available in our area — at least to operations like ours. Too many hurdles. Forget the chicken.

After realizing the difficulty with chicken, our attention turned to pork. Here again, the narrow buying spectrum raised its ugly head: only shoulders and a volume of three hundred to five hundred pounds a week. That was out of our range because it would require twelve to eighteen hogs per week. And we would have to move the rest of the pork elsewhere. I suggested that they try our hams along with the shoulders, to see if a blend would still be juicy enough.

Shoulder is juicier than ham. Steve agreed to try and, sure enough, found that our hams were juicier than the meat of their other suppliers, so we could use a fifty-fifty blend. That dropped our weekly hog numbers to six to eight, which was much more doable. Those numbers were still a stretch for us, but they were within eyesight. Our upscale restaurants were delighted to see more loins and bellies become available. The only problem then was the sausage. I joked with Steve that he needed to offer a breakfast in order to diversify his vendor portfolio, to take a broader range of product. But like any successful entrepreneur, he didn't want to mess around with what was clearly a winning combination by adding menu items or changing store hours. Eventually our family customers and hot dogs have handled the sausage, which is made from the trim and salvage parts of the carcass.

I joked with Steve, "Well, sure it works, but only as long as you can cherry-pick parts and pieces from a warehouse supply chain and truck things long distances." That's the conundrum facing any narrow-spectrum use venue like a fast food place. It works in the current context. Is the current context sustainable? I would argue that it is not, as illustrated by these stories.

I am certainly not trying to downplay Chipotle's efforts — our farm has a wonderful working relationship with Steve and the whole outfit. But I also don't shy away from nudging and pushing and educating. This has been a delightful dance, I think for both of us, and it's not over yet.

Beef has been on the negotiating table for a while, but we haven't yet been able to get together on price and volume. Again, Chipotle only uses about 18 percent of the carcass, so any supplier needs to find a home for the rest of the critter. The bottom line is that the lack of variety in the fast food simple-menu model creates an inherent inaccessibility to small-scale local producers who need to move the whole animal. The only way a narrow-spectrum fast food place can exist is to be able to cherry-pick from a big enough inventory pool.

In this regard, the specialization, simplification, and routinization of the fast food model discourages access by nonindustrial local farms. While we smaller local farms may produce a significant volume of product, we don't normally do enough of any piece of an item to supply such a narrow protocol in such volume. In this respect, the fast food industry has been a driving force in changing the landscape of the food system.

The old combination diner, offering a wider spectrum, nests better into a local food landscape. Another option would be for a couple of narrow-spectrum restaurants to collaborate in a locality, so that one could take a couple of items and the other could take complementary items. This would offer the local farmer a symbiotic marketing option.

If Chipotle, for example, could get Shoney's to offer local pigaerator sausage and bacon, then more of the animal could get used. On another corner, if a TGI Friday's would offer the loin, that would just about take care of the whole animal. That's the kind of collaboration that is really necessary to increase local food penetration in the marketplace — and that's just one animal.

Old-style diners that often served liver and onions or braised short ribs or chicken and dumplings used a much greater variety. They weren't afraid to nibble around the edges, to help salvage peripheral items. I'm thinking stewed tomatoes (a great place for blemished produce) and heavy soups. Squash bisque — that's where the blemished squash goes. Have you ever seen squash on a fast food menu? Squash is a wonderful, underutilized food.

Intensive farms serving local markets tend to be multispeciated, like ours. This was the problem we had dealing with Whole Foods. They only wanted our eggs. At Polyface, our animals are in balance. We can't have more eggs than we have cows to mow ahead of the Eggmobiles. The pigs turn the compost behind the cows. Everything needs to come up together to leverage the gifts and talents of each. This intricate symbiosis only works if it stays in balance. Whole Foods didn't want anything but eggs. They wanted to turn us into an egg farm. We don't want to just be an egg farm. The eggs are a by-product of chicken function, biological sanitizing under rabbits, behind cows.

The same is true for vegetables. Intensive farms achieve their hyperproductivity partially due to planting a variety. Cool-season vegetables in the spring double-cropped to hot-season vegetables in the summer. If the season is long enough, and with tall tunnel extenders, perhaps the same ground can go back into a cool-tolerant vegetable in the fall. That's three crops to make the system work and achieve the yields necessary for small acreages to be profitable.

That is exactly what industrial monocropping systems can't do as well. The unfair advantage, to use a business term, enjoyed by the smaller local producer is this ability to achieve higher productivity per square yard through synergistic crop variation. That requires lots of varieties. How many varieties are in fast food? Let's see, tomato, lettuce, pepper, onion. Did I miss something? That's not much variety. And therein lies the mismatch between today's fast food industry and the local food system.

You see, historically normal food systems were not only local; they were also diversified. The whole notion that a region grows only one thing has always doomed itself to fail. The Irish potato famine and King Cotton in the South were historical aberrations. Historically normal farming systems were highly diverse, with mixed animals and plants — such as we see in vibrant natural ecosystems.

Farms selling locally will naturally gravitate toward a more diversified portfolio in order not to oversupply the area with one thing. Fast food, because it does not flex well with this diversity, becomes aberrant. What does a fast food place do when local tomatoes or peppers are not available? It does not change its recipe. What about when lettuce isn't available? If a restaurant wants to use pastured poultry, what does it do when three feet of snow are on the ground and nobody in the area can raise chicken?

I'm reminded of one time when I was introducing our pastured eggs to a chef. It was spring, when we always have extra eggs and they also happen to be the best quality. In the winter, we put the laying hens in hoophouses on deep bedding — we call it a carbonaceous diaper — to keep them warm and comfortable through the cold and snowy winter. I began explaining to the chef that the egg quality would fluctuate throughout the year due to these changing conditions.

He stopped me in midsentence and said, with his sophisticated French accent, "Oh, no problem. In chef's school in Switzerland we had recipes for March eggs, recipes for July eggs, and other recipes for September eggs to take advantage of the nuances throughout the seasons." By this time I was standing there with my mouth hanging wide open. Can you imagine this in America?

Can you imagine McDonald's offering a March McSpring McEgg and then changing it completely for the July McSummer McEgg and the yet more glorious September McFall McEgg? And then taking it off the menu entirely in the winter because chickens don't normally lay very well in the winter? They could offer a local food initiative called "Get in touch with your local chicken. And then make her your inner chicken."

The ad copy could read like this: "When do chickens sleep? If you laid five eggs per week, wouldn't you need a break? The chickens in our county that have been working hard to bring you McEggs all season deserve a break. In fact, we're going to let them rest, like they normally do once a year in nature. It lets them build energy, go through a molt to get bright shiny new feathers, and catch up on the latest community gossip. In deference to seasonal chicken recuperation, we're pulling McEggs off the menu for one hundred days until our gals crank it up again. As we toast our hardworking gals, let's enjoy more toast, sausage, and hash browns for breakfast: The Vacation McCelebration!" Wouldn't that be a hoot?

Oh, hold on a minute. The phone is ringing. "Hello? Yes. Oh, you're the McDonald's ad agency? You like my jingle? You want to change? Well, glory me, that does beat all..."

The whole point of a fast food restaurant is the same menu, the same ingredients, every single day of the year, in Chicago as well as Tallahassee. Only a handful of bioregions could even attempt to support that kind of consistency. The result is that fast food has to come from a large inventory pool, produced nonseasonally and far away, where the ingredients can be warehoused.

My congratulations to Chipotle for trying to do better, but even an organization as with-it as Chipotle can only do so much with that model. Although they are sourcing local vegetables, it's hard to get enough tomatoes in Chicago in February. The business reality is that industrial suppliers like consistent sales. They don't like on-again, off-again buyers. If a buyer like Chipotle buys tomatoes locally for six months of the year and then moves to distant sourcing during the winter months, for example, it loses clout with its suppliers. And make no mistake, suppliers cater to their consistent buyers, leveraging the periodic dependency to keep alternative local sourcing out of the equation. It's a war out there in the food vending landscape. Historically, the price and logistical nightmare of long-distance transportation made all restaurants patronize local and seasonal products. They changed their menu accordingly. Consequently, people ate that way, realizing that the dining scene necessarily nested into the seasonal production landscape.

I wish a simple solution existed. Here are some thoughts.

1. If we were cooking at home and eating leftovers for lunch, we wouldn't have as many fast food places. We could still eat in the car, but it would be an extension of our kitchen rather than circuitous, narrow-variety, distantly sourced. Perhaps in the big scheme

of things, we really don't need this many fast food places and their diminution would signal a return to normalcy. Sorry, fast food stockholders.

2. Hearty soups and bisques are extremely nutritious, quick to dip out and serve, and offer a truly wonderful alternative to typical fast food. Don't forget bean soups and lentils.

3. Beef and pork are generally available year-round without compromising seasonality. Chicken is more problematic due to heat and cold on pasture. Cows and pigs are hardier. Fast food places could change their menus seasonally to reflect this, but that would fundamentally change their model. Great idea, but tough to implement.

Disodium Ethylenediaminetetraacetate — Yum!

Have you tried reading the labels on industrial supermarket food lately? You have to be a chemist and love multisyllabic science-speak to even decipher the labels. Folks, this ain't normal.

To return to Prince Charles's point, a culture is identified by its architecture, religion, and food. What differentiates groups of people primarily is not skin color, but how they live, how they think, and how they eat. These are the defining characteristics of any culture.

The language used to describe religion, architecture, or food should be a common one. People need to be able to talk about these things, and the more able they are to talk about these things, the better. A specialty language reduces the conversations, stratifying the community into a hierarchy of those who know the language and those who don't. How can the average person discuss the relative merits of one food over another when half the items on the label are a scientific-speak mishmash of unpronounceable lab concoctions? Reading the label on most modern American foods is more like wading through a science experiment than Aunt Matilda's Sunday dinner.

Whatever happened to simple language on labels? Peaches, sugar, water. Or for sausage: pork, basil, nutmeg, salt, pepper. You can pronounce all of that and everybody knows what it is.

I'm reminded of nearly twenty years ago when our customers begged our farm to make them pork sausage without monosodium glutamate (MSG), a taste enhancer. The abattoir we were using had it in their spice blend for pork sausage. It came prepackaged and they could not take it out.

I set out on a hunt to find a mix that did not contain MSG. Pork sausage starts out as simply ground pork. A butcher breaks down the hog carcass into tenderloin, from the back. You can feel your tenderloin right now by reaching onto your back and feeling those two long, round muscles that connect the back of your ribs to your buttocks, with the backbone depression between them — that's your tenderloin.

Those of us who work in meat constantly find ourselves touching our own bodies when we describe the animal parts to customers. It's an instinctive response when you live with it every day, and makes communicating the otherwise obscure parts easy and understandable. A lot of people don't realize that our anatomy coincides with that of lambs, pigs, and cows.

When I was a boy, one of our neighbors would run his hand down our backs and announce our lamb grade. At the sale barn where farmers sold their lambs, the carcass graders would feel the loins for firmness and finish. They had a four-compartment paint container with blue, red, yellow, and green colors. A round ring stayed submerged in the paint, attached to a short screwdriver-type handle so the grader could reach in and grab the appropriate color paint and stamp the back of the lamb with that ring. The colors coincided with typical competition ribbons: blue, red, yellow, green. Obviously, the farmer wanted to see his lambs get stamped with a blue ring, known as "Blue-O" (not zero, but the letter O). That was the common language.

So this neighbor's little compliment on a boy was to run his hand down your back, squeeze those two muscles on either side of the backbone, and pronounce triumphantly, "Blue-O!" Of course, we boys knew exactly what he meant and loved him for it.

The shoulder, of course, coincides with our shoulder, and a ham comes from the rear leg — equivalent to the top of our legs. If you really want this to make sense, get down on all fours like you're going to take your kids for a horsey ride and it will be obvious. The butcher, then, breaks down the carcass into the various cuts that he pretties up into rounds and squares. In doing so, he discards corners and odd pieces into what is called trim. He runs this trim through a grinder, creating ground pork. Adding spices to that ground pork is what makes it become sausage. Isn't that profound?

As soon as we put anything in that ground pork, according to the food regulations, it becomes a processed product and enters another whole level of oversight. Every additive — even salt — must be approved by the food police, and each addition must be noted on the label, in a certain size, in a certain font, in a certain order. Interestingly, the food regulations do not specify or care about the volume of the additives; all they care about is that the additives are delineated on the label and that they are legal for human consumption.

I'm sure some of you reading this are wondering, "Well, why didn't he just ask the abattoir to get a different blend without MSG? Or why not just formulate our own spice mix and take it in and have them put it in the sausage? Folks make their own blends and mix it in all the time."

I'm glad you're thinking that way, because that's exactly what I thought — in my naiveté. But this was in the early days before I learned how devious the food regulations are. I called the abattoir and asked for a different mix. "We don't know that any mixes exist without MSG," the butcher said. No problem, I thought. I was supplying a fine dining establishment in Staunton — the first Polyface restaurant account. We had an extremely close working relationship with the couple who owned and operated this restaurant, so I called them up and asked them to formulate a spice mix for me. They were delighted and over the next few weeks experimented with different ratios and spices to develop the perfect blend.

I called the abattoir and said I'd get the spices, mix them together at home, bring in the bag, and they could dip out of it to make our sausage. They would pull out a quarter cup per ten pounds of ground pork and we'd be up and running. I was triumphant — our own blend, happy customers, life was good. But then the folks at the abattoir informed me that such a plan was illegal. They needed tamper-proof packaging to be legal.

Now dear folks, I need you to understand this clearly. Even if the food police approved my blend, my spices, and my labels, it had to be packaged in tamper-proof containers following a licensed protocol. I could not put them together at home. They had to be blended and mixed by a licensed operation, and there wasn't one anywhere in our state that I knew of. I could not have the packages in our home, on our farm. The food police said I couldn't even have it in my possession — legally it had to go straight from the blending point to the abattoir.

Did you know it's illegal for me to have one of my own USDA labels in my possession? Anyway, coming up against all this bureaucratic hassle terminated my little fantasy about a customized blend that I would carry down to the abattoir in a canister so they could put it in my ground pork. Forget anything that sensible and easy. No, we had to go back to the drawing board. The only doable solution for me was to try to find a blend that was already out there, approved and package-licensed, without MSG, that I could use.

I started researching companies that make spice blends and found that the one our abattoir patronized was really the only commercial supplier in the country — goodness me, I wonder why? I called the supplier and learned that they didn't actually blend the spices; they were a middleman and they didn't have a clue which, if any, of the blends were MSG-free. They gave me the number for their formulator. I called the formulator, which was the only outfit in the country. Perhaps more exist today, but at that time, before computers, one was all I could find.

After being bumped from secretary to underling to boss, I finally got someone who could give me an answer — after he did a few days of research. I waited several days and called him back. He had an answer: "We have four." Dear folks, I wish I could convey, through these words, my relief. At this point, I didn't care what they tasted like. I didn't care what the blends were. This half-year search just to find an MSG-free blend that I could legally put in my ground pork was finally coming to an end. Or so I thought.

He gave me the four product codes for these blends, and fortunately, one was a breakfast-type sausage, one a mild Italian, one a hot Italian, and one a bratwurst. Perfect. We were up and running...I thought. Even though this outfit would drop ship the spices, I still needed USDA approval on my label to put them in. Stay with me here: The blends would come straight to the abattoir, from the licensed mixing formulator, in tamper-proof baggies each containing enough for twenty-five pounds of sausage to preclude measuring, leftovers, or open containers.

These were USDA-approved blends, shipping, and packaging. But the abattoir could not put them in my ground pork until I had the spices enumerated on my Polyface label. That required a whole separate approval process through the USDA — label size, font, type size, order, etc. I wish I were making this up, but I am not. Truth is stranger than fiction — and people wonder why more local, small-scale, artisanal food is not available? Don't even get me started.

Desperate for an end to this sordid affair, I took a day and drove up — yes, drove up — to the USDA offices in Washington, D.C., and took my label paperwork in to a food policeman, who was indeed extremely congenial. The hilarious part of this otherwise nightmarish story is that the officer to approve my sausage label was Jewish, wearing his yarmulke, carrying his lunchbox of kosher food. What were the chances that of all the officers I could have encountered to put the necessary USDA stamp on my pork sausage label was a Jewish fellow? I felt like God had put that together just for me, to lighten up an otherwise unspeakably frustrating ordeal.

The whole meeting took less than fifteen minutes, and I was out of there, winding through the labyrinth of hallways to find a street exit into the nurturing embrace of our nation's capital. Yeah, right. During the three-hour trip home, driving down the interstate, my victory was bittersweet. Yes, I had an approved label. Yes, I was free to produce an MSG-free label. Yes, I was relieved. But this half-year ordeal that took countless hours, phone calls, and emotional toll was all for . . . what? In the end, what did we have?

The fact is that anybody in that abattoir, wearing a long coat, who wanted to adulterate our sausage could do it. Tamper-proof baggies. And these food police assumed I wanted to put something in the blend that would hurt people? Give me a break. In the final analysis, the guys in the cut room running the grinder could put anything in that sausage they wanted to — if they wanted to hurt somebody. They have to get a baggie, break it open, and pour the ingredients into the meat. Numerous hands handle it, hover over it, stuff the final sausage into links. At any stage in that process somebody could drop something into it.

How much local food artisanship is being denied by this foolishness? All to create the semblance of food safety. Remember, this whole effort began not to put MSG into something, but to get it out. Is that crazy, or what? Wouldn't you think this hassle would be required more to put it in? But the sad state of our food situation is that this was required in order to get something with dubious side effects, foreign to our internal bacterial community, something unpronounceable, out.

By the time the food processors get done with their unpronounce-ables, what we are eating is unrecognizable to our internal microflora and -fauna. Our three trillion internal digestive bacteria, enjoying opera and sunny vacations in our intestinal community, speak a funda-mentally simple language that they've developed over millennia. Those critters don't know about the liberal left or the religious right, or the Tea Party, for that matter. They don't know who's in the White House or who's on the British throne. Actually, they might care about that.

They have developed a recognition that we would do well to appreci-ate. When red dye 29 comes down there, they have to form a council of inquiry. They convene a committee and sit around in college confer-ence rooms to ascertain how to interact with this strange thing.

"We've never seen this before," says Professor G. I. Tract.

"How do we digest it?" queries one of the bacterial grad students.

"I think we have to let it pass," adds Professor Small Intestine.

And so it goes. They confer with each other and it upsets the whole smooth-running community, trying to deal with this foreign invader. This example of mine may not be scientifically correct, but it does put the reality into perspective. Our bodies have never, never, ever eaten things that were not pronounceable until the last few decades. Until then, it was understandable, egalitarian — anybody could learn how to cook and everything in food could be grown in a garden, a field, or a forest. It could be picked, threshed, cut. It was not manufactured in a laboratory.

Interestingly, our awareness of this bacterial world is growing expo-nentially as scientists probe the depths of DNA and genetics. In his wonderful book *Making Supper Safe*, Ben Hewitt writes about Justin Sonnenburg, assistant professor of microbiology and immunology at Stanford University, who questions the adaptability of our microbes to this new fare. A process called lateral gene transfer (LGT) allows organ-isms to share information. The research is clear: The dialogue I described above is not too far off. These bacteria actually do talk to each other, which should give us pause in putting a bunch of foreign substances down there.

My hero and raw milk evangelist Mark McAfee likes to open his presentations these days with a TED talk by a Massachusetts Institute of Technology microbiologist who photographs and describes the nonhuman microscopic world in and around us. The conclusion? We're only 15 percent human and 85 percent nonhuman. Her pictures of this microbial aura are profound. We all really do walk around like Pig-Pen in the *Peanuts* comic strip, a veritable dust cloud community of unseen critters enveloping our being.

Since the famous Human Genome Project fell far short of finding the 100,000 gene pairs scientists "knew" they would have to find to explain known protein and enzyme variations, the whole science of epigenetics has taken off. Founder of the Nutritional Therapy Association and author of *Pottenger's Prophecy*, Gray Graham says this new science explains how foods switch genes on and off. The bad news is that foreign substances play havoc up and down the genetic structure. The good news is that it can repair itself fairly rapidly if we introduce sound nutrition. Epigenetics is the new science that explains these additional variations.

It's as if every time we find a new invisible world that explains the bigger pieces we discovered sometime before, we eventually discover yet another, smaller and more multitudinous world that underpins that one. Rather than fill us with hubris, these discoveries and brand-new sciences should fill us with humility. Rather than dumping MSG into sausage and requiring a farmer to jump through a maze of hurdles to get it out, why don't we make processors at least break stride in putting these things in? What are we doing to ourselves? Does anyone really know?

Whatever happened to the scientific precautionary principle? Apparently as a culture we quit paying attention to that principle long ago. We wade into this world of unpronounceable food additives like a bunch of swashbuckling pirates, looking for profits and stuffing our treasure chests with swelling medical and pharmaceutical millions to keep us alive while we destroy ourselves with concocted chemicals. Does anybody besides me think this is crazy?

Each one of us, whether we like it or not, is utterly and completely dependent on an unseen community, an invisible world. We pamper and primp to make the visible body more appealing, but what are we doing to beautify our unseen world? In our Western Greco-Roman compartmentalized fragmented systematized linear reductionist individualized disconnected parts-oriented thinking, we tend to disassociate the seen from the unseen. We do so at our own peril. We are all, every one of us, simply a manifestation of this invisible world.

I find it strange that our supposedly developed culture speaks condescendingly of more primitive cultures that ascribe deity or mystical approbations to the physical world. In an effort to describe what is going on out there beyond the visible, many cultures affix titles and names to the inexplicable. Is it less barbaric or primitive to know more of this physical world, to see it through an electron microscope, and then turn away thinking that such a world can be separated from us? That what's going on in our bacterial world does not manifest itself in acne or infertility or Type II diabetes?

In the end, does it matter if we call Type II diabetes some mystical name like Sugar-Dragon who lives in caves and comes out to plague people with blindness, amputations, and seizures? If we call it by a scientific name, study its origins, continue to subsidize the substances that encourage it, and refuse the clear ways to stop it, are we any less barbaric? Whether we do a ritual dance to placate the Sugar-Dragon or go about our lives expecting the medical and pharmaceutical gods to ameliorate our sugar addiction, what real difference does it make? Each is just as ludicrous as the other.

Which brings me to the next permutation: We're eating food we can't even make in our kitchens. Have you ever tried making high-fructose corn syrup? In the wonderful documentary *King Korn*, the kitchen looked like a science lab by the time enough apparatus was assembled to make high-fructose corn syrup. With the new science of epigenetics, we're able to document that sweetener's damage to DNA and cells.

By creating unnatural taste, texture, and keepability that is beyond our kitchens' reach, the industrial food system creates an infrastructure and foreign substances that assault both our intuitive sense of normality and our inner bacterial community. It creates hunger for something that should never exist. Thirst for something that should never exist. Indeed, it makes people ask the question, "Why have a kitchen?" And that, of course, is the ultimate industrial food victory. Creating food out of things that can't be made in a home kitchen sends confusion into our physical being while sending confusion into our mental being.

Unable to make the stuff, we withdraw from food knowledge and awareness. How many times have you heard people respond to the question, "Do you know what is in that?" with this answer: "I don't want to know." This isn't simple denial; it's too arduous to understand. It's the classic escape from what is too complicated to learn. The more complicated a subject, the slower we are to embrace learning it.

With many of our farm customers wanting lard but denied by the government food police from selling it, we created a home kitchen recipe using the slow cooker. Sheri, my daughter-in-law, developed this technique into an art form and shared it with our customers. We could legally sell pork fat, but not lard. Lard is a processed product, requiring licensed kitchens and other hassles. Immediately many of our customers began making lard. It was totally empowering. No obscurity, no confusion. Open-source cooking and eating. Compare that with making hydrogenated vegetable oil. Again, it takes a laboratory in order to do that.

These huge food processing facilities where everything goes through miles of stainless steel and cooling towers are not the friend of an empowered food proletariat. They are the monuments to an elitist hierarchy that wants ignorant consumers, an industrial-dependent class too afraid and too confused to discover the joy and taste of their own kitchen.

We buy peanut butter from a Mennonite bulk foods business in the county. The ingredients? Peanuts, salt. And if you want, you can get it without salt. How simple is that? Honestly, it doesn't need anything else. Really.

Food does not have to be adulterated and prostituted. Food does not have to be veiled in scientific jargon. Food, this most common of substances, the one thing none of us can do without, should be understandable, pronounceable, and doable for every person.

Personally, I agree with Michael Pollan, food guru and author of *The Omnivore's Dilemma*, that a good rule of thumb is to only eat food that was available before 1900. We can all be thankful that hot dogs were introduced to the world at the Chicago World's Fair in the 1890s. Whew! Just under the wire.

Prior to 1900, we didn't have the sophisticated industrial processing capabilities we have today. While many people are enamored of *Star Trek* pill-meals, the more we learn about assimilation and elimination, the more we realize that food pills will not replace real food for a very long time.

I'm reminded of high school science fair projects years ago using live feeding trials on rats. Industrial breakfast cereals fed to rats gradually led to declining health, hair coat roughness, and cognitive problems. If the ingredients listed on the box were fed in their raw state, the rats thrived by all measures. Now what do you suppose the food scientists have in mind by taking perfectly healthful raw ingredients and manipulating them so that they no longer offer health?

I am not one to use the word conspiracy. I prefer calling it a fraternity of ideas. But in the end, I believe that America's food companies, for all their advertising to the contrary, could not care less about health. The be-all and end-all is about taste manipulation, shelf life, and cheaper product. Cheaper usually means you take out the good stuff and substitute with junk.

In the end, what you have is a combination that our intestinal community sees as a foreign invasion. Such a foreign language into our innards is a diabolical invasion. This is not politics; it's biological reality. Kind of a new way of looking at intestinal fortitude.

So what can we do?

1. Quit buying processed food with ingredients you can't pronounce. Just resolve to stop this patronage and assault on your intestinal community. Despite what you might think, you really don't have to buy this stuff.
2. Buy organic, local, farmers' market, Community Supported Agriculture — essentially, homemade or cottage industry items are purer.
3. Get in your kitchen.
4. Meditate for five minutes about what you think your intestinal community would like today. Feed it.

No Compost, No Digestion

Food that won't rot just ain't normal. Throughout history, our living food enjoyed the distinct ability to rot. Not until canning, and then freezing, did preservation develop beyond drying, smoking, curing (pork), or lacto-fermenting.

Even food preserved in this way will rot once it's taken out of its protected state. If you hydrate dried fruit, for example, it will get moldy, eventually sour, and then rot. Parched corn dried down in an oven or a solar drier, when rehydrated, will mold and then turn to sour mash.

If Teresa sends me to our basement stash of home-canned vegetables, venison, and pickles with a shopping list, a nonsealed jar will sport a healthy crop of white mold and we feed it to the chickens. If we leave frozen meat out too long in the thawing process, it will get slimy, then smell fishy, then begin rotting right before our eyes. Food's ability to rot is one of the historically normal protections to keep us from eating spoiled fare.

Curing bacon with salt and pepper became a mainstay of Virginia agriculture during the 1700s. Home-curing pork before refrigeration required temperature fluctuations that Virginia's fall climate delivered more dependably than any other bioregion. The fresh pork must stay cold enough to not spoil until it can absorb the salt. It can't freeze or the juices will quit flowing inside the meat. The juices are the cure's conduit into the muscle tissue.

North of Virginia the climate was too cold and freezing too likely to entrust the precious pork to natural curing. South of Virginia the cold was too unpredictable to keep the meat from spoiling before it absorbed the cure. That is why Virginia became the leading state for cured pork. It wasn't because pigs liked Virginia, or that Virginians especially liked pork. It was because in the days before environmentally controlled storage, Virginia's cool nights and warm days in the fall provided just the right mix to dependably cure pork.

But even that pork, if unwrapped and exposed for very long, would begin to rot. Rotting is decomposition, which is nature's recycling program. If something won't rot, or decompose, we usually call it something other than food. It's plastic or metal or stone. And while those things do degrade, they don't rot in a biological sense; they erode or rust or break down into a more basic molecular structure.

Many years ago I remember reading an article about a farm unable to compost feedlot manure because it didn't have enough microbes in it to decompose. The manure was rendered virtually sterile with all the parasiticides, antibiotics, and other additives in the cattle diet. To be sure, manure that won't decompose is entirely abnormal.

Many years ago we had extra grass going into winter and didn't have enough cows to eat it all. We negotiated a deal with a neighbor to winter his cows at our place on a per diem basis. Not wanting to cause us any problems, he wormed them with a parasiticide before bringing the herd over to our farm in the fall. Our normal protocol required following the cows with our Eggmobile, a portable laying hen house that allows the chickens to range free behind the herbivores. This biomimicry duplicates the natural pattern obvious the world over wherein birds sanitize behind herbivores, scratching through their dung, eating out fly larvae, and spreading out the dung for more rapid decomposition.

A cow pie doesn't last long in our pastures. Those chickens go for fat fly larvae like kids to gourmet gelato. Within moments of letting the chickens out of their Eggmobile in the morning, they find and obliterate cow pies in a mad dash to this delectable buffet.

When this new herd of cows arrived at our farm, I was concerned about what they might bring, so I decided to move the Eggmobile away from our small herd and run it behind these new arrivals. Just precautionary. I knew what was in our cow pies, but these foreign pies might have aliens in them. I certainly didn't want any of that. So I sent in the chickens.

They wouldn't touch the cow pies. Used to attacking these pies, they simply looked askance, cocking their heads from one side to another, clearly sizing up what looked fairly normal, but then invariably backed away as if the pies contained poison. Amazed, I assumed something was going on that I couldn't see. Give it time, I reasoned. The second day yielded the same result. And day three. All the way through the week.

I couldn't believe it. Had my chickens suddenly decided to express their chickenness differently? Had they suddenly forgotten the most fundamental principle of chickenhood? I decided on day eight to move the Eggmobile back behind our little herd and check out this unprecedented phenomenon. Wonder of wonders! The second I opened the doors, the chickens descended their ladders and attacked the cow pies, with more than normal vengeance to make up for lost time. Their exuberance was palpable as they scattered, scratched, and pecked. "Oh, goody, goody," they seemed to say, "we're back to edible pies."

After a couple of days, I took them back to the foreign cows. Same thing. I brought the Eggmobile back behind our cows — oh happy day! Welcome to the world of sterile poop. Now, folks, I'm no scientist, but I guarantee you that any cow pie that won't make a chicken salivate with delight just ain't normal. It makes me want to create a new farm mantra: "As for me and my poop, we will taste delicious to chickens."

Life is not sterile. Biology is not sterile. Things that won't rot, or won't decompose, or a disposal system that impairs decomposition, all characterize inanimate things, mechanical things. We are surrounded, inside and outside, with bacteria and decomposition. The entire principle of recycling hinges on the ability of something to decompose. Imagine if when things died they did not decompose. Leaves, grass, carcasses of bugs and animals. Trees that fall over. The life, death, decomposition, regeneration cycle is both physically and ecologically fundamental and profoundly spiritual.

When we masticate that carrot between our teeth, we are taking the life of that carrot, crushing it, flooding it with bacteria-laden saliva, and decomposing it in our own bodies, with our own microbial community, which extracts new life from it and builds cells in our bodies, bone of our bone and flesh of our flesh. The spiritual metaphor is powerful: Without sacrifice, life cannot exist. Whether it's plant or animal, something must give its life for life to occur.

That so many religious sacraments and rites revolve around foods indicates a historic appreciation for the death-life reality. It also reflects a deep-seated understanding that food is fundamentally living. It is not inert protoplasm, but a biological entity, fully living and life-giving. It is fragile. Leave it exposed to the elements and very shortly it will begin to rot, or decompose.

That our culture has landfilled millions of tons of food wastes, and continues to do so, without a respectful decomposition protocol bespeaks a great irreverence for life. In previous cultures, no peels, cores, or uneaten food would be disposed of in a way that denied that life the opportunity to become life for something else. We've all seen reports of drilling down through landfills. Hot dogs decades old and hundreds of feet deep rise to the bore surface and are perfectly edible. So far, nobody really knows how long it will take for these food scraps and decomposable waste to become life again.

If you include yard waste and wood products in the percentage of decomposable inputs to landfills, it accounts for roughly 75 percent. That is immoral. To deny all that life a chance to decompose and restart the life cycle is not only insensitive, it is ecologically reprehensible. That material, had it all been encouraged to rot, could have fed the soil and maintained fertility without the use of toxic nonbiological petroleum-based fertilizers. It's not that we don't have enough biomass to maintain life; we have simply squandered the treasures given to us by solar energy and photosynthesis.

I recently spoke at a foodie conference in a big city and a lady, visibly torn with angst and frustration, asked, "I'm in an apartment. Every day I fret over how to dispose of my kitchen scraps. Do you know how hard it is to get rid of kitchen scraps in a city apartment complex?" What is easy for us on the farm is quite another story in the city.

That is why I advocate getting rid of the parakeet cage and replacing it with a couple of chickens. They are much quieter and far more industrious. They wouldn't require any more space than a fifty-gallon aquarium. How many households have an aquarium? Every time I get on this soapbox people begin laughing, and I realize it's a bit out of the box, but I'm absolutely serious about this.

Barring the chickens, get a vermicomposting kit. They are not expensive and quite sophisticated. In a contraption no larger than half a dozen shoe boxes, you can feed your kitchen scraps to worms and enjoy pathogen-free, nutrient-rich earthworm castings for your houseplants. If you don't have any houseplants, store the sweet-smelling fertility in a breathable bag and wait for your next trip to a farmers' market. I'm sure you can find a farmer more than willing to take the black gold off your hands.

I think farmers' markets should have food scrap receptacles so their customers can deposit this waste. Farmers could take it home and feed it to their chickens, or add it to their compost piles. Please understand, never before in human history have food scraps been placed anywhere they couldn't decompose and add fertility to the soil. Never. Putting it in plastic, carting it all over creation, and finally depositing it in anaerobic landfills where it can lie in state for centuries is not only abnormal, it's an ecological travesty.

While we're on the urban challenge — which occurs in lots of areas, from children's gardens to this composting issue — it's easy to start spluttering, "But, but, but what about?" I confess, I don't have all the answers. I know that's disappointing, but in full disclosure, I don't purport to have it all figured out. When I talk about cooking, people invariably bring up the single working mom with no time. When I talk about buying nutrient-dense food, people challenge me with, "What if someone can't afford that kind of food?"

If I mention gardens, the response is quick: "I don't have any land." On this one, composting or worm bins or two chickens, some will argue that they don't have room or time or whatever. "I can't have pets in my apartment" puts the kibosh on the chickens. Are earthworms considered pets? I don't think so.

I do a lot of speaking and these peripheral "what ifs" always come up to challenge my harebrained solutions. Right here, right now, I admit that I don't have the answer to all the fringes. When farmers in Idaho who live a hundred miles from a Coke machine ask me about selling local, I don't have a cookie-cutter plan.

With all this in mind, though, instead of picking away at the edges and challenging with the most fringe possibility, why don't we focus on the great majority for whom the idea is doable? Instead of saying my ideas are stupid because not everybody has land or room for a chicken yard, how about realizing how many people living on city lots, in the suburbs, or rural farmettes don't do any of this stuff? The truth is that if the majority would do the innovative right thing, the culture would change so dramatically we probably can't even conceive what the next tweaking would look like.

If all the households that could afford nutrient-dense food grew a garden, discovered their kitchen — would actually do these things — it would fundamentally return our food system to a state of normalcy. At that point, answers for the fringes would be more apparent. Step four doesn't look as forbidding once we've taken steps one, two, and three. I submit that we haven't even taken step one on most of these solutions. I'm not suggesting we should plunge willy-nilly into the unknown without planning, but can anyone think of a reason why people in the suburbs shouldn't grow their own food? Or raise some chickens and rabbits? Or have a chest freezer for bulk purchases? These are not dangerous ideas — unless you're the CEO of an industrial food system. Then they are downright subversive.

My dad was quite an innovator, and when he'd design a new machine or a system, we kids would begin with the "what ifs." Rather than answering each one, I can well remember him laughing and responding, "Well, we're going to know a lot more in thirty minutes than we do right now." What a wonderful outlook. He was saying that although he didn't have it all figured out, the right thing to do is to proceed immediately with the best plan according to current information. It'll work itself out as we move and adjust, move and adjust.

If nobody can move until everybody can, we'll never move. If we have to know every contingency before we move, we have the proverbial paralysis by analysis. The truth is that if everyone who could do what is noble and right would do it now, the cultural shift would be like an epic earthquake. And that would make room for the next set of changes. Defending our own intransigence to change by pointing out the desperate state of those who can't is simply irresponsible at best and negligent at worst. We can make excuses until the cows come home.

What we need to do is be faithful with what we know until the cows show up. They may show up and they may not, but we have a job list right now. Let's get at it. Living food, decomposing kitchen scraps, and living soil should be incorporated into everyone's life. Let's get at it.

Lest anyone think life doesn't exist in the soil, let me explain the real world under our feet. This is not just inert material that elicits a "Yuck" and a capful of detergent in the washing machine. It is a living, vibrant community so populous that in one double handful of healthy soil more individual life exists than there are people on the face of the earth. And that's just one double handful.

Let's see this world come to life under the magnification of the electron microscope: Wandering into the viewscape, a six-legged grazing microbe, lollygagging along on hairlike cilia, comes into view. Without warning, a nautilus-looking four-legged predator rockets in from two o'clock, impales the grazer with the saberlike spear affixed to its head, and sucks out the juices from the soft belly of the grazer. Before the hapless grazer microbe can fall to the hairy pasture, however, another predator enters the viewscape from ten o'clock and lops off the grazer's head, devouring it contentedly as the now-decapitated and fluid-deflated carcass hits the ground. Within moments, other smaller scavengers enter the viewscape and polish off the carcass crumbs.

This is all in a normal moment of activity in the soil. It makes Steven Spielberg's imagination look like a kindergartner. Better than sci-fi, better than Dr. Seuss, this real world of microbial soil life plays out the life-death-life drama every moment of every day. Yet most of us go through our days never pausing to even contemplate that our bodies, our very existence, our breath and being, are absolutely and completely dependent on this unseen world.

Lest anyone think I'm heading toward a dissertation of animism or paganism, or even romanticism, I am not. Rather, I see a divine hand in this complex intricacy — this marvelous, mystical, microscopic world — and fall to my knees in humility. Traditional and indigenous Eastern-styled peoples around the world maintain this reverence that connects all of us to an ecological umbilical. Our complete powerlessness to live, to do, without the active participation of this unseen microbial recycling and regenerative community should infuse us with awe and respect toward soil and food as a living substance. The visible, touchable, hearable world is literally tethered to a vibrant, moving, communicating, interacting, relational invisible community foundation.

And so we come to the crux of the matter: Whatever happened to food that rots? A mere century ago, not only did all food scraps get reused through the chickens or pigs, but you couldn't place something on a table and have it sit there indefinitely without decaying. Even table wine, if exposed to the air, soon deteriorates. Root cellaring is an ancient preservation technique, but it only lasts a few months. Those vegetables, when brought into the house, will begin to deteriorate in a couple of days.

Reducing spoilage through fermentation, vacuum sealing, drying, or freezing is both normal and ancient. What is new is food marketed as edible that will not rot at all in its consumable state. I met a fellow at a conference who told me he had a burger museum in his house. He said he has purchased one burger every year for twenty years from a particular fast food chain that will remain anonymous for obvious litigious reasons. The burgers have not changed significantly in all that time. They don't shrink appreciably, don't mold, don't rot. They just sit there, looking perfect. Day after day after day.

Think about the things in your kitchen and your pantry. Will they spoil if you don't eat them soon? The most notorious offenders are junk foods. Many varieties of candy can last virtually indefinitely. How long do kids hoard their Halloween stash in their rooms? Months?

Several years ago we participated in a food fair and wanted to illustrate the differences between our meat and its industrial counterpart. We went to the supermarket and bought a pound of ground beef and cooked it into burgers. We cooked a pound of ours into burgers. We measured the grease, put it in jars, and took the burgers to the fair. The cooking loss on the industrial burgers was significant compared to ours. When people complain about food costs for real food, they don't appreciate how much more nutritious the real deal is.

The fair was outside and on a warm day. When everything was done for the day, we didn't want to throw the burgers away so we took them home. We had four cats at the time — our biological vermin control unit — and just for fun, I put the four burgers from the supermarket on one plate and the Polyface grass-fed burgers on another plate. The four cats came running when I set the plates down on the back porch.

I purposely put the supermarket burgers closest to the cats so they would come to that plate first.

The cats approached the supermarket burgers, sniffed, and then stepped right over them to the other plate with the Polyface burgers on it. They devoured every one of those burgers, licked the plate clean, and refused to touch the supermarket burgers. I tell this story partly because it's a good story, but mainly because most people feel powerless to really verify the claims about food integrity that people like me expound. Most people just can't believe that in our enlightened culture we could actually be consuming bad food.

After all, if it's junk, shouldn't it be illegal? I mean, if someone adulterates the gasoline going into our car, heads will roll. Nobody is going to mess up my engine. But when it comes to food, not only are we pouring junk into our bodies' engines, we don't seem to care when we blow a gasket. Like blowing a gasket is supposed to be common or something. If our car engine blows a gasket, all our friends come around sympathetically offering condolences and we enjoy being depressed together. But if our bodies have an equivalent breakdown, we assume we've been the victim of faulty genes or the disease fairies, sprinkling their disease whimsically from the heavens.

This cat burger story, then, is a simple way for you to check me out. Don't take my word for it. Go duplicate this with your own cats. They are not funded by industrial food conglomerates. They don't have political alliances. They are not peer-dependent or swayed by hours of TV advertising. They are just primal beings whose sensory safeguards still function. Indeed, your pets probably have a much better handle on nutrition than your doctor. So ask your cats. Do the test. Folks, cat-repugnant burgers are not normal. If the cats don't want them, what do you think about your intestinal bacteria? What about the decomposers?

Think about compost. You put in wood chips, manure, grass clippings, banana peels, and wood ashes, and in a matter of days it takes on a completely different look. You can't distinguish the parent materials. It doesn't smell like the individual components you put in. It becomes homogeneous, dark, earthy, full of worms, bugs, beetles, and creepy-crawlies. Where did they come from? How did the initial raw ingredients turn into this? It is a completely different substance. This, dear friends, is death come to life.

If you put raw milk on the kitchen table in the morning, it will spoil by evening. You can smell and taste the spoilage. Ditto for raw meat, poultry, or eggs. But what about ultra-pasteurized milk? Touted as a way to extend shelf life, this procedure inhibits life-giving, life-necessitating decomposition — could we even say it destroys the sacrifice necessary for life? I know this is flirting with profound spiritual truth, but one thing I believe very strongly is that truth, real truth, permeates and threads its way seamlessly through the physical and spiritual. If it doesn't work spiritually, it won't work physically. And if it won't work physically, it won't work spiritually.

A homemade pound cake, made with real raw ingredients, will only last at household ambient temperature for a couple of days before white mold spots start dotting its exterior. That is why I eat this pound cake quickly and aggressively — immediate consumption is my personal preservation policy toward pound cakes. But no, it is not preservation, it is death, decomposition, and new life. Especially around my love handles. But see how long an industrial supermarket pound cake lasts out on the kitchen counter. Days. Weeks. It just sits there.

Think about the difference between homemade bread and the industrial supermarket counterpart. Who puts white bread in the refrigerator? Nobody does. You just leave it out on the counter and it stays perfectly edible for days. But if you use real flour, or especially if you grind your flour and then bake the bread, it will begin to mold within twenty-four hours. That doesn't mean the bread is poorly made.

On the contrary, it indicates that the homemade bread is full of life. And only fully alive things can decompose with virility enough to then resurrect in us a fully vibrant life. We as people can only be as vibrant as the vitality in the food we've decomposed in our digestive system. If that food went in lifeless, it doesn't have anything left to give, to create in us new cells, new flesh, new bones. This is such a basic intuitive principle that corroborative science, while it may be interesting, should not be required to convince us of such an essential principle. And yet our whole food processing industry cranks out product after product that won't rot.

How long will a candy bar sit out before it goes bad? A pastry with a sell-by date of a year hence is not real food at all. It may be ingestible, but it certainly won't rot. Instead of ingesting things that won't rot, we should all be devoted to eating only things that will rot. Cooked whole foods and casseroles need to be refrigerated right away. Why? Because they will rot.

You can check the viability of foods easily this way. Cheese is a good example. I challenge you: Put slices of Velveeta or liquid cheese out on the counter next to artisanal cheese. The real cheese will get moldy in a day or so. The other cheese will sit there for days without growing anything. If it won't grow anything, can it grow cells for you? Folks, we shouldn't need dieticians or nutritional therapists to tell us, "No!" This is not hard to understand. Yet if you look into the average shopping cart coming out of the supermarket today, very little will grow mold if exposed to air and ambient temperature for forty-eight hours.

We can all be grateful that vegetables and fruits, in their whole, unprocessed, raw state can hold up as long as they do. Otherwise, our predecessors before refrigeration would have had a tough time. As soon as we break the skin, peel, rind, or whatever, exposure initiates the decay process.

As I think about these principles, it occurs to me that perhaps God — my preference, or if you prefer, nature, or Gaia, or the cosmos — designed things this way to give us a litmus test on what to eat. If we didn't know, how could we know? We could know by looking at the decay cycle. If it would grow mold quickly, it was edible. Stated another way, if it would decompose, it was food. If not, like a stick or a stone, it was not edible. If today we would return to such a test, it would eliminate way more than half of the food ingested by Americans.

To think that we can devitalize — you can read that as disrespect — food life to this degree and then have a healthy population is insane. No civilization can be healthier than the life energy in the food it eats. And even more fundamentally, no society can be economically or ecologically healthier than the soil on which it depends. A bankrupt soil policy will naturally create a bankrupt food system will inevitably create a bankrupt health reality. No nation can be healthier than its soil-food life.

Processing in modern America seems devoted to making food lifeless. Taking out nutrients and then adding synthetics creates what is euphemistically called shelf life. Not much life about it. More like embalming a cadaver and calling it body extension. If we're going to stay true to digestive bacteria, we need to eat things that will perish. In order to perish, they need to be living. If they aren't living, they can't perish. If they can't perish, they can't give life. Contrary to most popular thinking, perishability is really a good thing, not a bad thing. The next time you buy any food, just put it out on the kitchen counter for a couple of days. If it doesn't significantly change in appearance, taste, odor, or texture, you just wasted your money on dead stuff. Except for when it's dehydrated, living food at ambient temperature has a relatively short existence. Living food is normal food.

What can we do?

1. Resolve today to keep kitchen wastes on your premises with animals, worms, or compost. Don't send it down the garbage disposal or out onto the curb with the rest of the trash. Separate and nourish the earth with its own blanket of biomass.
2. Institutional food services have the same imperative. On our farm, we've tried to get our restaurants to separate their food scraps so we can bring them home — go loaded with edibles and return home loaded with animal food — but so far have made no real progress. This must change.
3. If in doubt about your food, set it out for a couple of days and see if it will grow mold. If it doesn't, quit buying it. Buy only perishable food.
4. The one stable food at ambient temperature is dehydrated items and nuts. Rehydrating the dried food should make it grow mold. Nuts are the best exception to all these rules — and delicious to eat.

The Poop, the Whole Poop, and Nothing but the Poop

The Green Revolution through chemical-based agriculture is universally worshipped as the umbilical that enabled half the world's population to live and not starve. Even many greenies and foodies deep down in the recesses of their souls adhere to this notion. The idea that without chemical fertilizer, herbicides, and pesticides we would have to decide which half of the world starves is accepted without debate. Why?

Imagine you're living in about 1910. America is in that disturbing cultural shift between the agrarian and industrial economy. The information economy is still nearly a century away. The hot dog is only a few years old. The typewriter is revolutionizing writing and duplication. Heavier-than-air flight is still a few years off and bicycles are primitive and hard to ride.

Metropolitan newspapers editorialize on one of the hottest topics of the day: the demise of the American city. Why? Horse manure. Clogging the streets, piling up at liveries. This nasty cusp of urbanization without electricity, indoor plumbing, and automobiles is literally suffocating cities in horse manure. It's everywhere. You can't walk down a sidewalk without getting it on your shoes. When you cross the street, piles of it greet every step. Pedestrians bring it into retail stores and fashion galleries on their shoes. Wiping, washing, kicking — everything revolves around getting that manure off your feet.

Daily mule trains hauling straw, oats, and hay into town to feed the insatiable appetites of the liveries can't haul the manure out fast enough. Open sewers running along streets get clogged with manure. Farms nearby, within mule distance of the city, can't supply enough hay to feed the crush of horses amassed in the city. Finding a hotel room is easier than finding a stall for the night. And everywhere piles of manure rot, drawing flies and creating a stench.

People are tired of manure. On the farm, half the workload is shoveling manure. Low, dark, damp stables in bank barns must be bedded with straw each evening to soak up the manure. Routinely, these stalls must be cleaned out, using crude forks powered by strong backs. The bedding, packed down by the horses, contains a tight pack of straw and manure. The straw binds the pack together. Shoveling requires ripping those threads apart, stooping over the pile, breathing in the musty aroma of manure.

In the city, in the country, manure dominates life. The outhouse, the chamber pot. Human manure. Animal manure. It's everywhere and it all has to be moved by hand, with crude forks and shovels. Mechanical manure spreaders have not yet been invented. In the time it takes to load a wagon of manure, the animals waiting patiently to tow that wagon to a field have already added several forkfuls of manure to the floor you're cleaning. On the way to the field, they add manure to the road. When you get to the field, you shovel the manure out. Always shoveling. Always smelling. Manure, manure, manure. It's everywhere. It draws flies. Big, black flies.

Flies land on your pies. Flies get in the pitcher of cream you have sitting on the kitchen counter because you have no refrigerator. Iceboxes are beginning to be used, but they are still a luxury item. You curse the manure that brings the flies that land in the cream. You wipe your brow, sigh, and wonder when this manure tsunami will ever end. Talk around the table is about manure. How much we shoveled today. How much is piled up at the corner of Third and Main. How much fodder we hauled into the city today. Life, in short, revolves around manure.

If there just weren't so many people, the manure wouldn't be as bad. All these people crowding together need food, and some don't even have gardens anymore. Why are all these people coming to the cities anyway? Why all these horses? Why this infernal congestion? It's the rumblings of a new era, the industrial era. People have just begun hearing about a horseless carriage. Henry Ford is still tinkering. The nation is poised, ready, but will change come fast enough to deal with these infernal mountains of horse manure? Many city editors did not think so. It all looked hopeless.

At the same time, the great fertile West that had sustained the culture, as it raped and pillaged deep healthy soils with overgrazing and tillage, was now gone. The great fertile West. The salvation for infertile eastern soils. People could always go west. New land. The new frontier. Now it was gone. The inklings of resource management began to appear. The Soil Conservation Service was launched amid universal paranoia over a single question: "How can we feed the world?" Australia had been populated. It had no more west either.

Dust bowls, *The Grapes of Wrath* by John Steinbeck, and the demise of American buffalo all signaled a new fear for the world: fear of starvation. Soil depletion, widening deserts, and burgeoning urban populations meant answers to soil fertility needed to be found, and fast. Two schools of thought dominated this quest. One held to a mechanical worldview, that soil was really a mechanical process. Disciples of Justis von Liebig, the Austrian who in 1837, using crude vacuum tubes, announced to the world that all plants are simple rearrangements of nitrogen, potassium, and phosphorus (NPK), sought the answer in chemistry. If we could just manufacture NPK cheaper and easier, they reasoned, we could solve this fertility problem, feed the cities, and free people from handling manure.

The other school of thought saw the answer as being fundamentally a question of biology. Early environmentalists were beginning to gain an audience. John James Audubon, Aldo Leopold, John Muir, and of course Thoreau's *Walden Pond* all spoke to a new awareness of ecology. They began shaping an environmental ethic, trying to describe the physical world in terms beyond mechanical.

This universal search for answers to soil fertility drove scientists in both schools of thought. The automobile, especially the Model T, began to answer the horse manure problem. Meanwhile, the fertility problem grew more acute. Henry Ford's factory lured people to the cities by the millions. By 1930, automobiles had largely replaced horses. Tractors were just beginning to show up on the wealthiest farms. Most farms would not receive a tractor until the late 1940s or early 1950s. Plenty of four-legged horse power was still used well into the 1950s. But I'm getting ahead of the story.

Into this disturbing period of cultural change came two violently disturbing events: World War I and World War II. Both of them needed explosives. Lots of explosives. As fortune would have it, explosives are made out of NPK. As a result, the war effort drove incredibly fast advances in the chemistry, manufacture, acquisition, and distribution of NPK. Soil scientists and bomb scientists worked side by side. The industry to efficiently utilize, manufacture, and distribute NPK grew at warp speed, financed largely by the war effort.

Fortunately for this manufacturing, petroleum was cheap and plentiful. Manures, plant residues, bacteria, ashes, and rocks had historically supplied NPK. Of course, the greatest inventory of nitrogen is in the atmosphere. But these elements, in their natural state, do not exist by themselves. In order to intensify them, acidulation and heat are used to break away their buffering partners.

For example, phosphorus, which exists in nature primarily in rocks, can be broken out by itself in a manufacturing process. Normally, a mixture of phosphate, rock, sand, and coke is heated in an electric furnace. If enough air is added, the burning compound forms phosphorus pentoxide in dense white vapors. Add some water and you have phosphoric acid, or chemical fertilizer. Such intense portions never occur in nature, and certainly are foreign to soil bacteria.

Likewise potassium, the K, is never found by itself in nature. An electrical current frees the potassium salts from the compound. That takes a lot of energy.

Finally, the big one, nitrogen, is in some form of ammonia, which is one atom of nitrogen and three atoms of hydrogen. Under high pressure and temperature, these elements can be combined and stored. The common denominator in chemical fertilization is cheap energy for the manufacturing process. While nature has always used bacteria and gentle chemical processes with intricate buffering combinations, it was now replaced by high-tech, energy-intensive laboratories and manufacturing facilities. Hold that thought.

Meanwhile, in a backwater village of British protectorate India, a humble agronomist in the biological school of soil fertility thought labored away trying to answer the question. He looked at indigenous systems of nutrient cycling. Without the benefit of the developed Western cities, in the experiment station of Indore, India, Sir Albert Howard labored away on his compost research. An entire twenty-seven-year career spent there culminated in 1943 with his worldwide blockbuster book *An Agricultural Testament*. It was fitting that this codification of scientific aerobic composting, a true gift to the world, would be born out of India.

By this time, the hand labor to do large-scale composting without machinery was already too expensive in Western cultures. Cheap, plentiful labor was the prerequisite for where the prototyping would occur. When the materials had to be hand-chopped and hand-forked, American industry was already paying too much to employ unskilled labor on the farm. Not until the advent of economical and efficient handling equipment did this kind of on-farm composting effort generate the income potential enjoyed by mechanically innovative factories. But I'm getting ahead of the story.

As we've already discussed, innovation never occurs across all fronts at a time. It's a point of epiphany, and then a lagging policy, knowledge, and infrastructure that gradually metabolizes, assimilates, or leverages the epiphany. That metabolism takes time, information, and capital. In 1943, the world had scarce capital to expend on compost. It was investing everything in NPK.

Besides, compost was not nearly as sexy as making bombs. Although I would contend that much more sex happens in compost piles than in bombs.

Anyway, the war effort moved NPK applications to agronomy forward much faster than otherwise would have happened. And the reason Howard's work fittingly occurred in India was because by the 1920s and 1930s, during the heart of his research, nobody in the West was interested in shoveling more manure. Front-end loaders, chippers, shredders, and power takeoff manure spreaders had not been invented yet. But in India, with cheap, plentiful labor, Howard could cut and haul carbon, chop it up with machetes, haul manure, add minerals carefully, by hand, and craft a fertility panacea: scientific aerobic compost.

Perhaps to help drive this point home, if you visit any living history farm in the United States, from Plymouth to Williamsburg to the Frontier Culture Museum in Staunton, Virginia, you will not see a compost pile. You may see piles of things. You may see crude manure piles. But you will not see the scientific manipulation of carbon, nitrogen, minerals, oxygen, water, and microbes that defines true modern composting.

The reason Howard's epiphany did not get metabolized quickly was because the infrastructure needed to construct a scientific aerobic compost pile efficiently was not invented yet. Farmers were still shoveling manure by hand. Let's be fair. Put yourself in the shoes of a farmer in 1946. You're looking at thin soils, poor crops, and anemic grass. You have a choice.

You can get a few hundred pounds of some cheap stuff in a bag and spread it through a simple dusting device. Or you can shovel tons of biomass, tons of manure, build a pile, shovel it again into a cart, then shovel it again out onto the field. Which would you choose?

See, dear folks, those of us on the environmental side, the biological side, of agriculture are prone to point fingers at our grandparents and other ancestors and decry them as horrible people for spreading those bags of NPK rather than making compost. But faced with the decision, most of us would have done the same thing. The truth is that when the starting gun went off in 1946 in a race to feed the world, in what would eventually become the chemical-based Green Revolution, the artificial chemical side had a two-lap head start.

The Pentagon financed the knowledge, manufacture, and distribution of NPK, giving an unfair advantage to the mechanical school of thought. The fledgling biological school of thought — which was far more historically normal throughout the world — had a lot of catching up to do. In fact, about thirty years' worth of catching up. It took that long for highly maneuverable, affordable diesel four-wheel-drive tractors with hydraulic front-end loaders to be universally available.

It took a while for highly efficient chippers and tub grinders to arrive on farms and in places where biomass accumulated. It took a while for roads, trucks, and transportation to penetrate rural areas with affordable raw mineral components. And efficient power takeoff (PTO) manure spreaders finally arrived en masse by the mid-1960s. This was a major development, because up until the PTO shaft, all farm implements were either ground-driven or stationary.

Hay mowers, manure spreaders, hay rakes — these all operated from the wheels of the implement itself. A series of belts, chains, and gears connected to the wheels powered the machine. The tractor or draft power simply pulled the implement. If the tractor or horses stopped, the implement stopped. Implement activity independent of ground speed, then, was impossible. But when a direct spinning splined shaft extending out the rear of the tractor drove the implement, it could whirr, beat, spin, or whatever without having to move anywhere. This offered infinite ground-speed adjustment without changing the function of the machine. Suddenly, windrow compost piles could be built with manure spreaders — this was impossible until the mid-1950s.

With all the pieces in place, large-scale commercial composting came on with a vengeance, not just on farms but in urban settings and backyards. Today, we have backyard composters, vermicomposting, inoculants, and a whole host of gadgets and knowledge to leverage Howard's epiphany to the world.

In short and with a little forgiveness to the technically correct, had we had a Manhattan Project for compost, not only would we have fed the world, but we would have done it without creating three-legged salamanders, infertile frogs, and a dead zone the size of Rhode Island in the Gulf of Mexico. We would still have the half of Iowa's topsoil that in a mere century has washed into the ocean. And Rachel Carson would not have had to write *Silent Spring*.

How did chemical-based agriculture become the dominant paradigm? By a confluence of factors that people could not have foreseen or perhaps even changed. Rather than getting bogged down in conspiracy allegations and diatribe, let's just accept the historical context and move on. By the 1920s and 1930s, people couldn't rid themselves of the manure fork fast enough. Cities couldn't rid themselves of that stench soon enough. Farmers couldn't free themselves from manure shoveling quickly enough. Bless their hearts, they were doing what they thought would be easier and better. But it wasn't normal in the great ecological balance sheet.

In the 1957 USDA *Yearbook of Agriculture*, notice the official government and agricultural assumption: "Ways of handling fertilizers also have changed. The farmer once had to buy and handle bags of fertilizer weighing at least 80 pounds. The use of liquid fertilizers, which can be handled in bulk, has helped to relieve him of some of this chore." If you think the farming community was excited to move from bags of chemical fertilizer to bulk liquids, imagine the yen to go from the manure fork to bags. But this convenience was an ecological shortcut.

After all, soil is fundamentally a living organism. It's a biological world down there under our feet. Yes, you can fool things for a while, but eventually the balance sheet will bleed red. And the soil microbes, the actinomycetes (bacterial decomposers that give the soil an earthy odor), the azotobacter (microbes that grab atmospheric nitrogen and put it in the soil to feed plants), the mycorrhiza (fungi that build plant immunity), the earthworms will scream for — even demand — proper nutrition. As Howard said, they will look for something that is not artificial.

The dominant chemical paradigm received prejudicial stimulus through the newly created extension service. Launched by the Smith-Lever Act in 1914, also known as the Agricultural Extension Act, this federal, state, and local partnership extended land grant university research into every hamlet of the country. This taxpayer-funded effort ensured that the dominant scientific thinking of the day would spread rapidly onto the farm fields of America. Had this government-sanctioned and -financed educational effort not existed, chemical adoption would have been slower and the biological side could have established itself as a legitimate alternative. But with such a government-sponsored effort dispensing seemingly free information, the deck was stacked against any alternative view. This unfair competition for the farmers' attention still exists today.

Shortly after Howard's 1943 treatise, at the end of World War II, a great chasm existed in America's agricultural sector. Perhaps the greatest proponent of the biological approach was a man named Louis Bromfield, whose Malabar Farm in Ohio became a rallying point for the biological approach. A wealthy novelist, Bromfield was able to purchase the latest equipment gadgetry to demonstrate the efficiencies of biological soil fertility. Along came Edward Faulkner with Plowman's Folly in 1943 (which sold 500,000 copies in six months — can you imagine?). A former extension agent, Faulkner exploded the myth that fertility had to be brought in from outside and postulated that, with proper management, soil-plant symbiosis could draw fertility out of thin air and rock.

Of course, such radical teaching made him a pariah to his former employer, the government extension service. He taught that vibrant decomposition was the key to soil fertility. This was revolutionary, because by this time it was agriculturally axiomatic that fertility required bringing in things from outside. That a self-regenerating system could exist was a strange notion indeed.

About this time J. Russell Smith wrote *Tree Crops*, which was an early foundational work for Bill Mollison and Dave Holmgren's Permaculture work. J. I. Rodale began publishing *Organic Gardening and Farming* magazine before 1950. Meanwhile, in Great Britain, George Henderson of *The Farming Ladder* fame developed lightweight portable pastured livestock and poultry structures. Newman Turner wrote *Fertility Farming* in 1951 and *Fertility Pastures* in 1955, outlining a biological approach to whole farm soil fertility and absolutely obliterating the notion of chemical-based NPK agronomy.

Then electric fencing came along, perhaps the next biggest Aha! moment since Howard's scientific composting. Livestock controlled with electric fencing enabled the Frenchman André Voisin to add a foundational classic, *Grass Productivity*, to the soil fertility mix in 1959. Until electric fencing, farmers could not efficiently handle their livestock like nature did with large herds, migratory patterns, and predators. It wasn't realistic to move physical wooden fences around.

The electric fence was the technology that allowed smallholders to mimic nature's patterns. The large migratory herds, along with their cohort of birds, predators, and other species, which were so foundational to soil development, carbon sequestration, and biomass accumulation, could not be practicably duplicated on a domestic scale. Nomadic shepherds had tried, with varying success, but generally that required portable living quarters and usually ended up with the tragedy of the commons — overgrazing. Without a formal agreed-upon grazing plan with adequate monitoring, land held in common generally doesn't receive long-term planning for biological renewal. Of course, most privately held land doesn't either. But with smaller private parcels, duplication of massive natural herds becomes more difficult. Enter salvation through duplication by electric fencing.

Rodale's *The Complete Book of Composting*, perhaps still the most authoritative tome on the subject, came out in 1960 and put the final nail in the excuse coffin of the naysayers who still believed chemical-based fertilizer was the answer to soil fertility. The culture's love affair with everything industrial and factory-made reached its zenith in the almost universal abandonment of breast-feeding, newly considered barbaric and Neanderthal. Something as historically common as breast-feeding, barbaric? Folks, this ain't normal. So we raised a generation of allergy sufferers and asthmatics on Enfamil and Similac. I've often thought that perhaps the greatest single resource squandering our culture ever did was during that roughly thirty-year period between 1945 and 1975 when all those breasts went unused. What a crying shame. And now, of course, research everywhere is showing a direct correlation between lower breast cancer rates and early breast-feeding.

Then came *Silent Spring*, the beaded, bearded, braless environmental movement, Woodstock, hippies, back-to-the-land, *Whole Earth Catalog* and *Mother Earth News*, and the gradual awareness and unraveling of the chemical fertility paradigm. By the mid-1960s, with electric fences, efficient manure spreaders, front-end loaders, chippers, shredders, rural electrification, and roads, the earth's jury had voted. It was obvious to all who could see and hear. Soil fertility is a fundamentally biological question. Even the USDA's soil scientists amended their pontifications to include a dozen other trace elements as necessary, along with the standard NPK.

But many did not want to see or hear. They were focused on short-term gratification and Wall Street objectives. They were focused on the latest pontifications of credentialed university scientists who by this time had been completely co-opted by the NPK crowd. I can remember as if it were yesterday attending a USDA-sponsored soils seminar in the early 1980s taught by a land-grant PhD agronomist, who started his soils lecture with this sentence: "The most common substances in the soil are carbon, oxygen, and hydrogen. But we're not going to talk about them; we're going to talk about nitrogen, potassium, and phosphorus."

The farmers in the room, on the edge of their seats, lapped it up like honey. I glanced around, suddenly very uncomfortable, realizing I was the only one in the room who thought the statement absurd. Can you imagine Dan Barber, chef extraordinaire at Blue Hill at Stone Barns restaurant in Pocantico Hills, New York, conducting a lecture about cooking forest-finished pork by saying, "The most important thing about this is the cooking heat, the diet of the animal, and care during the slaughter and butchering phase. But we're not going to talk about that. We're going to talk about the pepper you use for seasoning." Come on, folks, this is nonsense.

When it comes to the soil, if you take care of the carbon, hydrogen, and oxygen, the NPK will essentially take care of themselves. But you see, the chemical companies don't make money on carbon, hydrogen, and oxygen. Those are things the farmer can manage himself. And the agronomy professor's research is financed by a chemical company or some other industrial conglomerate, so the lecture will necessarily adhere to academic requirements and deal only with NPK. We're all good little boys here in this university, you know. The good ol' boy network must be held together, all for one and one for all, at all costs. The Three Musketeers have just morphed into university professors protecting King Chemical.

These classic soil texts predicated on biology are the foundation of today's host of high-tech options and infrastructure. The reason I've belabored these giants of the faith, if you will, is because the average American has never heard their names or studied them in school. We know about Liebig, Bosch, Faber, and the Green (Chemical) Revolution. We know about Tyson, Monsanto, and Cargill. But those of us who see agriculture and food as a fundamentally biological approach stand on the shoulders of giants who were generally vilified in their day and certainly don't merit recording in today's mainstream conversations. Yet these scientists and researchers paved the way for modern, viable, ecological, and biological farming systems. These people were speaking out before the environmental movement existed. They predated more modern environmental agricultural evangelists like Wendell Berry; Charles Walters, founder of *Acres U.S.A.* magazine; Allan Savory, founder of Holistic Management International; Stan Parsons, founder of Ranching for Profit; Allan Nation, founder of the *Stockman Grass Farmer* magazine; J. D. Belanger, founder of *Countryside and Small Stock Journal*; Mollison and Holmgren's Permaculture movement; Sally Fallon Morell's Weston A. Price Foundaton; and Carlo Petrini's Slow Food movement.

The list is growing daily as this movement toward ecological integrity gains momentum. Today we have RegenAG based in Australia; essential microbials and the soil-food web with Elaine Ingham; manure tea; Phil Callahan with infrared insect communication; Paul Stamets with fungal remediation; the Nutritional Therapy Association; and Jo Robinson's website eatwild.com. Goodness, now we can spray electromagnetized foliar fish emulsion on leaf stomata pushed wide open by music beamed from loudspeakers playing calypso music. Folks, this is a long way from shoveling manure.

In an expensive energy age, make no mistake about it, these are the epiphanies, the new leaders, and the resources that will fuel soil fertility into the next millennium. It won't come from heating chemicals and elements. It won't come from a Middle Eastern tanker. It will come from real-time solar biomass recycled on-site to feed the biology of the soil. I've belabored some of my heroes of the faith, if you will, both past and present, hoping that you will seek out these alternative voices. You have not seen these names in common American literature, in the media, or referenced in scientific journals. Yet these organizations, publications, and individuals are the backbone, the foundation, holding up and encouraging this fundamentally biological view of soil and food.

I'd be remiss, of course, to not mention Michael Pollan with his tipping-point book *The Omnivore's Dilemma*, Eric Schlosser with his dynamic *Fast Food Nation*, and Barbara Kingsolver's masterpiece *Animal, Vegetable, Miracle*. I hesitate to start on a list like this, knowing I'll miss people and regret it. But finding one leads inevitably to another leads to another. The point is that a whole world of philosophical and scientific support exists out there that is not receiving media coverage or credentialed recognition. This is Robert Frost's road less traveled by. And I guarantee you, it will make all the difference. I want to shout these names from the mountaintops. I want them on Oprah. I want the world to hear what they have to say, because it makes sense and is being empirically proven every day in countless fields and forests. This message spins circles around the old-school dinosaurs who still think the soil is inert and lifeless.

How does nature feed soil? It feeds soil with brown carbon on top of its head. Leaves don't fall until they are brown. Needles don't fall until they are brown. Grass doesn't fall over until it is brown. And nothing incorporates it into the soil through deep tillage. It is incorporated by periodic surface disturbance caused by herbivores or bird scratching, and earthworms that reach up and pull down materials.

If we step back and let nature teach us, we will learn all we need to know. The more we try to trick, shortcut, or adulterate these processes, the less productive and efficient nature will be. So on our farm, we do large-scale composting. It is all about biomass recycling, nutrient retention, and letting animals do the work. Here at Polyface Farm, this is our permutation on everything I've discussed in this chapter, and I hope it will illustrate this best of old and new. We embrace appropriate technology to leverage the wise tradition of nature's biology.

In the winter, when we feed the cows hay, after the pasture is eaten up, we move them to a simple shed where their manure can be protected from winter leaching rains and sun-induced vaporization of nutrients that are prone to oxidize. Every cow is dropping fifty pounds of nutrients out her back end every day. I've always thought surely this is the ultimate perpetual motion machine (not that a cow is a machine, mind you, but the phrase is too common to adulterate): She eats twenty-eight pounds of hay in one end and gives me fifty pounds of goodies out the other end. Of course, she also drinks seventy pounds of water, and much of the fifty pounds out the back end is nutrient-dense liquid. But in any case, she's pretty efficient at recycling.

During this dormant winter time of year, the soil life is hibernating, which means it can't metabolize nutrients. It doesn't matter whether they are organic or inorganic. When you're sleeping, you don't eat. We want to hold these nutrients in stable suspension until the soil life awakens and can eat again. But how do we do that? We do it with deep bedding, also known as a manure pack.

Using available sawdust, chips, leaves, old hay, and other sources of carbon — even occasionally peanut hulls — we bed down the cows enough to absorb all these nutrients. This carbonaceous diaper holds the nutrients, never freezes due to the anaerobic fermentation going on, and stays a warm and inviting lounge area. As we build it, we add whole shelled corn, which the cows tromp in with their hooves. It ferments. In the spring, this pack may be three or four feet deep.

When the cows come out to begin grazing again, we put in the pigaerators. Seeking the fermented corn, the pigs aerate the pile, turning it into aerobic compost. This takes no petroleum or machinery. The animals do all the work. We spread it on the fields in the spring, after the soil community has reawakened to the new season, and these microbes gobble down the compost nutrients and grow more biomass through photosynthetic activity.

This has been the heart and soul of our fertility program for decades. Composting, along with intensive pasture management using herbivores and electric fencing, has gradually taken our weedy and barren fields to arguably the most productive in the county. I have that on good authority.

A few years ago we began having an elderly neighbor mow our hay because he had a much more efficient machine and could cover the ground faster than we could. He was an old-timer who had mowed lots of hay fields all over the community in his day. When I saw that he was about finished mowing, I went to the house, got the checkbook to pay him, and walked out to the field to meet him.

Something you need to know about real farmers — they never turn off their tractors to talk. They either get off and step away from them to talk, leaving them idling, or they don't talk much, transacting their business over their idling engine. Diesels don't burn much fuel when they're idling, compared to gasoline engines. Well, he finished the last swath and drove up next to where I was standing. Then he turned off the engine. I thought to myself, "Ooh, boy, this is big."

I climbed up on the tractor to talk with him, and he did something else that people in farm country learn to heed: He moved his chaw of tobacco from one side of his mouth to the other. Now let me tell you, when a farmer in the Shenandoah Valley moves his tobacco from one side of his mouth to the other, you'd better pay attention because something very important is fixin' to be said. He slowly and deliberately moved his chaw to the other side of his mouth, got it situated, and then started with his exclamation: "I ain't never seen nothin' like this. I done mowed hay all over this county, but I sure didn't know you could grow hay with mulch."

He didn't know the word compost, so the closest vernacular he could think of was simply "mulch." He went on to say it was the thickest, nicest, most weed-free and groundhog-hole free hay he'd seen. That from the poorest, most eroded, barren farm in the county a scant four decades earlier.

Two years later, another fellow mowed our hay at one of the rental farms. This farm is highly visible from a well-traveled two-lane highway, so neighbors watch what we're doing — like hawks. I think chiropractors should put us on retainer for the number of whiplash cases we create. "They're doing what? Did you see that, Marvin?" I'd like to be a fly on the wall around some of these homes of an evening as these old-timers try to decipher what those crazy Salatins are doing.

Anyway, this fellow climbed down off his tractor when he finished and said roughly the same thing: nicest piece of hay he'd seen. Then he began asking questions: "You didn't put on any fertilizers?"

"No." Daniel was talking to him.

"What did you do?"

Daniel explained, for the umpteenth time, what this fellow had seen from the road: "We move the cows every day from paddock to paddock, letting the grass regrow and get tall before mobbing it down."

Shaking his head, the mower operator said, "Well, I'd sure like to take a soil sample to see what to put on to make mine like this." You see, dear folks, your heart determines what your head will believe. I can explain it, I can show it, I can demonstrate it, but as long as you're stuck in that NPK paradigm, you'll never believe it. Not until you have your own come-to-Jesus epiphany that soil is fundamentally a biological community, not a mechanical blob, will you be able to understand anything about true soil fertility.

Feeding the soil reconfigured chemicals just ain't normal. And neither is viewing it as an inert pile of dead material. I hope that as a result of this discussion, everyone who espouses soil as a biological community, and who may feel a bit intimidated by the credentialed agronomists in our culture, will hold your head high and realize the historical context of our soil chemical dependency. It's also a high-energy dependency.

I have a hard time faulting those 1920–1940 farmers for reaching for that bag of NPK. But I have little sympathy for those after 1950, less for those after 1960, and none whatsoever for anyone after 1970 who continued down that path. By 1970, everything was in place to leverage biological integrity. Anyone who refused to jump from the chemical

soil ship by that time deserved to go bankrupt, lose their farm, or whatever. That sounds hard, but it's kind of like saying a pedophile just can't
help it. I'm sorry, a soil abuser that can't help it? No way. They can all
help it.

During the toddling stage, back in the 1920s and 1930s, even early
1940s, I can appreciate reaching out for something abnormal. I'd have
been tired of shoveling manure too. But we're not in 1930 anymore,
Toto. This is an unprecedented time of biological infrastructure. Not
only can the biological approach feed the world, but it is the only one
that can do it regeneratively over the long haul. Sunlight. Biomass. Soil
community. That's been the recipe for millennia, and anything else
just ain't normal.

So where do we go from here? Let me suggest a few positive things.

1. A national commitment to quit landfilling *any* biomass. If it will
   decompose, it should not go in a landfill. It should rot where it
   can be returned to the soil.
2. All manure must be leveraged to greatest advantage. Quit burning it for electricity. Quit putting it in lagoons.
3. Crank up the chippers and begin converting diseased, crooked,
   and junk trees and other biomass into compostable pieces. Begin
   systematically growing and harvesting biomass in interstate medians, along expressway ramps, and other public rights-of-way.
4. Quit feeding herbivores grain. Period. That alone would so fundamentally change fertility cycles that we can't imagine all the
   ramifications. Herbivores would once again be spread out across
   perennial prairie polycultures managed with electric fence
   instead of lightning and predators. Poop would fall on biomass in
   real time, without any energy required for transportation.
5. Begin dismantling water-based human sewage and move to
   methane digesters, composting, and red wriggler decomposition.
   We must quit throwing away manure — it's the secret of fertility.

Park, Plant, and Power

Peak oil. Only people with their head stuck in celebrity magazines have never heard of it. The debate surrounding oil supplies and peak oil can make your head spin. I well remember in the late 1970s when I was on the intercollegiate debate team in college, quoting authoritative experts predicting the end of oil by 1990. This, folks, is why I never prophesy. The one question I will never answer in an interview is this: "What do you foresee twenty years from now?"

Some people I respect even say oil is still being made; perhaps not as fast as we're using it, but being made nonetheless. I actually don't know if it is or isn't. I don't know if we're about to run out of oil or not, but I do know that hockey stick charts never go on indefinitely. They also always crash. I don't want to rehash all the oil debate nuances here. Again, plenty of great books already exist to get your mind thoroughly engulfed (pun intended) in this subject.

In keeping with the theme of this book, I want to go back, to think about energy in a primal sense. When you flick on that light switch, or hear the thermostat cut the furnace on, or the air conditioner on, what is that? I think if we're ever going to be really creative about solving issues, we need to reestablish what is historically normal. Until we have some sort of benchmark, we don't know how to measure progress. We may think we're going forward and actually we're going backward. The fact is that many of us concerned about finite energy, or energy footprints, or carbon footprints, still live in air-conditioned homes, patronize energy-intensive industrial food, use a clothes dryer instead of a clothesline, and have two cars when one would do. And it's not always simple.

In the early 1970s during the Arab oil embargo my dad was in his early fifties and worked at a welding and metal fabrication shop thirteen miles away. He read blueprints, made the estimates, and was the in-house accountant. It was on the other side of Staunton, a town of 20,000 roughly eight miles away from our farm. You may recall that Jimmy Carter was president and vowed to break our dependency on foreign oil. Yeah, right. A Department of Energy and billions later, we're sure weaned off foreign oil, aren't we? I can't believe people still think government agencies are the answer to much of anything.

Gasoline became so tight that by law filling stations could only dispense fuel into cars with license tags that ended in an odd number on calendar days that were odd; evens went on the even-numbered days. Dad decided to wean himself from foreign oil by buying a ten-speed bicycle and riding that thirteen miles to work, so he did. He couldn't figure out why everyone wouldn't just do that and show the Arabs who was boss. But very few people who complain actually want to inconvenience themselves on the way to fixing the problem.

In full transparency, I was in high school and thought he was insane. I was a teen, and of course was supposed to roll my eyes and be embarrassed. Without getting into all the familial dynamics of the situation, I can assure you that now I am awed by such conviction. I wonder how many environmentalists would have done that or would do it today. When he arrived home, sweaty and breathless from the trip, he had a real understanding of energy. Prior to the industrial age, the average person had this level of understanding about energy.

I live smack dab in the middle of Virginia's Shenandoah Valley, which stretches north and south between the Blue Ridge Mountains on the east and the Allegheny Mountains on the west. The valley runs north and south from roughly Woodstock to Natural Bridge. The trough rises in the middle and falls toward either end. On a map, of course, the easy thing is to say that from here in the Staunton area, in the middle of the valley, we would drive down to Natural Bridge and up to Woodstock. But old-timers say down to both areas. Why? Because in the days before mechanical transport, that thousand feet of elevation change in fifty miles made a big difference.

In a car, of course, you don't notice the slightly downhill grade. But a team of horses or mules certainly could tell it. This visceral understanding of energy was normal not too long ago. Today, if you say you're going down to Winchester, people look at you like you're crazy. "Winchester isn't down," they correct. "Winchester is north — it's up."

But it's down in terrain. The water that runs off our farm goes north to Harpers Ferry, where it intersects with the Potomac and then flows out past Washington, D.C. Just two miles to the south of us, the water flows south until it intersects with the James and flows to the Atlantic via Richmond. These subtle nuances of terrain, energy, and effort used to be part of normal awareness. Things are different today.

People have had a much closer relationship with energy throughout history than we do today. We pump gas into our vehicles from a nozzle. We pay for it with a plastic card. We hop back in the vehicle and zoom off down the road, giving nary a thought to whether it's uphill or down and the relative energy it takes to get there. Ditto for electric lights, the furnace, and the air conditioner. Not to mention the entertainment center and the computer.

Go back a little bit. Not long ago, that drive down the road required owning a horse. A horse that needed feed, water, and grooming. We needed to check his hooves, train him, rub him down with a curry comb after a ride. We couldn't just put the carriage in "Park" and leave it for a week while we vacationed in the Bahamas. In fact, the Bahamas were not reachable in a jet. It took weeks by train and steamer, or sailboat, to get there.

Today, on a whim, we can grab a cab and hop a jet to the Bahamas. Not very long ago, such a trip would be reserved for the extremely wealthy and require months of planning. I'm not saying we should ground all the jets or park all the cars. I am saying that this is not normal. We are the first generation in human history to have this kind of energy at our disposal. To think that our minds and our worldviews are not shaped by this cheap energy, this easy energy, is to disregard the influence that such profound changes create in a cultural psyche.

Perhaps I should explain a bit about how I grew up. Remember, my dad rode a bicycle. Dad, though extremely conservative politically, was an early and avid reader of *Mother Earth News*. I remember marijuana-reeking hippies in our house when I was growing up, a far cry from our conservative fundamentalist Christian leanings. But our family found a wonderful camaraderie with these left-leaning folks, a reverent view toward resources that we did not find among our friends in the religious right.

Earth stewardship, to my family, was not some cerebral thing that you recited in catechism class and threw out the window at the first mention of dominion. If it meant anything, it meant living differently. It meant a new awareness. So as the 1960s wound down and my brother and I got big enough to cut and tote firewood, Dad disconnected the oil furnace. To heat this big rambling farmhouse required more than a thousand gallons of fuel oil a winter.

We purchased a woodstove before they were in vogue. The Riteway company began building woodstoves in Harrisonburg, about thirty miles north of us, and we went up to look at them. The shop was tiny, employed a couple of guys, and they were cranking out one or two a week. About half a dozen sat on the floor in varying stages of fabrication. We bought one. Within two years, Riteway was one of the big players in the national woodstove boom.

Our family was always thinking about independence, about earth stewardship, about how to keep resources in the ground for as long as possible. If we want raindrops to stay where they land as long as possible, shouldn't we also want energy to stay in its deposit for as long as possible. Why extract it as fast as possible? Why not be as conservative as possible?

I find it amazing that the conservative/liberal mantra, when it comes to resource stewardship, has flip-flopped. You would think the liberals, who can't give other people's money away fast enough, would be the ones wanting to strip out all the energy. But that's not the case. The conservatives, who correctly think people should keep what they earn, are the ones seemingly least interested in conserving natural resources. These stereotypical political agendas always get squirrely to me. That's why I call myself a Christian libertarian environmentalist capitalist lunatic. It seems to cover all my important bases.

We installed that big Riteway in the front foyer, shoved a flue pipe up into the chimney, and began heating with wood. Although it had a fairly large firebox, our big old rambling, leaky house sucked up the heat. To keep from freezing, I would wake up every morning about 2 a.m. and restoke the stove. We burned that thing harder than it was designed to, I'm sure, trying to heat the big old house. I still can't believe we didn't burn the house down, because many times, in the dark, the rear of the stove and the flue pipe glowed red. That's how hot it was. It's a wonder they didn't melt right off. Fortunately, it had a thermostat on the back that would eventually close down the oxygen. Then it would pull such a hard vacuum that it eventually sucked the side steel plates right off the mounting bolts. I would definitely plead guilty to abusing that stove.

A few years later, we bought a newer and bigger Riteway, moving the first one to the dining room. It being a smaller room, that stove just smoldered and kept the room cozy. But the big stove upstairs had all it could do. I shoveled wood through that thing day and night. Over the years, I rebuilt all the steelwork inside three times because it would eventually deteriorate to nothing.

Every week I spent half a day with a wheelbarrow bringing wood into the house and stacking it next to that stove. Unless it was single-digit cold, that cord would last a week. Although the wood was a fair amount of work, we figured that was some of the best money we made on the farm, displacing fuel oil expenditures to the tune of $3,000 a year. The stove required no fan, no electricity. If the power went off, we were cozy as could be. We could even cook on the flat surface if we needed to.

I've sold mountains of firewood over the years, and still do. It's a renewable resource, makes very different emissions than petroleum, and actually creates atmospheric particles necessary to encourage condensation and rain. Some scientists say we need more smoky fires to encourage proper weather patterns. When you consider how the Native Americans routinely burned the landscape, you can appreciate how much less burning is going on today. From what I've read, the idea is that woodsmoke particles offer the necessary microscopic-sized piece of dust that encourages moisture to change from vapor to something heavier.

Today, we've graduated to an outdoor water stove that heats both our house and my mother's, saving a total of close to $10,000 a winter in energy costs. The water stove also heats all of our domestic hot water. Water stove technology was developed in the early 1980s as one answer to the energy shortages. It's a way to have a central heating system without the fire and associated wood mess in the house.

Face it, wood fires are high-risk in a domestic heating situation. Even if you have a wood furnace in the basement, for example, a spark could jump out of the door and ignite the woodpile you have stashed nearby. The water stove uses a firebox encased in a water reservoir. The fire heats the water to about 180–190 degrees — below boiling. That's one of the beauties of this technology; it uses no pressure and is in fact completely open to the air — a pipe hooked into the water reservoir eliminates any pressure, even if something happened and the water began to boil. A thermostat controls a fan to blow air into the firebox when the water temperature drops below 170 degrees.

The idea is to shut off the air supply between fan cyclings, in order to turn the wood into charcoal, which burns more efficiently than wood. In the house, thermostats on the wall, just like any thermostat, connect to heat exchangers and circulating pumps on the back of the water stove. When the thermostat calls for heat, the water pump sends water into the house and it goes through the heat exchanger, which is like a big car radiator on the end of a huge squirrel-cage fan. The fan blows ambient air through the radiator and it heats up as it goes through. That hot air then comes into the house just like any central heating system. No mess, no fire danger, and it keeps all the far reaches of the house toasty warm.

I still personally cut most of the wood and enjoy it immensely. I find it quite satisfying to deny the oil barons a few thousand gallons of oil sales a year. If we as a people were still personally involved in acquiring energy, we would be more aggressive about extricating ourselves from the oil stranglehold. If our whole economy depends on cheap oil, what happens when it becomes expensive?

Now, for those who think it's heinous to cut down the trees to fire this stove, I would respond that our cultural fixation on trees as a nonrenewable resource shows just as much ecological disconnection as thinking a chicken is a human child. While it's true that many trees, especially in the East, were cut during early settlement, we used trees unbelievably wastefully. With a crosscut saw, cutting four feet high on every tree wasted the best part of the butt. Now, with chainsaws, we can cut right down on the ground and even cup out the base to get all of that high-quality butt wood.

Think about the wood used in a log cabin compared to modern-day studs and roof truss design. The technology for domestic heating is as different from fireplaces as a hybrid automobile is from a Model T. A fireplace sends most of the heat up the chimney. But today's modern stoves, with catalytic converters, double combustion chambers, and all sorts of snazzy designs, achieve extremely high levels of efficiency.

Look what we've done in milling efficiency. Until half a century ago, all lumber milling machinery created a kerf (the amount of wood removed by the blade) a quarter of an inch thick. That means every four cuts, or four boards, removed an inch of wood. That's a lot of wood. But today's bandsaw mills only remove an eighth or a tenth of an inch, which means much more of the log can be used in boards instead of going out in sawdust. Small-dimension wood can now be used that would never have been profitable just fifty years ago. The science of milling has come as far as heating and construction.

The truth is that we need to cut far more wood. The horrendous Yellowstone fires were a result of a no-cut policy that allowed too much fuel to build up. The Shenandoah National Park is a silvicultural travesty. A forest is a living thing, just like a vineyard, and it needs to be pruned to keep it healthy and productive. Just because a forest is pretty today does not mean it will be pretty tomorrow. That we have locked up millions of acres of forest and denied them the massaged care that would keep them healthy is terrible domestic resource policy. Healthy, growing trees far more efficiently sequester carbon and create oxygen than old, mature trees.

I know some of you will disown me as a raving forest rapist for saying these things, but I enjoy taking people up to our woods to see thirty-year-old clear cuts (all less than an acre in size) and how they are now beautiful, productive forests again. I don't like massive clear cuts any more than an environmentalist does, but a one-acre cut is a wonderful management tool to maintain a vibrant forest. Unfortunately, the excesses in the industry have created an overcorrective backlash that is just as inappropriate as the initial problem. I love trees, especially healthy trees. That's why I cut old ones, sick ones, crooked ones, and unproductive ones.

I can't imagine that someone who runs a lawnmower to maintain a healthy, pretty lawn can't appreciate the same principles on forests. Trees go through the birth, fast growth, and death stage just like any living thing. Thinning concentrates the available solar and soil resources on the most healthy, productive biomass. That is not environmental rape; it is environmental stewardship. Denying the forest the benefit of human stewardship actually harms the ecology. With today's forest products technology, applying this care can yield far more use while upgrading the forests' ability to achieve their environmental magic.

When I walk around our old house, realizing that for a hundred years it was warmed by five fireplaces in a time without chainsaws, without front-end loaders, without tractors, it makes the energy issue more critical. Before petroleum, people acquired their own energy. Not very long ago, the average person was responsible for his own energy.

Here was the historical energy path. I had to maintain a horse to travel somewhere. That horse required care and feed. I had to cut wood with an ax and crosscut saw to feed the woodstove and, before wood-stoves, the incredibly inefficient fireplace. Waterwheels often powered grain mills and sawmills. Later, steam engines powered these things, as well as trains. Coal gradually replaced wood. Lights came from candles made from animal fat. All of this took lots of time. I suppose someone has computed the amount of labor involved in supplying energy. A huge amount of every person's day was spent hauling water and generating energy.

Because energy was precious, people tended to live close to their work. Driving to the office was too expensive and laborious. Expensive energy drove cultural design. Craftspeople tended to live over their shops. Commuting in to work was not only impractical, it was undesirable and inefficient. Suburban developments only became possible, and will only remain so, as long as energy is cheap. The day energy returns to normalcy, suburbs will collapse. Or they will become much more self-sufficient by converting lawns to gardens and mini-forests, and by attaching solariums to the sunny side of the house.

Food had to be grown close to consumption because transporting it was too expensive. Feedstuffs for animals, whether it was grain or grass, had to be grown and consumed on the same farm; nothing else was possible. For the first time in human history, the Transcontinental Railroad made the economical transportation of grain and livestock possible. But the railroad boom largely followed the coal boom, which preceded and set the stage for the petroleum boom.

As energy became divorced from daily activity, and as it became cheaper, other interdependencies and economic relationships fell apart. What had been a highly interconnected economic and social community became highly stratified. The energy disconnection, with a lack of appreciation for energy's value, opened the door for other disconnections. Indeed, it allowed the community-based and tight-knit village culture to fragment into economic apartheid.

The butcher, baker, and candlestick maker, formerly embedded in the village, were summarily removed from the community because with cheap energy, their businesses could grow beyond local energy carrying capacity. Prior to cheap energy, all industry stayed naturally within the community's energy capability. But as cheap energy fueled non-community-reliant business scale, the butcher, baker, and candlestick maker became less neighbor-friendly.

We could certainly spend a long time discussing what is appropriate human scale. I won't delve into it here because I really don't know. I am not opposed to big business per se. But it seems to me that when a majority of people lived where they worked and were dependent on local resources for their crafts, whether it was leather for the shoes they made, wood for the furniture they made, wax for the candles, or wool for the fabric, such close bioregional dependency created boundaries to size. Cheap energy broke down those boundaries, and with it the village-scape model that had been normal for centuries. Ordinary industries that had been shackled to a village scale could suddenly grow unimpeded, whether it was leather tanning or furniture making.

These huge industrial factories could not be nestled into the village. In fact, the owners didn't want them nestled in villages. In fact, villagers didn't want them nestled in villages — how would you like to live next to a huge factory? These monstrous facilities were different from the former cobbler, spinner, and furniture maker.

These mega-industries actually became repugnant to neighbors, so much so that the businesses erected large security fences to keep out curious eyes that could testify about pollution or worker abuse. Whenever an economic sector cloisters itself behind opaqueness, it will begin taking environmental, social, and economic shortcuts. Integrity occurs when people can see what's going in at the front door and what's coming out the back door. Absent that accountability, you lose integrity.

Accountability is a direct result of transparency, and transparency is a direct result of neighbor-friendly scale that allows the business to be embedded in the community. The present economic apartheid expresses itself in many ways, one of which is strict zoning. As we created business districts, commercial districts, industrial districts, and residential districts, we kept parsing the restrictions, until today we even restrict people who can only afford a 1,200-square foot-house from living in the same area as people who can afford a 1,500-square-foot house.

Talk about snobbery. I actually like foreign countries where peasant shacks surround business district skyscrapers. I think it's healthy for these high-powered businesspeople to walk past shacks on their way to power brokering. Economic segregation protects the haves from seeing the needy, and prevents the needy from seeing possibilities.

Landscape requirements are another form of this apartheid. Many residential estate–type developments restrict farming and other noxious land uses. Farming suffered the same problem as untethered industry. Free to expand without local energy restraints, farms expanded to the point of nasty odors and water pollution. The bucolic farm became repugnant to the average person. A "not in my backyard" (NIMBY) mindset developed even against farms — and rightly so. Who wants to live next to a Tyson chicken house?

The farm industry fought back with "right to farm" laws that I refer to as "right to stink up the neighborhood" laws. As all of this progressed, paranoid people began demanding protection and enforced integrity through government regulation. Of course, that never works, because every time government injects itself in the marketplace, the biggest businesses have the wherewithal to curry favor with bureaucrats and politicians. What has happened, of course, is a regulatory climate that protects the huge opaque anti-human-scale businesses and bullies entrepreneurial innovators who would dare compete.

The reality is that bonanzas don't survive for very long, and that is what cheap energy is: a bonanza. I don't know how long it will last, but the way to bet is that we will return to a more normal energy cost sometime in the future. That's as close to a prophecy as I can handle. The whole point of this book is to show just how abnormal our last century has been. Any data that looks like a hockey stick when plotted on a graph will always crash. Always. Energy use certainly looks like one right now.

This abnormal cheap energy petroleum age may appear to be a bonanza, but in the long run it has shredded boundaries and proximities that defined economic and social normalcy for centuries. In the continuum of human history, this petroleum age is a mere blip. Cheap energy, on a timeline, is scarcely a speck on the chart. Yet we have the audacity, the irrationality, to plunge forward with building designs, suburban designs, transportation designs as if this cheap energy blip will last forever.

My friend Martin Payne, founder of Anvil Energy LLC, wrote me the following recently:

> I have been a student of oil supply since the mid-1980s. My father first introduced me to the works of King Hubbert in the 1970s, but I didn't pay much attention to it for many years. Sometime after 2000, Peak Oil really gripped me. I became fascinated by the magnitude of the problem, coupled with the fact that most folks had never heard of it. Further, of those who had heard of it, most were disbelievers. I tried hard to find a reason not to believe in it, but only became more convinced that it was real.
>
> In short...I believe Peak Oil is an "Industrial Revolution-sized" disruption. It's a planet-sized "fire on the mountain," or buffalo stampede. Many believe it will lead to total collapse, die-offs, etc. I choose to believe that we can avoid total collapse.

Payne believes we crossed the peak in 2008 and the result is being delayed due to the economic downturn. In one of his postings on the website Energy Bulletin, Payne adds the following:

> The reality is — although there is a long ways to go, there is also "a lot going on," much of it over the last five years. None of these steps, taken alone, will "save the world." Symbolically, however, they represent

changes in behavior and belief that if continued and extended, will have meaningful effects:

- Vegetable gardening — interest has blossomed in the last few years (just ask the folks in the garden department of Home Depot).
- Local food movement — it's on fire in various cities, all over the country. Farmers' Markets are popping up everywhere.
- Grassfed beef, pastured poultry, pork — healthier, less energy intensive, can provide a scalable starting place for new family farms.
- Backyard chicken movement — is growing everywhere, it seems; keeping chickens is "cool," now.
- Vehicle choices — in 2000, in Texas you would see Suburban after Suburban, truck after truck, even in the city. The vehicle population and preference is substantially different today.
- Reusable grocery bags — a small but important and symbolic step; much more of it is going on.
- Smaller, more efficient houses — witness the plethora of news coverage, books about smaller or "tiny" houses; the McMansion is no longer cool.
- Small energy production — in addition to the large commercial efforts, much tinkering is occurring with small wind, PV, woodgas, alcohol, algae, biodiesel, and more.

This looks like a pretty cool list. In fact, it looks a lot like America a century ago. And indeed, that's my whole point. Be ready for this as we return to normalcy.

Payne sent me the definitive work commissioned in 2005 by the Department of Energy, titled *Peaking of World Oil Production: Impacts, Mitigation, and Risk Management*, prepared by project leader Robert Hirsch. The DOE would not release the report initially. According to the report, two-thirds of the twenty million barrels of oil consumed in the United States every day are in the transportation sector. In the introduction, here is the first sentence: "Oil is the lifeblood of modern civilization."

I would like to rephrase that sentence to this: "Nothing about modern civilization is normal, ever, in human history, because it runs on oil." That puts it in perspective, doesn't it? Suburbs. Little League games requiring parents to travel two hours to watch the kiddos play. Pizza delivery. Jetting to the Bahamas. Jetting anywhere. Skyscrapers. Ignorance about the cost of energy.

Again, looking at this definitive report, in the period 1973 to 2003, which saw a 140 percent increase in gross domestic product, oil consumption in the industrial sector remained flat due to conservation technologies and high-tech efficiencies. "In sharp contrast to all other sectors, U.S. oil consumption for transportation purposes has increased steadily every year, rising from just over 17 quads in 1973 to 26 quads in 2003," the report says, adding that "67 percent of personal automobile travel and nearly 50 percent of airplane travel are [sic] discretionary." Which begs the question: What if we had as much excitement going on in our kitchens as we think we might find doing some discretionary traveling?

I'm not opposed to travel and I'm not a hermit, but do we really have to move around as much as we do? I think the reason we need to travel more is because we don't have anything exciting to do at home anymore. But if we're gardening, cooking, and cottage-industrying — home can be as exciting as any discretionary destination. We've divorced our own homes as the centerpiece of life, and that disunion manifests itself in running elsewhere looking for satisfaction. That takes a lot of energy. What can be more exciting than watching kitchen scraps turn into eggs via a couple of intermediary chickens?

Interestingly, the DOE report also notes that "on average, developing countries use more than twice as much oil to produce a unit of output as developed countries." In an uncommon show of humor in a government report, it says this: "What used to be termed the 'not-in-my-back-yard' (NIMBY) principle has evolved into the 'build-absolutely-nothing-any-where-near-anything' (BANANA) principle, which is increasingly being applied to facilities of any type, including low-income housing, cellular phone towers, prisons, sports stadiums, water treatment facilities, airports, hazardous waste facilities, and even new fire houses." Isn't it fascinating how closely this assessment mirrors my analysis of how cheap energy created this economic apartheid?

As I see it, cheap energy enabled people to separate. It enabled communities to fragment. It eliminated transparency in business. And it created universal snobbery. Heretofore, snobbery was limited to the extremely wealthy. They were the only ones who could afford it. Now everyone can be a snob.

How else do you explain the story a lady told me when I spoke recently in Texas? As she told it, she was fined for a landscape violation because she had a tomato plant in her flowerbed. A neighbor turned her in for farming, and the judge agreed. "Roses and nasturtiums only, ma'am. On second thought, no nasturtiums. They're edible. We wouldn't want anything edible around here."

How could anyone think a tomato plant in someone's backyard is an eyesore? Only someone who hasn't thought about energy for a long time. The snooty neighbor probably thinks taxes should increase, too. All to help the disadvantaged, of course. What if the gardening neighbor is trying to save a couple of bucks by growing some of her own food? What if she's trying to reduce food-miles on her plate? I wonder if the snob ever thought about that? Maybe she just lost her job and is trying to grow something to eat.

For all the snobs out there, let me present several shifts that I think would occur if we returned to a more normal environment.

1. Living where you work. Whether this be telecommuting, which is certainly a burgeoning trend, or locating businesses in residences, this is the starting point for a more normal culture. Licensing agencies and zoning departments need to encourage amalgamated living/business arrangements because this consolidation is one of the first steps toward recreating the human-scaled entrepreneurship that can be embedded in a community within walking distance.

One person starts baking cookies; another one begins a wedding cake business; another a fabric shop; another an appliance repair shop. Before you know it, you have what looks like Williamsburg in 1750. Most of the things in your life, most of the skills necessary to augment your lifestyle, would be located nearby. Zoning snobbery is what is keeping this from happening — and cheap energy.

2. Passive solar gain on all houses. Solariums are not expensive. As far as I'm concerned, building anything today without enough of a solarium on the sunny side to heat the building is immoral. With as much knowledge as we have now about energy costs and depletion, I can't believe that anyone, anyone, anyone could build a house today and not put a solarium on the sunny side. It's cheap to do and can literally eliminate winter energy needs.

Coupled with that is the shade structure on the north side to pull air through the house. I'm a fan of underground and earth-sheltered houses. That keeps things warm in the winter and cool in the summer, without any supplemental energy, just by using constant earth temperature. We cannot afford to run air conditioners.

3. In-home entertainment and recreation. Playing board games, backyard games like badminton, and home-run derby can provide all the entertainment-recreation opportunities you need. I can't think of any reason to visit theme parks or resorts as a normal pastime. Enjoy your family and nearby friends. Play music.

Write books. Read books. Start a community discussion group. Have a spelling bee, a community variety show, an art contest. Our compartmentalized world is so segregated that we've come to think that entertainment can only come from industrial entertainers. My family has never had a TV in our house and still don't. About the only TV I see now is when I travel and turn it on in a hotel room. Localize your entertainment, leave the car parked and the jet on the runway.

4. Edible landscaping. Why have a monstrous lawn? I can't believe the number of people who call themselves environmentalists, join the Nature Conservancy, and then drive a half-ton mowing machine over an acre of lawn every week at their residential estate. Come on, folks, get real. Plant a garden; plant some fruit trees; plant some bramble fruits like thornless blackberries.

Reduce your food-miles by growing some pastured chickens and rabbits. Cook the food you grow and quit patronizing that energy-hogging industrial food system where every morsel travels fifteen hundred miles. Not only is that abnormal, it's borderline immoral when energy is as precious as it is.

With that said, one of the best uses for oil is plastic to cover tall tunnels and greenhouses. Put a couple of them in your yard, or better yet, affix one to the sunny side of your house. Grow lettuce in the winter and heat your house. If we'd quit squandering our oil on industrial food and discretionary transportation, there would be more left to make the plastic to grow our food in our own yard all year long.

This can be as classy as glass with redwood framing (you can get a kit) or as simple as some cattle panels (sixteen-foot-by-four-foot welded wire rectangles) bent from the ground to about eight feet high on the edge of the house and covered in plastic. Might not look perfect, but how does a zero heating bill sound? Even if you couldn't grow vegetables in it year-round, these things should be installed for the energy-saving potential. Again, as a culture, think of all the high-tech energy programs we're throwing billions into, but nobody is saying, "Just attach a solarium to the sunny side of your house." Simple, yet so profound. Just do it. And you don't have to cotton to every building inspector either. If you think the one your neighbor installs is unsightly, shut your mouth and be grateful he's enabling you to drive another day.

5. Abolish the cheap energy policy by getting the government out of the business. We shouldn't be committing billions of dollars in military action to ensure a cheap supply of oil. Oil companies should pay all costs; no sweetheart deals, concessionary tax provisions, or government help cleaning up oopses.

The day America walks away from a cheap energy policy will be the day innovation explodes. My automobile mechanic says fifty-mile-per-gallon carburetors existed in the late 1960s but never saw the light of day because big corporations bought out the fledgling enterprises and shut them down. I've read about these high ratings for a long time. For anyone to purposefully keep these innovations sequestered is — dare I say it? — evil. It's morally reprehensible.

Along with this, I'd suggest eliminating the gas tax and instituting a mileage tax. One of the reasons the gasoline tax is not keeping up with highway infrastructure needs is because higher-mileage vehicles occupy the same square footage of road, but use far less fuel per square foot of road coverage. When the gas tax was originally envisioned, nobody was thinking about higher-mileage cars and expensive fuel. The cost of transportation is the square footage of road surface occupied by vehicles. As fuel efficiency accelerates, the gas tax will become more obsolete. A Prius occupies the same road surface as a Suburban. A mileage tax would be a much fairer means of financing transportation infrastructure. To me this is such a simple concept, it's a no-brainer. And yet if you suggest it at a highway department public hearing, they'll practically rule you out of order. Taxing the square footage of road surface occupied by your vehicle, to me, is the only commonsense way to fairly tax the use of the infrastructure. Why is this such a hard concept?

6. Abolish the Bureau of Alcohol, Tobacco, and Firearms. Stay with me on this. The Model T Ford could run on either alcohol or gasoline — it was a hybrid vehicle. Alcohol was everywhere on the American landscape, from apple brandy to corn squeezin's, and it served several purposes. It was an antiseptic, an anesthetic, and a preservative.

Because alcohol was ubiquitous at the time, Henry Ford envisioned his automobile running on community resources. The country didn't have filling stations at the time. The only way to gain wide acceptance was with an alcohol-burning vehicle. He installed a dashboard switch to change carburetion and a switch on the engine to change the spark calibration.

A little cultural disturbance upset that energy independence. It was called the Woman's Christian Temperance Union (WCTU), which culminated in Prohibition. I've read that John D. Rockefeller, a teetotaler Presbyterian who of course was the first oil baron, desperately wanted that alcohol button removed from the Model T. And so he helped finance the WCTU, increase its political clout, and finally won the day with Prohibition. I don't know if that's actually what happened — makes a great story, though.

At any rate, although Prohibition lasted for only a decade, that was long enough to eliminate that pesky alcohol button on the Model T because it destroyed community-based energy production in the United States. Today, thousands of backyard alternative energy enthusiasts are making alcohol and biodiesel but are held back by these ridiculous alcohol regulations.

I could add hemp to this. Hemp was a major farm commodity in those days, providing much-needed fiber for rope and other products. Henry Ford made a car body out of hemp. The material was stronger, lighter, and more durable than sheet metal. Today's prohibition on hemp growing in the United States keeps such innovative solar-driven solutions away from the imaginations of innovators. Criminalizing hemp in the name of drug wars is an incredibly anti-environmental policy.

The answer to energy is not taxpayer-subsidized mega-alcohol facilities or government-sponsored wind turbines. Let energy costs run to wherever they need to like any other business and let private entrepreneurs enter the marketplace. Big anything is still big anything. Industrial alcohol plants will enslave the culture into using them whether we need them or not. Capital-intensive, single-use infrastructure costs so much money and emotion to build that it enslaves the culture economically and emotionally for the foreseeable future. Whether we need the energy or not; whether it's appropriate or not; whether it destroys the surrounding land with monocrop corn or not — nothing will stop us from putting corn through that megalithic plant because, by gum, we built it and we're going to use it.

I suggest that we allow hundreds of thousands of innovators to bring their skill and passion to the marketplace. For me, it's wood-fired steam. I'll plug into the grid and run it a few days a month. A neighbor with a fast-flowing, fast-falling stream can put in a pelton wheel microturbo generator and plug it into the grid. Another neighbor who grows pigs can make corn alcohol and feed the distillers' grains to the pigs. They'll do great on that by-product. Somebody else with a windy hill puts in a windmill and hooks that into the grid. The point is that between the bunch of us, the community gets its power from an embedded, transparent, participatory source.

Someone may ask, "But what about big cities?" First of all, if everyone who did not live in big cities would do as I suggest above, more energy would be left over for cities. Second, in the big scheme of things suburbs have a larger energy footprint per citizen than cities, and many people in the suburbs could do many of the things I've discussed in this chapter — at least put on a solarium and plant a garden. Suburbanites are the people with land for whom edible landscaping, kitchen chickens, and solariums are really doable. Again, just because everyone can't do everything doesn't mean someone shouldn't do something.

Third, perhaps some cities are too big. People who decry big business, as if bigness is wrong, should apply the same thinking to their big-city living. Maybe that's wrong, or maybe a big city would be better if it were a little smaller. This is a discussion that's almost taboo in urban sectors, but I'm not afraid to at least mention it. The amenities and vibrancy of a 50,000-person city are not much different than those of a

500,000-person city. I would argue that perhaps one is more ecologically livable. People who love small farms and want to protect small
business, who think small is beautiful, should realize that in order to be
consistent, perhaps such thinking should apply to cities.

Fourth, most cities have a tremendous amount of space to do things.
I've already discussed that in this book. Farming the edges, the rooftops
is doable. Let's take an extreme example: New York or Los Angeles. I
don't have the figures in front of me, but what a difference it would
make if in those cities household chickens ate every single scrap of
decomposable kitchen waste so that it did not go down the garbage disposal into the sewage system or out into the garbage to be picked up by
sanitation crews. That one thing would eliminate truckloads of eggs
transported into and around the city and eliminate tons and tons and
tons — get the picture? — of garbage to be collected, toted, transported,
and either composted or landfilled. All that stuff takes energy to move
and handle.

What if everyone in the city ate properly and exercised enough not to
be fat? Today our newspaper carried a story about how municipal buses
are looking at reducing their carrying capacity because people weigh so
much more that they are overloading the buses. When our buses can
only carry 80 percent of the people they've been carrying, that's energy.

I recently spoke at a sustainable living symposium held by our local
community college and one of the other speakers was a professor who
had recently returned from a trip to China. He showed a picture of a
250,000-person city recently built in China. The way he told the story,
they went out into a rural area and just built this city — I guess you can
do that if you're a communist. Anyway, the stipulation was that the city
could not decrease the crop production on that footprint.

It was an amazing aerial photograph. The buildings were all about
five stories high and you could barely make out some of the upper-floor
windows through the foliage. All the roofs were flat and growing luxuri-
ant plants. Vines even hung down over the edges and between the
buildings. The living roofs sponged up rainfall, which reduced or eliminated storm sewers. It takes energy to build storm sewers and drainage
systems. The foliage kept the buildings cool in the summer, eliminating air-conditioning. That's energy. The crops fed the people, eliminating hundreds of trucks that had to enter the city bringing food. Dear

folks, we can do this. It's not high-tech; it's high normal with modern adaptations.

Okay, so the food is not dangling in the top of a smoky Native American Powhatan village; it's up on the roof of a five-story apartment complex. Do you see the normalcy with modern adaptation? I submit that this is the future, and a far more doable future than gene splicing and industrial-sized midwestern corn alcohol plants.

For example, I'm amazed that confinement dairy operations that received government money twenty years ago to put in manure lagoons received conservation awards. Today, these same outfits receive government money to cover those lagoons with bladders to collect the methane and receive awards for suddenly joining green energy. That's not green energy. Green energy finances itself and grows out of the ground, from the bottom up, not from the top down. A confinement animal facility is an anti-ecological, anti-animal, energy-guzzling facility from the get-go.

Putting a methane bladder over an improper manure handling system in order to capture the gas to run the myriad inappropriate energy-consumptive motors in such a facility and then calling that green thinking is simply madness. Green thinking is eliminating the confinement facility to begin with, eliminating the motors once and for all, turning the cows out onto pasture, using a simple composting system, and eliminating the need for 90 percent of the energy in the first place. That's green thinking.

The energy answers are not going to come from others. The solution that resounds with normalcy is one that involves each of us, doing something. The cumulative effect of those thousands of small actions is huge. The answer to energy is not some magic high-tech, big-industry bullet. It may be, but that's not the way to bet. It's participatory energy connectedness that occupies a significant amount of our time and capital, like it has for millennia until this petroleum blip. This cheap energy anomaly, folks, just ain't normal.

What can we do, individually, to ease our energy use?

1. Grow as much of your own food as you can.
2. Patronize your home and community for entertainment and recreation.

3. Patronize cottage industries located within walking distance.
4. If you're building a house, incorporate the ideas in this chapter.
5. If you're a building inspector, kick, scream, and demand that building codes accommodate innovative techniques more easily.

Roofless Underground
Dream Houses

For the first time in human civilization, you can flip on a switch or clench a nozzle to get energy from who knows where, turn on a faucet and get water from who knows where, send the sewage out a pipe that goes to who knows where, and build a house from materials that came from who knows where. Folks, this ain't normal.

One of the reasons religion, food, and architecture define culture is because all of this was locally based. The logistical ability to import materials from afar didn't exist for common substances. As a result, bioregional differentiation rather than homogenization was both pronounced and normal.

Until recently, construction materials were locally sourced. They couldn't be hauled from Timbuktu. In a nomadic culture with few trees, like Mongolia, yurts were the domicile of choice. The people had yak skins and they needed something portable to move around with their herds. Bedouins in the Middle East had similar needs and dwelt in tents.

Carved rocks became the material of choice for the upscale in Europe, while wattle and daub between post-and-beam skeletons sufficed for more common folks. On the largely treeless American plains, the soddy functioned as a starter home, while in the Southwest adobe made sense, since good red clay was everywhere. The log cabin signified the ability of a family to pull themselves up by their bootstraps. In eastern America, with abundant wood, it made sense to build from things available a few feet away.

I've always been enamored of the Native American houses in the mid-Atlantic region, built from bent-over saplings, cordage, animal skins, and branches. They lasted about fifteen years and then com-posted. That's about the length of specific housing requirements. A couple gets married and only needs a tiny house. Kids come along and they need a bigger house. Kids move out and they need a smaller house. Those time frames are about ten to fifteen years. Seems like a pretty good idea to have compostable houses. They're cheap and easy to build, and the whole thing returns to the earth. Native natural resources, therefore, defined local building materials and design, and birthed local economies. Local construction sourcing created value for the local resources. You could say the homes and buildings grew out of the earth, almost an organic expression of available materials.

Intimate knowledge of available building materials and design fea-tures that fit those materials were fairly universal until very recently. In my father's World War II generation, every man knew how to make at least a rudimentary shelter. Or at least how to hammer a nail. In our internship program at our farm, I am amazed at how many twenty-year-old males do not know how to hammer a nail.

I fear that manliness is being eroded. When boys know how to play video games but not how to drive a nail, where does masculine self-esteem go? Confidence to tackle historically normal activities doesn't even exist. I'm certainly not suggesting that a woman can't hammer a nail — our female interns hammer right along with the guys — but something about a man coming to adulthood unable to hammer a nail seems downright unnatural.

Scavenging materials and building shelter — having an intimate knowledge of what's available — that is primal masculine responsibility. The skill to cut, shape, and attach scavenged materials into at least a minimal structure has been part and parcel of growing up since time immemorial. When we remove ourselves from this process, we lack appreciation for how the process fits with the landscape. Does the pro-cess support our community or someone else's? Does the process make ecological sense? Is the process appropriate?

As I travel the country and see countless complicated McMansions being built on five-acre estates on parceled prime farmland, it begs the question on several fronts. First, who needs a house that big? Many of these are being built by midlife couples who have finally put together enough money for their dream home. Just so we have full transparency here, let me share with you my dream home idea.

First, it would be earth-sheltered. Why does anyone build above ground in climates that have snow? At least build into a hillside with the open side facing the sun. This is naturally cool in summer and warm in winter. If you only have to heat the house from earth-constant 50–55 degrees in the winter, that takes much less energy than heating it from single-digit temperatures. In a hot climate, earth sheltering provides natural cooling, reducing air-conditioner requirements. In either case, exterior temperature has to go through both earth and wall, which is difficult. In our old farmhouse, when the winter winds blow, the window drapes stir on the billows of seepage. For insulation, summer cool, and winter warmth, nestling the house into the earth yields lots of benefits.

Second, since one of the biggest costs of a house is the roof, I'd dispense with that and just build a hoophouse as the roof. Hoophouses probably qualify as the single most important modern eco-techno architectural design breakthrough. Using a simple bent pipe as an arch, called a hoop, these simple rounded structures covered in plastic are cheap and quick to build. The plastic acts like poor-boy glass, allowing ultraviolet solar rays in and trapping the heat inside. Essentially, the hoophouse is a series of these arches, set about six feet apart to look like a rib cage. The covering is the skin. If they have no supplemental heat they are often called tall tunnels. If they have supplemental heat, they are called greenhouses.

On our farm, we currently have four hoophouses for pigs, chickens, and rabbits to live in during the winter. The engineering and cost are such that now huge hoop structures can be purchased, covered with UV-stabilized poly material, and used for storing hay, machinery, grain — anything. Because they don't entail much mass (weight) they are extremely simple and cheap. All the material for a 3,000-square-foot structure could fit inside a pickup truck bed. I'm a fan of hoophouses, in all their stripes. The roof of my dream house, then, would be a simple hoophouse with plastic covering. The covering is cheap enough that when it falls apart in a decade, you just buy a new one. In that amount of time, perhaps it won't be made out of petroleum plastic. Maybe it will be made out of buffalo hides again. Who knows?

Obviously I need a ceiling separating the earth-sheltered living quarters from the hoophouse roof. The ceiling would serve two functions: ceiling on the living area and floor to the hoophouse. This ceiling would have a couple of air holes and maybe small squirrel-cage fans in them to help move air above and below. In the winter, during the day when the sun shines and warms up the hoophouse, a fan would suck that warm air down into the living quarters for heat. At night, the warm living area would be a heat sink, slowly giving off warmth that would naturally rise back through the holes into the hoophouse at night.

Because the earth-bermed house is built into a hill, it has two ground-floor entrances: one into the living quarters and the other one into the second-story hoophouse.

The south-facing living quarters (in the Southern Hemisphere, you'd want to turn all this around and face it north) would be a glass wall for solar gain. The toilet would flush into a methane digester. Digested nutrient-dense effluent would drain out to the yard to keep trees and flowers watered. The methane would come off the digester in an air hose into a barrel half full of water with an inverted garbage can inside that could move up and down like a sleeve to trap the methane as it bubbled into the bottom of the barrel. A simple brick or rock on top of the garbage can sleeve would provide the pressure to send the methane over to the kitchen range.

I saw this demonstrated beautifully in Perryville, Arkansas, twenty years ago at the Heifer Project International Guatemala house project. Heifer Project is an international agricultural development and food sustainability nonprofit that I have had the distinct privilege to work with over the years. The United Nations could learn a lot from these folks. Simple, regenerative, locally appropriate systems always work better than high-tech bureaucratic know-it-all Western dumping. Anyway, they had the system I've described above and it worked beautifully. If I have one skill, it's the ability to see a good idea and then steal it.

Every human's daily excrement can produce enough methane to cook all of their own food. Behind the kitchen, into the hill behind the house, would be the pantry and root cellar, as well as a special room for the refrigerator. This cool area would greatly reduce refrigerator energy because the unit would not have to cool down from living-quarter ambient temperature. It would only need to cool from earth temperature — about a dozen degrees instead of 30.

Upstairs in the hoophouse, of course, I'd have chickens to eat kitchen scraps and rabbits to eat the lush vegetation grown by the digester efflu-ent in the yard. Fresh cool-hardy vegetables could be grown year-round, and of course daytime solar heat would keep the downstairs living quar-ters warm. At night, natural rising heat from masonry mass downstairs would keep the plants from freezing upstairs.

A solar water heater in the hoophouse would gravity feed down-stairs to run showers and hot water faucets. A clothesline in the hoop-house would offer plenty of space for a clothesline (solar clothes dryer) even in the winter. Most Americans today don't know the distinct finger-numbing joy of hanging clothes on a line when temperatures are below zero. They freeze before they dry, hanging there stiff as a board. The clothesline is still one of the most ecological appliances that exists.

I was in Comox, British Columbia, recently doing a seminar for a natural foods initiative. It was a great group of people and the area had thriving farmers' markets. But it was illegal to have a clothesline in the whole city. Why? Because they are unsightly and make the community look impoverished. This kind of disconnect, unfortunately, is more common than not. People seem to understand the importance of nor-malcy in one area, but then have no clue in others.

Gray water would irrigate vegetables and fruit. A gutter along the edge of the hoophouse would catch all the rain runoff and send it into a cistern. Self-contained water, self-contained heat and cooking, supple-mented with a small woodstove as necessary, and self-contained cool-ing through earth berming make this house nest into the landscape using the best modern technology with the greatest resource leverage. A solar array or windmill obviously could supply electricity.

That's my dream house. I don't understand the fascination with expensive, fancy corners and rooflines, multijointed dormers, and the like. Many of these modern McMansions look like somebody is playing a Let's-Stump-the-Carpenter game. Don't we really have better things to spend money on than trying to have a more crazy-angled exterior than the neighbor? Our nation's luxury is financing ostentatious structures that stick out of the landscape like architectural cacophony. Why not see how blended, how camouflaged human buildings can be?

Most of these McMansions are multiroom affairs built within a couple years of the children leaving home. They are energy-guzzling, lumber-greedy stick houses that require massive upkeep not only on the outside, but also on the inside. Who wants to grow old in a massive castle, by themselves?

I love the tiny house concept. This fairly broad architectural genre includes both self-contained homes that are simply tiny and modulars that hook together. A core self-contained house, with all the necessities for living crammed into a hundred-square-foot structure, can be a starter unit. Then if marriage or kids necessitate more room, another unit can be attached to the initial one. Essentially, a bedroom unit, living room unit, and kitchen unit can be hooked together as needed. In one concept, as the first child leaves to go on her own, her bedroom is detached and becomes her core starter unit.

Some people put them on a chassis, like a mobile home, except they look more like a regular house or cottage. Mixing and matching rooms like a glorified puzzle is a great idea. As the family grows, add another compartment. As the family contracts, sell off the compartments to a younger expanding family. That makes a lot of sense. Who wants to enslave themselves to a monstrosity for the rest of their lives?

In our county, of the five hundred to eight hundred homes being built every year, not more than five use any local lumber. It's imported from Canada, the Pacific Northwest, or foreign countries. Meanwhile, nonindustrial private forestland in our own county is terribly mishandled because it carries no value. If these homes being built used local lumber, it would inject millions of dollars into the local forestal economy and provide an incentive to better steward these woodlands.

Stewardship derives from value. The reason we have jewelry boxes is because diamonds are expensive. The value drives the care. The same is true with natural resources. We can wring our hands and ask for legislative relief all we want, but in the end, what really drives stewardship is value. Our forests will be managed in direct proportion to economic incentives that justify better management. Pruning, thinning, release

cuts, salvaging diseased trees — these are all part of a forest management plan that must pay for itself.

Getting building crews to use local lumber is a lot like trying to get
local eggs into Kroger or Wal-Mart. The fraternal web that protects the
insiders from upstart competition is quite impregnable. And what really
makes it difficult are the building inspectors who want people to use
graded lumber, who define what kind of construction will be allowed.
I guarantee you that my dream house would never pass the building code.

When our son Daniel began building his house on the farm, we cut
the trees, milled the logs on our bandsaw mill, dried them in our hoophouse when the chickens went out to pasture, and did the construction
ourselves. Originally planning to go with a small house concept, we
found it was illegal to build a house of less than nine hundred square
feet. Why? By what authority can anybody tell me what kind of house
I have to live in?

The house police said it was to protect a future buyer in case the
house was ever sold. Again I ask, by what authority? If I want to build a
house that nobody will ever buy, isn't that my prerogative? Since when
does a government bureaucrat have the right to tell me what I can and
cannot live in? If I want to live in a yurt of yak skins, what's wrong with
that? If I want to build and live in a house that nobody would buy, isn't
that my problem?

If I want to live in a house that's different than standard construction, why shouldn't I have a right to innovate? Believe me, buildings
constructed long before building codes will far and away outlast the
buildings built since the codes went into effect. Our house was built in
1750. I'm so glad some bureaucrat checked to make sure these timbers
were joined correctly. People have been living in houses for thousands
of years before any inspectors came around. This bureaucratic penetration into the marketplace creates a political market for the regulated
entities to wine, dine, and schmooze the government oversight officials
in order to curry favor. Since the biggest private industries existing at
the time of regulation have the greatest ability to wine and dine, those
businesses win the special concessions game to the detriment of smaller
and more innovative sectors that have not yet become the status quo.

I was discussing this with a visitor here at the farm recently and he
said, "I wouldn't walk into a structure that didn't have a building

permit. An uninspected building is unsafe." We had just walked through our house, built around 1750. At the moment, we were standing in our sales building that our church group helped us build twenty years ago, without any plans, no blueprints, and no inspectors. Does anyone really believe buildings collapsed more throughout history before inspection bureaucracies?

How did people survive before the building inspection department? Could it be that builders were responsible for their buildings, and their pride kept them true to engineering necessities? Could that possibly be? How do we encourage personal responsibility in craftsmanship? I submit that we encourage personal responsibility like we encourage it in our children. If my child's homework becomes somebody else's grade, my child won't put the effort into it that she will if the grade is her responsibility. If a building collapses and a builder can say, "It's the inspector's fault because he didn't tell me," we won't encourage personal responsibility. Creating a climate of performance excellence requires personal responsibility.

The fewer skirts there are to hide behind, the more personal responsibility we engender. Today, if a house has a problem, and things eventually wind up in litigation, more often than not it comes down to the judgment call of the inspector rather than the builder. "He saw it. He signed off on it. Not my fault," the builder says. As soon as we remove that protective cloak, builders will become more careful.

How vocationally secure would a negligent or poor-quality builder be if he and only he had to shoulder the responsibility for construction problems? Word would spread like wildfire and he'd be out of business. That's called the power of the marketplace, and it has guided artisanship's integrity for centuries. And that is normal. This bureaucratic oversight has done more to standardize construction and stigmatize innovation than any other single factor. Why does modern construction look similar everywhere? Because the building police all went to the same boot camp and read the same code book. Try something innovative and they shut down the project.

The building police have grown up alongside the lack of understanding and involvement that people have with the construction of their homes. Again, the enigma breeds distrust, and distrust drives government manipulation. When building a home, do you think about where the lumber comes from? Or did you think it just grew down at Lowe's or Home Depot? I have news for you: That lumber doesn't grow there any more than eggs grow in a supermarket.

The eggs and lumber come from somewhere. Where is that somewhere? What kind of values govern that somewhere? What kind of local economy, or local ecology, is that somewhere creating? Most forests in the United States are in dire need of upgrading through strategic harvesting. Forests are living organisms. They grow, age, then die.

The Native Americans kept the cycle vibrant by massive burning. Today, we have chainsaws and tremendous silvicultural knowledge. We can take core samples to determine vigor, health, and age. We can use small pieces in plywood and OSB board, glued together. We can ease into an area on rubber tires and surgically remove individual trees without damaging the residual stand. Unfortunately, this is not as common as it could be, but where it's practiced, it reflects a value system that honors the surroundings.

Using horses to log, to minimize impact, is enjoying a bit of rejuvenation in the logging industry. This is an attempt to match the machinery and technique to the place.

Our county has designated wilderness areas that are turning into forestal nursing homes. The carbon these dying, decaying forests are pumping back into the atmosphere is unprecedented. They should be harvested to restart the carbon sequestration cycle. The oak forests of the Appalachian region are dying due to lack of disturbance — fire and buffalo. By running pigs through them to create periodic disturbance and strategic harvesting, we can return these forests to their primal status. Locking them up in no-burn, no-cut parcels is not normal, and it destroys their health. Opening them up enables the trees to fully reach their genetic potential.

In his comprehensive book *Fire in America: A Cultural History of Wildland and Rural Fire*, Stephen J. Pyne notes: "It may be said that the general consequence of the Indian occupation of the New World was to replace forested land with grassland or savannah, or where the forest persisted, to open it up and free it from underbrush." The thick forests encountered by European settlers were limited to marshes and other wetlands, where burning was more difficult. The great and important point Pyne makes is that the magnificent forests of American legend sprang up with the demise of the Native American. Said another way, the Europeans brought the forests; they were not here prior to European settlement.

To be sure, plenty of large trees existed, but they were scattered across the landscape as part of a silvo-pasture. Thick forests developed only after the collapse of the Native American populations. While it may seem like environmentalist heresy to call current thick forests abnormal, the reality is that rich North American soils developed during centuries of widely spaced trees surrounded by grasses.

In his wonderful book about preindustrial food systems, *The Moving Feast*, Allan Nation describes this in more detail:

> The net effect of all this burning over thousands of years by the Indians was to turn the landscape from a continuous forest into an open, grassy savannah. Only the fire-resistant oak and pine survived in great numbers on the region's uplands. The fire-resistant swamps were said to resemble California redwood forests where huge cypress and gum trees soared some 120 feet into the air. Many early explorers used the term 'Cathedral-like' to describe the effect of these mature trees. Some revisionist historians are now saying that the upland eastern forest followed European civilization rather than preceded it because most Europeans stopped the Indians' fire regime.

Strategically grooming local forests to acquire building materials is a key component of returning America's cathedral-like forests to their pre-colonial splendor. Rather than importing wood from offshore, we should be massaging our own community forests with cutting and disturbance (ideally with ranging hogs) to heal and rejuvenate the precious forestal resource. Conspicuous dead, downed, and dying trees, stunted growth, many crooked stems — all these characteristics indicate a forest in decline.

Here in the Shenandoah Valley, while our own forests plead for attention, we're using imported monoplantation poor-quality softwood to build McMansions rather than our own regenerative resource. We're exporting those dollars to faraway places while our own local woodlots die for want of attention. The forest is ultimately one of the best renewable resources. Realizing that each of us can connect to it with our construction projects should drive us to consider its health and benefits.

Our cavalier attitude toward getting building material from somewhere else begs the question: Why not here? Why not indeed? Here are some ideas that would help us build responsibly, that would link accountability between our desire for ecological soundness and the board we're about to nail. Allow me to build any house I want to, constructed out of anything. It's my house and I'm going to live in it. If I want it to look weird, that's none of your business. This would encourage local building material scavenging and pump much-needed money into the local forestal economy.

1. Allow ungraded lumber to be used in construction. If the homebuilder says it's okay, then it's okay. If he wants to hire a grader to come and certify it, that's fine. But it's up to the homebuilder's discretion. Studs do not need to be dressed down. They can be full-cut and rough-cut. More wood sequesters more carbon.
2. Encourage hogs running in forests. Using electric fencing, this can be done easily and actually stimulates the trees to grow better.
3. Release to strategic silvicultural management public areas currently locked up and unhealthy due to blanket no-cut policies.
4. Demand local lumber in your construction projects. This is as important as buying local food.

Grasping for Water

If we made a list of resources Americans take for granted, the top spot would go to water. Water is so essential for life that throughout history its availability dominated decision-making and community planning. Its acquisition required a heavy investment.

When was the last time you looked at the water flowing out of the kitchen tap and contemplated its presence, in your house, at the whim of your fingers? That water condensed somewhere around little particles in the atmosphere and formed mist that gradually increased to the point of forming a cloud. When the particles got big and plump, they obeyed gravity and began to fall.

In a perfect world, those particles strike thick vegetation and not the earth directly. The vegetation breaks up the drops into a fine mist again, which trickles down stems and gently embraces the soil. After filling pores between soil crumbs, the water percolates into the subsoil and gradually fills aquifers and underground cracks and crevices. Seeping downhill, this base flow maintains springs, which start streams that gradually morph into rivers.

The water falling from the kitchen faucet has migrated there from real droplets from a real rain event, through someone's permeable and hopefully vegetated ground cover, and eventually made it to your sink.

Think about that journey. That circuitous path is the sum and substance of your ecology. If you do not have that water for a day, you could die. We are utterly and totally dependent on that condensation up in the atmosphere, that cloud fog formation, that droplet falling, and eventually the moisture percolating through the soil and maintaining the water cycle.

In our day, the most basic necessities to maintain life receive scarcely a thought. Water, food, shelter, energy, clothing — as a culture, we don't give these any thought. Somebody else takes care of all that. Just let me go shopping, or watch my wall-sized flat-screen TV. Our visceral relationship with life's fundamentals has been severed, and the result is an arrogance, a cavalier attitude toward the foundations of life.

Imagine how most people throughout human history have dealt with water. Indigenous peoples cultivated almost a spiritual ability to locate water. They weren't driving cars between filling stations with drinking fountains. They didn't even have a thermos to fill. This is of course why all civilizations have sprung up near water. Las Vegas would not have existed a couple of centuries ago.

Throughout history, water availability was a limiting factor in the development of a community. Not just total water availability, but conductivity as well. The Roman aqueducts, of course, illustrated early attempts to engineer a way to move water from one spot to another. But these took massive investments of labor and materials.

In the American experience, many frontier homes and certainly forts were built over or around a spring in order to have a steady source of water. Potable water has been far more valuable than gold throughout human history. The notion that we can turn on a tap and effortlessly receive potable water would be considered magical, even fantastical, for most of our predecessors. They could not have conceived of such a thing.

In earlier times, even if you located your domicile next to a spring or stream, or dug a well, you had to carry that water to the house. Indoor plumbing is a fairly recent invention. Several years ago we were digging around a spring on our farm, trying to develop it a little better, and uncovered about twenty feet of old wooden piping. Drilled with an auger, this section probably dated to the early 1800s. Our house was built around 1750.

Imagine drilling a hole through the center of a straight six-inch log, perhaps twelve feet long. I've seen these long augers in museums, but what I can't imagine is the skill and patience it took to drill that hole straight enough that even halfway through — six feet — the auger would not come out the side of the wood. To line it up that straight, within an inch of tolerance over the course of six feet, is completely beyond my imagination.

The sheer craftsmanship and time it would take to slowly drill out pipe from straight logs…inconceivable to me. Water was so precious that people committed large parts of their lives to figuring out how to capture it and move it to places where it would be more useful. Imagine lying in your log cabin with your beloved, talking in hushed tones about how to get the water from that spring a hundred yards away closer to the house so you wouldn't have to trudge back and forth carrying heavy wooden buckets of water. Goodness, no wonder people only took a bath once a winter.

Thomas Jefferson loved cisterns, and he designed his Monticello to collect as much water in underground storage pits as possible. He even guttered raised walkways to increase water collection for his cisterns. Throughout history, cisterns have been an integral part of water accumulation and storage. In our area here in the Shenandoah Valley, every old barn has a cistern on one corner. The roof gutters all flow to a cistern. At my father-in-law's farm, the cistern holds about 20,000 gallons of water. It's round, about ten feet in diameter, dug out by hand and lined with brick and mortar, and extends twenty feet into the ground. Just imagine the investment in these cisterns. They were massive undertakings, occupying days and weeks of hand digging.

The biggest digging job I ever did was during summer break from college. During college, I spent my summers here on the farm where I most loved to be. June was haymaking month. July was devoted to one big project. Then in August I cut the firewood to heat the house for the winter — and in our old leaky farmhouse, that's a pile of wood. For those of you who know wood, we needed about twenty cords a winter (a cord is a tightly stacked pile four feet by four feet by eight feet). Dad would split it as he burned it, but I cut it and hauled it to a bay in the shed. I'll never forget coming home one Christmas and seeing the sledgehammer he used to pound wedges into the big pieces for splitting. We'd gotten into some willow and sycamore, both of which have a corkscrew type of grain and are therefore incredibly hard to split, even though the wood itself is light in weight. The sledgehammer head was a mushroom, literally peened over with all the pounding on those blocks of wood. My admiration grew.

For most of human history, people have toted water, dug cisterns, bored wooden water conduits. They have invested, viscerally and personally, in their own water issues. They didn't have a phone to call the utility company. They had to get down and wet with water. They had to understand access, gravity — since they didn't have pumps — and domicile location relative to available water.

When you have to carry all your water, it becomes precious. You don't waste it. You shepherd it and reuse it. Hence the biblical reference to vessels unto honor and vessels unto dishonor. Water used to wash dishes, for example, was put into a vessel unto dishonor — nonpotable. This used water tended to be carefully directed to vegetables and other plants adjacent to the house. Even bath water was carefully saved for reuse.

The greatest insult to water in modern days, of course, is using potable water to flush toilets. This reprehensible squandering of water could never have occurred before modern times. This luxury of unlimited potable water is already coming to a screeching halt. In 2009 when Atlanta's reservoir fell to a capacity of fewer than thirty days, the Georgia governor held a prayer vigil on the Capitol steps to implore the Almighty for a hydration reprieve.

Meanwhile, Georgia was fighting Tennessee to get a bend of the Tennessee River close enough to the Georgia line to stick a pipe into it and suck out water. Georgia battled with Alabama for water, but Alabama refused. Many books are being written prophesying future water wars that will eclipse the oil wars and the salt wars. I spoke at a xeriscaping conference in Arizona last year and heard a lecture about water use around Las Vegas.

In that desert location, where water is more precious than elsewhere, the conflict between developers and farmers is most acute. In order to justify water being routed to Las Vegas urbanization, government officials analyzed the economic impact of a gallon of water used in the city versus that gallon used in agriculture. I have no clue how these numbers were created, but the bottom line was that a million gallons of water for resorts generated $100,000 and a million gallons used to grow crops generated $2,000. Guess who will win the water wars?

For me, it was an epiphany just to know that important, credentialed government officials actually make these kinds of calculations. I don't know enough to come down hard on one side or the other, but that people are valuing water based on hot tubs compared to broccoli seems surreal to me. With most comparisons like this, probably the real value lies way upstream (pun fully intended) where nobody wants to look. I suppose as long as the rest of the world can grow food and fuel stays cheap enough to ship it to Las Vegas, things will be fine. What happens if energy doubles? With apologies to Marie Antoinette, "Let them eat chips — roulette chips, that is." The thinking that created the thinking that thinking people think water use should be allocated based on its gross dollar returns is thinking reflective of jaundiced thinking that indicates improper thinking in the first place.

Our land, blessed with plenty, has unfortunately moved from a water conservation policy to a water squandering policy. Perhaps the best way to deal with the cheap food policy and the cheap energy policy is to start eliminating the cheap water policy. Of course, at this wonderful xeriscaping conference, we were exposed to all sorts of water conservation systems: green roof, native landscaping (rather than high-water-demanding landscaping in a desert), gray water plumbing for toilets (one of my favorites), insoak landscape retentions to reduce surface runoff, and my personal favorite, cisterns of every shape and size.

Perhaps no state has a more wrongheaded, antiwater environment than Colorado. In Colorado, filling a five-gallon bucket from a roof gutter and downspout is illegal. According to official Colorado government idiocy, if you impound water, you're hoarding a public resource. Impounding water from your rooftop keeps it from flushing downriver where it can be used for municipal supplies and irrigation on farmland and golf courses. This is completely foolhardy as I will now explain.

Let's get some historical and hydrological context. Holistic Management International's founder, Allan Savory, whom history will vindicate as one of the greatest ecologists of all time, has identified the differences between the temperate and brittle environments. The dividing line between the two is around twenty-two inches of rainfall. The most pronounced difference between the two ecologies is rainfall. But other differences are equally profound. One is that in brittle areas, soils tend to accumulate minerals, whereas in temperate areas, mineral leaching is an ongoing limiting factor. Decomposition in temperate areas occurs at the ground level (fenceposts rot at the soil line and fall over); in brittle areas, decomposition occurs out at the tip, where oxidation gradually works its way down the stem. Grasses in brittle environments tend to be bunch types; in temperate, they tend to be spreader types.

P. A. Yeomans, Australian water genius, author of *Water for Every Farm*, and originator of the keyline system, saw his native brittle environment's challenge as being fundamentally a hydration issue. That idea, refined now by other thinkers, has cast yet another huge difference between brittle and temperate ecologies: hydration versus drainage.

Obviously western Europe is temperate. "One misty, moisty morning when foggy was the weather" does not describe a desert. It describes England, Wales, Scotland, Ireland, where peat bogs and dampness define the ecology. Wellingtons originated there for a reason. In these areas, if you read their farming history, you will see constant references to drainage. In order to get the land into workable condition for crops — remember, grain is queen — it had to be drained.

From a water standpoint, these Europeans developed a culture of viewing hydrology as a giant plumbing problem. Long before the flush toilet — indeed, maybe that is why the flush toilet was developed — the overriding view toward water in the culture was to get rid of it. Ditching, trenching, tiling, and canals predominated. The problem was too much water for arable farming.

With that paradigm fully entrenched, Europeans migrated to America and Australia. Indeed, marshes and sloughs (remember the *Little House on the Prairie* books?) greeted early Europeans in these new worlds. Land around the seacoasts was often too wet for arable agriculture. You can't plow a bog. And so this drainage mentality proliferated.

But in both Australia and America, and to a lesser extent New Zealand, large portions — indeed more than half — are brittle environments. The Shenandoah Valley is the only area east of the Mississippi that borders on brittle, with our thirty-one-inch rainfall. Just a dozen miles outside the valley in any direction, the rainfall jumps ten inches and the frost dates move three weeks on both ends of the season. That is why our growing environment is similar to South Dakota's, and why these tallgrass prairies gave way to the Breadbasket of the Confederacy. The Shenandoah Valley, unlike much of Pennsylvania, Maryland, Massachusetts, Wisconsin, Indiana, and Iowa, did not need draining. It was ready for the plow from day one.

Peter Andrews in Australia has spent a lifetime trying to convince policymakers that the brittle landscape needs hydration, not drainage. The maddening thought process goes like this: "I'm a farmer downstream. I need irrigation water from the river. In order for me to get more irrigation water, I need more water flowing. Therefore, we need to drain the water away from the highlands in order for me to have adequate water."

But as any Permaculturalist will tell you (and by the way, I consider Permaculture practitioners true deep ecologists, as opposed to mainline radical enviromentalist advocates for a hands-off approach), the goal for water is to keep the raindrops as close to their initial point of fall for as long as possible. Imagine the landscape like a huge sponge, obviously with seams and folds and ridges. The faster the water moves down into that sponge, the drier the ridges will be. The more water we can hold up in the ridges, the more total water the sponge can hold.

What we're after is base flow. That is the continual, regenerative movement of water through the soil substrata, gradually moving down from higher elevations. Remember that one pound of organic matter holds four pounds of water. The most efficacious way to hold raindrops where they fall is to increase soil organic matter so that a cubic foot of soil, rather than holding only a gallon of water, can hold four or five gallons.

The higher we hold water in the terrain, the more useful it is. Ideally, we will use water multiple times on its way to your municipal tap. Louis Bromfield, writing in the 1940s, said the answer to the flooding Mississippi was not huge Army Corps of Engineers projects along the river, but rather millions of farm ponds from Pennsylvania to Iowa, holding billions of gallons of water. Some of that water would evaporate into the atmosphere and encourage cloud formation and rains in the area. Some of it would seep into the ground below the pond, feeding aquifers, springs, streams, and maintaining base flow. Some of it could be used for irrigation in a dry time, to maintain solar biomass formation, organic matter accumulation, and percolate into the ground, joining other seeping water. Some of it could water livestock, which would prune the forage to restart newly excited biomass accumulation. Much of that drinking water would go back onto the ground as nutrient-rich urine, to again percolate through the ground, to be purified in the soil as bacteria grabbed the nutrients out of the liquid.

Those nutrients, in turn, would feed soil bacteria that would team up with plant microbes, which would feast on them and in turn stimulate the plant to grow. A growing plant creates more biomass that can decompose to add more organic matter to hold more water to transpire through the leaves to stimulate cloud formation and therefore rain. Straightening the Mississippi is the worst water policy imaginable because it takes billions of gallons of water capacity away from the channel. The mighty Mississippi has lost a huge amount of water-carrying capacity because it is so much shorter today than it was a couple of centuries ago when it meandered more.

This all brings us back to Colorado and the illegal rain barrel. Colorado is not temperate; it is brittle. Its weak link is not drainage, but hydration. How do you hydrate a sponge? You do it by filling all of it with as much water as possible. You don't do it by standing the sponge up on one end so all the water drains out fast. If you want the sponge to stay hydrated, you drip water slowly to the highest point. That drip keeps the sponge fully hydrated all the way to the bottom. That provides the most water for the most possibilities for the longest time.

Even in extremely brittle environments like Phoenix or Tucson, if you could eliminate surface runoff in a downpour by impounding it and metering it out gently later on, you could literally create an oasis in the desert. I've seen it numerous times. Hoarding water is exactly what you want people to do. That water, held high up on the sponge, will hydrate the whole and keep the base flow running continually. The worst thing is to let the rain get away quickly by running downhill fast, unimpeded. Then all you have is a giant flush and nothing left in the tank.

A rain barrel under a downspout offers water for a garden. That water makes plants grow, which in turn creates more leaf area to transpire more water into the atmosphere and stimulate rain events. Some of the water will not be used, and it will percolate into the subsoil and begin its long journey downstream, to keep springs and rivers flowing at a constant rate rather than cyclical flood/drought fluctuations. Water held high is always useful, and finds its way downstream over time rather than in one big flush gush.

As I look at the landscape of our farm, I am always thinking about water. How to slow it down. How to hold on to it. How to get more use out of it. How to hold on to it so it doesn't create a flood problem to neighbors downstream. In fact, if all the energy tilling the native prairie grasses to plant grain in the Shenandoah Valley had been devoted instead to building catchment ponds in the ravines of the surrounding hills, today this 1,600-square-mile valley would be droughtproof and floodproof. We would have created a veritable Eden. That ought to be our stewardship mandate, to create Edens wherever we go. That's why humans are here. Our responsibility is to extend forgiveness into the landscape.

Landscape forgiveness, or redemption, through pond building did not happen because we were lazy. It did not happen because we didn't want to move soil. Goodness knows, tillage moves billions of tons of soil. It didn't happen because we were brain-damaged. As a culture, we came to this place brain-damaged. We were thinking about drainage instead of hydration. We viewed water as a plumbing problem. And way too many policy officials still view water as a plumbing issue rather than a landscape hydration issue. The indigenous peoples knew better. The Incas, Aztecs, Pueblos, and others, carving out vast civilizations in arid conditions, on mountains, building terraces and carving irrigation canals that still defy modern engineering — those people understood the gravity of the situation. They knew they were dependent on water. They revered water as more valuable than gold or casino hot tubs.

To treat water with such modern American disdain, such disrespect, just ain't normal. With that in mind, here are some things I think we need to do to restore an historically normal reverence for water — to rebuild a connection, to show that we've spent some time meditating at the blessing of the domestic water faucet.

1. Encourage water barrels. Every new house should have a cistern that holds all the water that comes off the roof. In fact, I think it would be a good idea to eliminate public water to all suburbs.

Every home should be water self-sufficient. If the homebuilder is not willing to be water self-sufficient, then he doesn't care enough about the ecology to have a house. After its 2009 brush with calamity, wouldn't you think Atlanta would rethink and overhaul its water policy? Instead, it's business as usual. Atlanta's suburbs are growing, with extended pipes. It's unconscionable. I'd say it's certifiably insane.

Any home that wants to install a cistern big enough to hold all its roof water should be given a tax credit. Of course, I think the Internal Revenue Service should be abolished, but that's another topic for another book. The Fair Tax is a much better solution. Go check it out. In the final analysis, if we give tax credits for college savings funds, why can't we do it for water care? What good is a degree if you don't have any water to drink? Come on, let's get our priorities in place here.

2. Give 100 percent tax credits for rerouting plumbing to take gray water into flush toilets. That would save billions of gallons of water a day. The answer is not low-flush toilets that have to be double flushed many times. In Australia, they have an ingenious system with two different buttons: one for No. 1, and one for No. 2. They dispense different amounts of water for the two different uses. For sure, every new structure should use gray water to flush toilets. Any building inspector or health department official who balks at reusing gray water in flush toilets should be fired. Get it done, folks.

3. No recreational water from public sources. Period. If you want to water your flowers, you have to figure out a way to do it that doesn't require piping potable water from a municipal reservoir. I've learned recently that all the golf courses around Phoenix now use second-use water. Wonderful. That's a step in the right direction. Now if they'd put some cows on those courses to graze them instead of mechanically mowing them, they'd really be on to something. Homeowners can put cisterns in their basements to catch gray water and take it out to the flowers. Cisterns under the roof downspouts in many cases can gravity-feed water out to the vegetation surrounding the house. I hate to say lawn because ideally the majority of the landscape surrounding a house would be

edible. Water dispensed to raised beds growing vegetables is far more valuable than water dispensed to turf grass. Look, somewhere, somehow, people need to appreciate how precious water is before we don't have enough to drink.

4. Alternative toilets. The number one user of potable water, after lawn irrigation, is the flush toilet. Think about that. More than drinking. More than washing cars. More than showers. More than laundry. I don't care whether we go with methane toilets, composting toilets, moldering toilets, chamber pots, Johnny houses, or a combination of these. But our culture's fixation on flushing everything away just ain't normal. There is no away. It always goes someplace. The fact is that if you Google "Humanure" you'll find a host of possibilities.

Recently I was at a farm conference center and the men's urine went down a pipe into a barrel. Each day, the urine went into a spray rig hooked to an all-terrain vehicle. As a foliar pasture fertilizer, the urine went right onto the grass just like the urine out of a cow. Beautiful. Red wigglers in large vented garbage bins handled the rest of the goodies. The bins were wheeled under the toilets. No odor. Perfectly safe. Worms completely sanitize the excrement. This could be done in airports, resorts, restaurants. We haven't begun to tap the amazing benefits of worms.

Composting toilets have been around for some time. The problem with them is that most of the domestic ones have too small a composting chamber to handle special events. Am I saying this delicately enough? Whether the event is a bad case of the runs or a party in the house, these small holding chambers can easily be overrun. Large ones with big chambers work much better. I ate in a restaurant in Saskatchewan with a composting toilet. I'm sure it was expensive, but it kept all that excrement from going into a water-based system, whether on-site or municipal, and generated lots of compost for ornamental flowers around the restaurant.

Moldering toilets are yet another alternative. They use a large chamber, at minimum three feet by three feet by three feet, big enough to maintain a functional static compost pile. Each toilet is positioned over one chamber, or in the case of several toilets, they are situated over one longer chamber. Each chamber is designed to handle about one year's excrement. An adjacent identical setup is for year two. After not using the first toilet-chamber setup for a year, the excrement is completely composted, odorless, and ready for use as fertilizer. In this way, the two setups are flip-flopped back and forth from one year to the next.

The beauty of the moldering toilet is that the chamber is big enough to handle events. It's all about volume. Of course, worms and bacteria in the chamber constantly decompose the poop and toilet paper, reducing the volume. Once the pile is big enough to sustain a community of decomposers, they hold the volume virtually steady. It's quite remarkable.

I looked into the holding bin of a huge moldering toilet in Massachusetts, designed to handle 30,000 student visitors per year. No odor. Waterless. Wonderful. The technology is here. There is no reason on God's green earth why we can't have a more environmentally friendly, respectful way to handle our own human manure without wasting water. Our antipathy toward its yuckiness, to not see it or deal with it, is completely abnormal.

The goal in handling excrement is to get it out of the water, not put it in the water. Sir Albert Howard knew, and prophesied, that by the late 1950s the world would realize the folly of water-based sewage systems. He designed what he called diamond cities, in which twenty-five houses would occupy a diamond formation so that all of them would have unimpeded solar exposure. In the middle of the diamond, the twenty-five householders would have a one-acre garden/farm. The twenty-five householders would employ one full-time master gardener, who would handle the excrement generated by the twenty-five homes and grow all their produce and fruit, with perhaps eggs thrown in. The chickens would eat the kitchen scraps. Unfortunately, his optimism about human common sense far exceeded reality. His wonderful ideas were not adopted.

The raging battles in our culture between developers and land preservationists could be eliminated by policies that encouraged these kinds of living arrangements. If we dispense with water-based toilets, we cut per capita water needs by more than half. If we recycle gray water to grow vegetables to feed ourselves, we eliminate the trip to the supermarket. Just think of what a difference it would make to have a fairly urban community without a water line, without a sewer line, and food-independent. The only things left are electricity and heating. With a sun-facing solarium, we eliminate the heating problem. Now we're down to electricity, which of course has lots of possibilities from photovoltaics to windmills to bicycle-powered generators. Instead of driving to town to exercise, why not hook your exercise machine up to a generator and store all that exercise energy to run your computer? This self-sufficient type of living would completely change the land impact of development.

5. Encourage farm ponds. Back in the 1950s the old Soil Conservation Service used to design and help farmers build ponds. Now the USDA views ponds as liabilities instead of assets. Insurance companies view them as attractive nuisances. Food police think Canada geese and ducks will land on them and bring avian influenza to factory chicken concentration camps.

    Farm ponds are actually one of the best returns on investment in basic ecology enhancement and hydrology cycling. They retain sediments that would otherwise run off during heavy rains. They provide drought irrigation protection. They offer landscape beauty and diversity. They attract wildlife — which, unlike the USDA, I think is rather cool. And they maintain base flow rates because no pond is completely impervious.

There you have it. I encourage you, when you next turn on your kitchen faucet, or get in the shower, to think about the journey of that water. Imagine carrying all of it in buckets to a tub for a monthly bath. And when you sit — or stand — over the porcelain fixture bathroom centerpiece and do your duty, ask yourself, "Is this the best use of this water?" When you start connecting mentally, spiritually, and viscerally with water like this, you will begin getting an inkling, just an inkling, of historic water normalcy.

Mob Stocking Herbivorous Solar Conversion Lignified Carbon Sequestration Fertilization

Perhaps nothing illustrates modern farming's departure from normalcy as dramatically as beef feedlots. These sprawling corrals containing thousands of beef animals, with nary a place to stand or lie down except in their own excrement, and fed a candy bar diet of starch — primarily corn — to grossly and quickly fatten them, epitomize a system worthy of the exclamation, "Folks, this ain't normal."

The joke goes something like this: A fellow goes by to see his friend at the feed yard and spies him across the sea of steers, only head and shoulders sticking out above the manure. "Hey, Mac, how you be?" he yells.

"Oh, I'm okay, but my horse is struggling a wee bit." If you don't get the joke, it's this: The manure is as deep as the horse, so all the friend can see is the cowboy astride the horse. Yes, now you can laugh. Just a little feedlot humor there.

Feedlots are the most poignant expression of a food production system that has departed from historical normalcy on several fronts. The first is the diversified farmstead. While farms, like any business, tend to gravitate to an area of expertise that becomes the mother ship, or most important component of the business, all farms used to have a menagerie of plants and animals.

Many farmers today don't even grow a garden. I remember the first time I learned that many of our beef-cattle-producing neighbors bought their meat at the supermarket. I was just a teen, but intuitively I couldn't imagine raising all this food and then not eating any of it. I well remember a vegetable farmer telling me his conversion to biological farming was the morning he picked a green bean and realized he wouldn't eat it until he'd thoroughly washed it. "I couldn't even eat my own green bean in my own field. This ain't right," he said.

Until very recently, the homestead formed the nucleus of the farm. Sometimes called the farmstead, it included all the components of a diversified food stream. We recently rented a farm nearby, and the old farmstead is one of the best-preserved examples of this practice. The large, rambling frame house is at one end of a lane lined with little outbuildings. Next to the house is the summer kitchen, a two-story affair that allowed cooking and canning to be done outside. That kept the heat outside during the summer and reduced fire risk in the main house. The two-story summer kitchen has plenty of storage for dry goods, canned goods, and cured meats upstairs.

Next to it, a small piggery offered a garbage disposal for kitchen wastes, soured milk, and whey left over from cheesemaking. The small pen probably only housed three or four hogs at a time — these were for the household use, not primarily to sell.

Next to the little piggery is a chicken house, distinctive with its windows to let in direct sunlight. Birds are highly responsive to light. The chicken house is big enough for maybe fifty hens — again, enough to eat kitchen scraps, garden weeds, and rotten vegetables and fruit. Across the lane and along the house is a large fenced garden area.

The next building in the summer kitchen, piggery, chicken house line is the granary, with a slatted corn crib for ears of field corn. A hand-cranked corn sheller still sits there, waiting for Grandpa and grandkids to chuck ears of corn into it and watch the cobs spit out one spout while golden corn kernels pour into a bucket at the bottom. This corn, of course, was handpicked, usually into a wagon pulled by a team of horses.

It wasn't that long ago in 1980, when I was writing feature stories for the local daily newspaper, that I wrote an article about a farmer in the county who still used horses. I got up early on a frosty November morning, drove to the farm, and walked out into a six-acre cornfield near his house. The team of Belgian draft horses stood patiently in their traces while the farmer, using a little metal hook, shucked the ears and jerked them off the stalk, tossing them into a wagon. The wagon had one low sideboard and one high sideboard to catch the incoming ears. It was magic, that frosty morning in the Shenandoah Valley, smoke wisps rising out of some chimneys, and variegated farmland stretching out toward the Allegheny Mountains to the west.

Picking two rows of corn at a time, every twelve feet or so, he'd gently cluck to the horses, "Move up." They would obediently pull forward until he said, "Whoa." Then they would abruptly stop. He never missed a beat picking off those ears. This beautiful dance between man and beast, carefully choreographed through years of practice and trust-building, was both peaceful and graceful. No engines. Just the steamy breaths spurting from big Belgian nostrils, ears twitching, ready to hear the next command. I was mesmerized. Truly, I had stepped back to yesteryear. This was serene, magical — but highly inefficient. Or so everybody said.

Once the wagon was filled, which took all morning, the farmer drove the team to a corn crib. With a scoop shovel, he shoveled the ear corn into the crib, a narrow slat-sided holding container about five feet wide and twenty feet long. He shoveled the corn through a doorway cut into the crib side. The slats allowed lots of air to circulate, thwarting mold and encouraging the kernels to continue drying. A shed roof over top protected the precious crop from rain.

The granary also has holding compartments for barley, wheat, oats, and rye. These are roughly five feet wide and eight feet long (or deep) — going away from you as you stand in front of it. The front is open except for a slot down both edges to insert garner boards. This allowed the farmer to shovel the grain in but raise the front retaining wall as the pile grew. Obviously as he shoveled it out later on, he would remove the garner boards to allow as easy access as possible. The grain was used for household flour milling as well as animal feed — primarily for poultry, pigs, and horses. It was a supplemental treat for sheep, dairy, and beef cattle.

Beyond the granary, on this farmstead, is the barn. A hay mow on a floor above the ground level allowed the farmer to throw hay down into a manger where the animals were. Across the lane from the barn is a shop and another toolshed, no doubt for hand tools like hoes, shovels, and rakes. Now we've walked the entire farmstead compound, ending up back at the garden and house. With few alterations, this was the basic configuration of the farmstead. A smokehouse for curing pork, even a washhouse for laundry, were also common. The point is that the heart of the farmstead centered around self-sufficiency. The home economy provided the nucleus of the family's enterprise. First you fed the family and its associated workers. Then you produced stuff to sell. In a day before supermarkets, domestic success required a diversified group of people, plants, and animals working in harmony.

Today, this has largely given way to a single item, whether it be fruit, dairy, pigs, vegetables, grain, or cotton. The house and farmyard, histori-cally, have always been a seamless continuum of production, processing, and family life. This diversified farmstead provided entertainment, voca-tion, and craftsmanship. Today, most farmers shop at the supermarket just like anyone else. For all their surrounding abundance, the farmstead is sterile, almost antiseptic, and certainly devoid of people. Machines sit patiently in their sheds, waiting for drivers.

This is progress, we're told. Before tears start rolling, nostalgically reminiscing about what was lost, let me make the first huge point: Throughout history, grain was dear. Even the prophet Hosea, in the Bible, talks about buying a beloved harlot and making her his wife, for the price of about nine bushels of barley. Barley was expensive.

Think about grain prior to mechanization. Tilling the soil, or tillage, required a team of oxen or horses pulling a sharp stick or crude instru-ment through the ground to break it up. Then you had to sow the seed, by hand. Hopefully the germination was good enough and thick enough to stay ahead of weeds, but some hand weeding was always nec-essary along with hand hoeing. As the grain grew, it finally set a seed-head and then gradually turned from green to brown. Once it was brown, you scythed it off at ground level and stacked the cut stalks with seedheads (grain heads) in a shock to encourage further drying.

As soon as it was all cut and shocked, you began stacking it on wag-ons to bring in to a threshing floor. This was a hard floor, often made with heavy wooden timbers, where you could beat the grain heads to dislodge the grain from its husk. This could be done with beating sticks, animals treading across it, or simply stomping it. Then you tossed this heap of flailed grain and plant material up into the air, called winnowing, and the breeze would carry away the chaff. The heavy grain, or seeds, would fall to the floor. After a day of this hard work, you might have a few bushels of grain.

But now came the hard part: storing it so that rats and mice wouldn't consume it all. Before the advent of modern extruded steel siding and mesh wire, this was a major problem. Spring rat killin's in and around granaries were a necessary farm survival activity. In ancient days, of course, clay pots were the favored rodent-proof vessel for storing this precious grain. Here's the point: Throughout history, grain has been too expensive to waste on animals.

Priced in relation to other food items, bread was expensive. It was not cheap. Every kernel of grain needed to be preserved carefully for human consumption. Not until mechanized tillage, harvesting, and rodent-proof storage has grain become cheaper than vegetables and fruit, and cheap enough to feed to animals. Historically, grain was reserved for human consumption precisely because the tillage required to prepare a seedbed to grow it was too laborious. Grain was precious because tillage was hard.

Because tillage or cultivation, which are fancy terms for stirring the soil, were so laborious, a farmer could only cover a little bit of ground in a day. Tillage is a generic term for lots of specific types of soil stirring functions. The whole point of tillage is to eliminate vegetation already growing on the soil to create a receptive environment to plant seeds. Discing is a slicing and stirring tillage that uses narrow saucer-shaped circles (discs) that don't penetrate very deep into the soil. Harrowing is the finest tillage, using a toothed machine almost like a large garden rake to break up clumps and create a fine seedbed. A chisel plow penetrates deeply with curved tines and does not invert the soil. A subsoiler goes up to two feet deep with a shank that simply cuts a slit in the soil to encourage water and air movement. Both the chisel plow and subsoiler have only been widely used since the advent of mechanical power; it took too many horses to pull one. A moldboard plow inverts the soil, bringing what's on the bottom up to the top and burying the top layer, along with the vegetation.

Historically, a man with draft animals — either mules or horses —

could moldboard plow up to an acre in a day. Today one person can plow more than a hundred acres in a day. The sheer ability to move that much soil practically effortlessly is perhaps one of the most abnormal things about the days in which we live. The historic difficulty of stirring soil created a natural protection against more rapid ecological devastation. Tillage was laborious to the point of being painful.

That's actually a good thing, because tillage is actually painful for the soil. It superoxygenates the soil, exposes it to the weather, and burns out organic matter. In order to compensate for the soil degradation tillage causes, farmers developed numerous techniques to rebuild soil between years of tillage. Historically, multiyear rotations were necessary in order to preserve fertility. Lest I be accused of stating what ought to be obvious, nature does not do tillage. This is one of the big flaws in vegetarianism, which tends to replace perennials with annuals. Annuals require tillage to prepare a seedbed to plant and germinate the seeds. Some wonderful techniques are being developed to minimize tillage, and I'll address them later, but for now stick with me as I discuss the natural template.

Nature builds soil with perennials, herbivores, and periodic disturbance, or pruning. Plants are solar collectors. A plant is 95 percent sunlight and only 5 percent soil. That means if you pick up one hundred pounds of plant material, ninety-five pounds was created out of sunlight and thin air, so to speak, and only five pounds came from the soil. This is obviously a magnificent process in which the earth, if properly managed, should be gaining soil, indeed gaining weight, every day.

All indigenous tillage systems revolve around a healing fallow. Even swidden systems, commonly known as primitive jungle-type slash-and-burn agriculture, only till for a couple of years and then let the land go back to native perennials for restoration. One of the reasons is because annuals put all their effort into growing seed; perennials put all their effort into accumulating root reserves. That is a huge difference in the energy flow and the objective of the two different kinds of plants.

Annuals tend to concentrate all their energy in the seedheads rather than in what's below the soil. Perennials want to maximize their energy below ground, storing carbohydrates in their root bank account against cold, drought, flood — any kind of unfriendly weather. Annuals know their seeds will lodge somewhere, take root, and grow. Maximizing seed production is the annuals' goal; maximizing below-ground energy storage is the perennials' goal.

Wes Jackson, at the Land Institute in Salina, Kansas, has devoted his life to selecting a perennial that will offer a seedhead big enough to compete with annual grains. He's made a lot of progress, and all of us in the biological community applaud the goals. This is groundbreaking research and should be encouraged on all fronts.

Equally amazing is the work of Colin Seis in Australia, whose Pasture Cropping systems now have two thousand farmers aboard. He combines grazing animals, tight seasonal planting schedules, and perennial pastures to grow conventional small-grain crops. All the major small-grain crops (wheat, oats, barley, rye) are cool-tolerant. In the fall, Seis grazes down a perennial pasture, lets it come back some, then grazes it again to weaken the perennial sward a little bit.

He plants into that weakened sward, using either a simple disk coulter (kind of a heavy metal pie plate with zigzag edges) to open up a slit, or a narrow shoe ripper (a narrow metal foot attached to a shank; yes, it looks much like your foot and shank, hence the similar terminology) — in any case, a slit only an inch or so wide — to receive the seed. No herbicide, no chemicals. The grain crop germinates and jumps ahead of the perennial forage, already retarded by the grazing and fall temperatures. The annuals stay green and grow slowly when winter days are above 40 degrees Fahrenheit, but then jump rapidly in the early spring and stay ahead of the grass, even smothering it a bit.

The grain plants outcompete the pasture in the early spring and shade it out. But the pasture is very much alive, an understory below the towering grain plants. When the grain is ready to harvest, he runs through it with the combine, clipping off the seedheads but leaving the pasture plants unscathed. Afterwards, he grazes the robust perennial pasture with the animals again, and in the process they stomp and shred the straw into the soil to provide a shot of lignified carbon to the soil biota. The little rips for the grain planting actually provide miles of edge effect to colonize soil bacteria, which in turn stimulates the perennials to grow better. Seis crops only once every five years, allowing four years for grazing and perennials to recuperate from the single cropping year. Even without tillage, the soil recuperation between grain crops is four years. Interestingly, his yields per acre are the same as with clean tillage and chemicals. Is that cool or what?

Both Jackson and Seis are seeking answers to the age-old dilemma of regenerative cropping systems. The Rodale research farm in Emmaus, Pennsylvania, has been researching this conundrum for years and through the use of judicious cover crops and complex planting successions, along with newly designed machinery, is demonstrating success as well. The point I'm trying to make is that grain production — annual cropping — is unnatural at today's volume. Historically, it has always been practiced sparingly, held in check by the sheer difficulty of stirring the ground. In areas where it was not used sparingly, deserts generally follow — like the Sahara in Africa and the Rajputana in India, documented quite well in Reid A. Bryson and Thomas J. Murray's book *Climates of Hunger.*

Of course, many more grains exist than just the common four. Spelt, amaranth, rice — in the Western world, however, we just don't think of these as much. And we typically don't feed those to livestock, so for the purposes of this discussion, I want to hold it to traditional Western grains that are used for livestock feeds.

Herbivores in nature act symbiotically with the perennial plant to mow it and stimulate it. Here's how. All plants go through a sigmoid growth curve, like many biological curves. You don't see many straight-line graphs when dealing with natural systems — they tend to cycle in gentle waves.

Like all plants, grass grows in a sigmoid curve which resembles an S. Using your imagination, think about a sprout coming out of the soil. It's delicate, a bit yellowish, tender, and not growing very fast. As leaf area increases, photosynthesis kicks into overdrive and the plant shoots skyward, accumulating energy momentum and biomass rapidly.

Then it shoots a seedhead as it slows down in growth, putting energy into the seeds but greatly slowing in biomass accumulation. This is the top of the S, or the senescence stage. I call the rapid mid-S growth the juvenile or teenage years, as opposed to the earlier sprout, or diaper, phase. The nursing home phase rounds out the top of the S, as the seedhead sets and pollinates. Then the plant begins to die. It begins turning brown as the cellulose lignifies and complexes. It's no longer accumulating solar energy, but rather begins to oxidize, giving off CO_2 as it bends under the weight of the seedhead and structural deterioration.

At this point, the plant has pumped lots of carbon dioxide — CO_2 — into the root zone through sequestered carbon, with literally miles of root filaments extending down and out from the plant crown. In fact, nature maintains biomass bilateral symmetry at the soil horizon, so there is as much carbon under the soil as on top. In natural grazing systems, whether they be wildebeests on the Serengeti, Cape buffalo in Botswana, or bison on the North American landscape, these herbivores are the restart button for biomass accumulation.

A decaying plant releases CO_2. Only an actively living plant inhales CO_2 and exhales oxygen — O_2. Sequestering carbon requires active growth. But brown plants aren't actively growing. And so in nature, herbivores act as restart buttons to take off that oxidizing, dying plant material and restart the rapid green growth period. In fact, due to their more rapid cycle, grasslands are more efficient at CO_2 accumulation — carbon sequestering — than trees. That doesn't mean we should kill all the trees, because they do some things grasses can't, like bringing up deeper minerals and scattering them through leaf drop, pumping water to stimulate the hydrologic cycle, and acting as nesting sites for birds that sanitize behind herbivores by eating insects and bugs.

To use another metaphor, most people are familiar with pruning. Vineyards, orchards, and ornamental shrubs all receive periodic pruning to help them grow better, to be more productive, and ultimately to set healthier fruit — at least in the case of the edible plants. The herbivore is nature's grassland pruner to stimulate far more production and health than could be achieved if the plant were left alone. Since trees don't have this natural pruning relationship, grasslands have historically sequestered more carbon and built more soil than forests. Hence the deepest soils in North America, for example, are not where forests are most thick; they are where the buffalo and prairie grasses lived.

For you agronomists out there, I'm well aware of the differences between soils and the fungal versus bacterial properties that stimulate forestal or grass-type vegetation. I don't want to get bogged down with glaciation and agronomic detail. The main point is to understand the dramatic soil-building capabilities of the grass-herbivore relationship, and the symbiosis between the two. The other point is that properly managed grass will outcompete forestal carbon sequestration, at least on the best soils.

Let me inject here my little "lawn isn't the grass I'm talking about" lecture. We modern Americans are brain-damaged when it comes to understanding grass. Typically, we think of grass as a lawn — short and a bother to care for. But when I say grass, I mean native prairie. One of the most spiritual experiences I ever had was in the two-acre native prairie maintained by the University of Nebraska at Lincoln. I was there speaking at a conference and went out into that grass during a break. It was twelve feet tall and nearly an inch thick at the base.

Just walking into it a few feet obscured all the buildings. To stand there, dwarfed by the sea of grass, and imagine the hundreds of miles of undulating prairie just like it used to exist overwhelmed me. When Ma and Pa in the Laura Ingalls Wilder books wouldn't let the girls go more than a few feet from the homestead lest they become lost, we modern-day Americans have a hard time imagining such a thing. The sheer volume of biomass, standing there as thick as the hair on a dog's back, twelve feet tall — it defies imagination. When I say grass, that's what I'm talking about.

In a very practical sense, grasslands are the lungs of the earth. They are the rapid cycler, the rapid breather, if you will. Without herbivores, grasslands are lethargic and anemic. Some would even argue that grasses would not exist without herbivores because it is the periodic grazing that freshens up the plant. If not for periodic pruning, the grass plants implode and gradually wither away. Perhaps no person in our world has done more to bring this to light than Allan Savory, founder of Holistic Management International. The symbiotic relationship between herbivores and forage is one of the most powerful ecological principles we know. New evidence even suggests that when the animal tugs at the plant to shear off the grass tillers, it excites the roots into renewed productive activity. Kind of like exercise builds new muscles.

This periodic grazing disturbance has its own formula for efficacy. It is not a random, haphazard occurrence. The herbivores are always clustered together in a tight herd due to either human or animal predation. That clumping of the animals creates a fluid organism rather than a group of individuals. The herd moves across the landscape as one entity. The individual competition to stay up with the herd tends to weed out weaklings and the elderly. Within the herd, then, the social and physical dynamics create their own disturbance that maintains a freshness, a virility, in the group.

The herbivore is a four-legged portable fermentation tank, a sauerkraut vat, if you will, turning biomass carbohydrates into meat and milk. This fermentation, or digestion process, gives off less CO_2 than the biomass would if it were allowed to simply decay on the stalk. And we now know that North America contained nearly three times as many pounds of herbivores (bison, elk, antelope, deer) five hundred years ago as it does today — even with all the petroleum-based fertilizer, corn, and tillage being practiced. Clearly, cows aren't causing global warming. That junk science is sponsored by a thought process that blames the cow for ecological degradation.

In fact, the cow, or domestic herbivore if you will, is the most efficacious soil-building, hydrology-cycling, carbon-sequestering tool at the planet's disposal. Yes, the cow has done a tremendous amount of damage. But don't blame the cow. The managers of the cow have been and continue to be the problem. The same animal mismanaged to abuse the ecology is the greatest hope and salvation to heal the ecology.

Mom and Dad purchased our farm — a worn-out, gullied rock pile — half a century ago. I've witnessed the difference between soil-building capacity from pasture versus forest. We had large scallops, like shallow plates or discs, in the fields, some as large as fifty feet across, in which the soil had eroded to bare rock. Completely bare rock. With herbivores, controlled grazing management, compost, and care, all of those saucer-shaped bare rock scallops now have several inches of soil covering them. In fact, I'm the only one now who remembers where they were.

In the early days, this farm did not have enough soil to hold up electric fence stakes when Dad began developing the portable electric fencing system. For the uninitiated, an electric fence stake is a metal or plastic rod less than half an inch in diameter that you shove six to eight inches into the ground to hold up a tiny strand of wire. It doesn't take much soil to hold one. But we didn't have enough. So Dad poured concrete in old car tires, then pushed two pieces of about six-inch-long half-inch pipe, one straight up and one on about a 10 percent angle, to receive the fence stakes. When we would build fence, Dad would pile these standards (like volleyball standards) on a platform behind the tractor. My older brother and I were barely able to heave these off as Dad drove slowly along the field. He would then come back and stick the stakes into the pipes. I have yet to meet anyone anywhere who started out with soil so thin it wouldn't hold up electric fence stakes. Yes, we have kept a couple of these around to show the unbelievers.

One field was a bit more inaccessible, and rather than trying to nurse it back to pasture, we abandoned it to the forest. It has been left to its own devices, growing trees, for the same half century. Trees have found crevices and spots for toeholds, and now that seven-acre field, from a distance, is completely forested. But underneath, the same rocks I saw as a child are still there, on the surface, just as exposed as they were decades ago. I'm sure some soil building has occurred, but it's precious little. Under those trees, the rocks are not covered over with anything. They lie there in stark exposure and the healing we've seen on the pastures has not occurred. The difference in healing is so obvious that I've decided if we're ever going to build soil on that seven acres, we need to cut down the trees and get it into grass. Nothing builds soil like intensively managed grazing on grasslands.

To achieve these natural grazing intensities and patterns like the multimillion-head wild herds, we use high-tech portable electric fencing. Since we don't have lions or wolves and bison, with this nifty fencing we can achieve the same results. Cows wandering over a field ape the natural and normal wild herd grazing model. On our farm, lightweight, highly portable electric fence allows us to define each day's grazing block, called a paddock, and concentrate the herd onto that spot like bison corralled by wolves. High-tech electric fence allows us to duplicate this traditional, normal herbivorous pattern. By denying the herbivores access to a paddock until the grass has rested enough to go through that middle rapid growth period of the S curve, we metabolize far more sunlight into biomass than would otherwise occur.

We call this "mob stocking herbivorous solar conversion lignified carbon sequestration fertilization." And if every farm and ranch that has cows in the United States would practice this biomimicry, in fewer than ten years we would sequester all the atmospheric carbon generated since the beginning of the industrial age. For more information, visit Holistic Management International and Carbon Farmers of

America — two groups doing the empirical analysis and demonstrating the efficacy of these principles.

On our farm, we do this type of grazing management because historically it is the most normal way to build soil. What a delight to learn that it is also the most efficient way to sequester carbon. When any system returns to historical normalcy, benefits begin showing up that often we can't imagine. If we just do what is right, everything else seems to fall into place. Good nomadic grazing management uses the same principles — one is extremely low-tech while our electric fencing control is extremely high-tech. But this is not about technology; it is about ecological normalcy.

The critical thing to understand is that grazing can be done in a way that builds soil and heals the land, or it can be done in a way that destroys the land. Grazing is not inherently good or bad. It is the grazing management, the pattern, that makes it ecologically positive or ecologically negative. Nomads have certainly destroyed plenty of land through overgrazing, as have American farmers.

The abuses, however, do not change the fact that worldwide soil building occurs most dramatically with herbivores, perennials, rest periods, and periodic disturbance. This is why all indigenous agriculture systems include herbivores. Even Eastern systems use yaks and water buffalo for power. Prior to the internal combustion engine, draft animals injected a grazing component into every hamlet, every farm, every industry. Prior to the Industrial Revolution, grazing animals dominated the landscape and farmscape. Embedded in every civilization is the pastoral imperative. Pastoral scenes tugging nostalgically at our senses actually demonstrate the land-healing reality of herbivore-perennial-rest-disturbance. That these landscapes soothe the human spirit may indicate a primal connection with historical human normalcy.

An agriculture without animals just ain't normal. Animals generate the magic elixir of agrarian wealth: manure. Anyone who farms with integrity realizes the value of manure. Gene Logsdon's recent book *Holy Shit* elevates this most mundane substance to its rightful place as steward of the planet. This is why indigenous cropping systems utilized a multiyear rotation, with only two of five, or two of seven, years in cropping and the balance in soil-building, land-healing pasture. Old-timers spoke reverently of the "new ground" effect following the pastoral fallow. The biblical seven-year fallow certainly fits this historically normal recipe for building soil.

Now let's bring these threads together. What dominated farmscapes for centuries was not tillage, poultry, or pigs: It was perennial pastures and herbivores. Indeed, even Jesus's parable of the prodigal son, in which the forgiving father commanded his servants to prepare the fatted calf to celebrate the wayward son's return home, did not imply a grain-fed beef. In a day when tillage was difficult and grain as expensive as prostitutes, no one would think of feeding grain to an herbivore.

In nomadic situations, because the animals had to walk a good distance every day to pasture, fattening occurred in corrals. To reduce daily exercise and coddle an herbivore with easy gorging, farmers had two options. One was to confine the animal in a corral or stall and bring forage to it — called green chop, which is fresh-harvested forage, like fresh lawn clippings. Forages would be scythed and brought in on a cart once or twice a day. The other option was tethering, which involves attaching the animal to a rope, usually on a halter, and tying the rope to a stake affixed in the ground. The animal grazes in a circle, to the reach of the rope, and the next day the farmer moves the stake to another spot. Both of these options utilized land near the homestead that was especially fertilized and set aside for fattening purposes.

Stall feeding required about three acres nearby to grow the forage. An oxcart provided the transport for the fresh-cut forage into the corral and the shoveled manure back out to the pasture. Sometimes called ley farming in Great Britain, this method created an intensive forage area with high fertility because the manure was constantly hauled out and applied to it. This fattening methodology was normal until the advent of cheap grain. The only way to efficiently harvest solar energy in bygone days was through a grazing animal. Right at the end, when it was fattened for slaughter, it was confined and doted on with human-harvested feedstuffs. But still no grain.

Because of the need for draft power, the inefficiency and luxury of grain, and the dominance of pasture for land healing, grazing with herbivores, including sheep and goats, has formed the centerpiece of agriculture since the dawn of civilization. I'm belaboring this point because many people today think we can have a viable regenerative agriculture without animals. And many people think that domestic livestock, especially the cow, has no place in ecological stewardship. These people don't know what they're talking about. Such thinking just ain't normal.

The acceleration of environmental degradation in the last century is not because we have too many cows. It is because we have too few cows and the ones we have are too often locked up in massive feedlots eating chemical-based annual grains (corn and soybeans) rather than out grazing on perennial forages like their predecessors. The abnormal acceleration of cow-induced ecological degradation is symptomatic of widespread disregard for historical ecological normalcy, which required that grazing animals do just that: graze.

Lowly grass, however, gets no respect in a culture dominated by expensive grain. When grain is queen, and grass is simply a healing mechanism between queen crops, grass never achieves high status. It is always a means to an end, just a necessary step in order to ready the ground for another round of tillage. After all, grain is diamonds. The digging is just a means to an end. The real quest is for the diamond. The lowly digger is just the lowly digger.

For centuries — arguably for most of civilization — expensive grain's status had a concomitant depressing effect on the value of forages. While the universal understanding that grasses (pasture) were necessary to enhance fertility encouraged farmers to grow grass, it was just a lowly servant on the way to true wealth: grain. Throughout history, you don't see many statues to honor grass. I use the word here loosely to describe perennial forages: grass, clovers, forbs, herbs, even weeds. The nomadic and animal-herding cultures are the only ones that had much appreciation for grass. In the Bible, the Kenites are mentioned as leaving their pastures better than they found them. Must have been an awesome tribe, I'd say.

Because a grazing animal could self-harvest pasture perennial biomass, herbivores became the backbone of nutrient-dense diets the world over. The herbivore concentrated nutrition with minimal human effort. Compared to acquiring and storing grain to make bread, cheese and meat required less effort for the nutrition generated. A couple of village children could take thousands of pounds of animals out to the pastures, sit with them all day to move them along, and bring them back to the protection of a corral at night. The amount of human labor necessary to till and plant grain for a given amount of nutrition was astronomically higher than that required to move animals around grazing perennials.

I well remember when Teresa and I received a conservation award many years ago when Daniel was only eight years old and Rachel was three. We had to travel to the ceremony in Washington, D.C., and left the children in the care of their grandmother (my mom) and the livestock in the care of our eight-year-old Daniel. We had a hundred cows at the time. I set up electric fences for the two days we would be gone and he moved them, by himself. An eight-year-old moving a hundred cows — no problem. They were used to the daily move and simply came when he called them into the adjacent paddock. This is a lot easier than controlling a plow behind an ox, throwing out grain, hoeing it, scything it, gathering it, flailing it, winnowing it, and storing it. Herbivores have been the backbone of agriculture and food not because people didn't know better, but because energy, labor, and ecology demanded it.

The main point of all this is that omnivores, which cannot survive on self-harvested perennial forages, tended to be a luxury. The two most common domestic farmstead omnivores, of course, are chickens and pigs. When President Herbert Hoover envisioned a "chicken in every pot" it was because chicken was a luxury. Historically, chicken was the food of royalty. Peasants could not afford chickens whenever they wanted one. The common person could only eat chicken once in a while as part of some festive occasion.

Omnivores were primarily scavengers around the farmstead. Remember the buildings I described around the normal farmstead at the beginning of this chapter. The chicken house and piggery were both located closest to the house, garden, and summer kitchen because that was the farmstead garbage disposal. Raising poultry or pigs for commercial sale was not an option in a time of expensive grain. Commoners ate beef and had a milk cow not because they liked beef more than chicken, or milk more than pork, but because the herbivore was the land fertility link in a chain of objectives with grain production at the end.

To be sure, people preferred poultry, primarily because it was a small enough animal that a family could consume all of it in one meal. In the days before refrigeration, smaller animals were preferred because they could be eaten in one sitting.

In its day, jousting was equivalent to car racing today, with sponsors and wealth dominating the players. Only the wealthy could afford the grain required to increase the octane in a horse enough for it to grow big enough to carry a mounted knight clad in steel and the heavy armored tack involved with the competition. The mounted knight was the Sherman tank of its day, and it took centuries of metallurgy, breeding, and finally enough wealth to afford enough grain to grow a horse big enough and strong enough to hold all that weight and still be able to gallop.

Until cheap grain, farmers in Virginia could only grow as many pigs as their chestnut and acorn crops could feed. They couldn't afford to dump grain into troughs. Pigs ate whey left over from cheesemaking. In those days, it was cheaper to feed soured milk to hogs than it was to buy grain. The soured milk came from an herbivore that could convert nontillage perennials into nutrient density. Grain required the farmer to get out there and walk all day in the hot sun at the west end of an east-facing mule. Are you starting to understand the ramifications of expensive grain? Good grief, I hope so. I've analyzed this from every angle I can think of to help people understand the profound implications of expensive grain and the role that the perennial-herbivore relationship played in sustaining a grain-valuing agricultural paradigm. Without the herbivore, the grain could not be sustainably grown.

Cows, sheep, and goats — herbivores — were common. Pigs and poultry were luxuries. Grain was expensive. Pasture dominated the landscape not because people preferred herbivores, but because it was the only way to heal tilled land and maintain fertility in tillage-based, or arable, farming.

All that changed with mechanization and petroleum. The combination of machines and cheap energy, both to power equipment and to make fertilizer, completely changed this intricate balancing act of diversity. Suddenly draft power was unnecessary. Suddenly tillage was relatively cheap. Suddenly a pasture rotation was not necessary to maintain fertility because farmers could simply restore lost fertility with an injection of chemical fertilizer — at least that's what the USDA said. Suddenly grain could be cheaply fertilized, cheaply harvested, cheaply transported, and cheaply stored.

Cheap grain enabled a complete reversal of historical normalcy.

Farmers began feeding herbivores grain because for the first time in human history, it was cheap enough and abundant enough to feed. And herbivores grew fast on it. Talk about octane. They pumped up like blimps. That took the craftsmanship out of forage finishing. No longer was finishing a beef an art form; now it could be done by any dummy strong enough to dump grain into a feeder.

Not only that, but with cheap grain, omnivores were no longer constrained to scavenge forest products or kitchen and garden scraps. Now farmers could pour grain into feeders and grow chickens and pigs for market. In turn, this cheapened chicken and pork to something common people could eat every day. Since pigs and poultry convert grains to meat more efficiently than herbivores, cattle had a decided disadvantage economically.

In general, a pig converts about three pounds of grain to one pound of animal, a chicken two pounds; but a beef requires about five to seven pounds of grain to gain a pound. With this new grain-based livestock paradigm, both pigs and poultry had a decided economic advantage over beef. During the last several decades, as the full import of this cheap energy/cheap grain situation expressed itself, poultry became the cheapest meat, pork next cheapest, and beef the most expensive.

In just a few short decades, the production/consumption ratios in place for millennia completely inverted. With the advent of drugs, these animals could be pulled off pastures and confined in tight quarters under a roof. Folks, this ain't normal.

If any piece of this abnormal model breaks down, it can't function. If energy became expensive, grain transport to these animal factories would be too expensive. If energy became expensive, the chemical fertilizer would be too expensive and fertility maintenance would revert to long rotations of pasture between cultivations. If drug development can't keep up with increasingly adapted and virulent pathogens, the animals will get sick and die. These are all very real scenarios and show the fragility of this system that most people think is efficient and expresses a rock-solid model that can feed the world. Nonsense.

The only, and I repeat only for emphasis, reason that the current grain-fed beef and dairy factory system works is because petroleum is cheap. Take that out of the equation, and the whole thing collapses. Indeed, if all herbivores returned again to perennial pastures using the biomimicry outlined above, not only would the meat and milk be of superior quality, but farmers would make more money and soil would build instead of eroding. And carbon would be sequestered in the soil instead of being pumped into the atmosphere via cultivation and petroleum use.

I asked Allan Nation, editor of *Stockman Grass Farmer*, what would happen if farmers universally understood the economic superiority of grass-based herbivore production. I naively assumed that a sudden shift to grass production would create a glut of grain that would be even cheaper. He is older and wiser than I am, and responded, "When farmers realize how much more money they can make growing grass instead of grain, they will stop growing grain. When that happens, grain prices will soar due to grain shortages. Grain prices would have to rise substantially to induce farmers to rip up their valuable grass and plant grains." His logic is perfect.

Indeed, if and when that happened, grain would become expensive — like normal. That would drive up the price of poultry and pork. Beef would return to being the least expensive meat, as it has been throughout history until cheap energy. At that point, grass would return as the dominant crop and our agriculture would begin building soil instead of destroying it.

In my book *The Sheer Ecstasy of Being a Lunatic Farmer*, I describe in more detail the economic benefits, to the farmer, of shifting from grain production to grass production. To be sure, this return to normalcy maintains production, ecology, and economics. The only losers are the petroleum, machinery, and confinement animal feeding operations — essentially, industrial agriculture. But everybody else wins. Don't worry, the losers will find something else to do that doesn't hurt the earth as much.

Now a word to those who think they are doing the environment a favor by eating chicken. Actually, I don't think we should eat so much chicken. If you really want to do something environmentally healing, eat forage-finished beef. And I don't mean beef fed some grain and some forage for thirty days. I mean forage-finished, period. Ditto for dairy.

I wish I had time in this book to go into all the whys and wherefores of how this can be done, how nutritious it can be, and how the economics work, but I've already addressed that in my other books. The point is that eating poultry from a cheap grain basis doesn't do the planet any favors. One of the most poignant and active environmental decisions you can make is to patronize 100 percent grass-based herbivores: beef, dairy, lamb, chevon, yak, bison, deer, antelope, elk, moose... you get the picture.

One final thought for those who are reading this, bewildered that I have concentrated on animals and pastures, who shake their heads and ask, "But what about tofu? What about vegetables?"

Tofu is from soybeans, and I don't have any problem with soybeans per se, but they are an annual. That requires tillage, or herbicide in a no-till situation. Of all the grains, soybeans are probably the most ecologically devastating. I realize that some people are working on no-till mulching systems. But no matter what system, soybeans require either animal manure or several years of pasture between plantings in order to keep the fertility up. You cannot escape the problem of tillage.

For all the soy milk and tofu lovers out there, historically normal ingestion of soybeans requires lacto-fermentation and eating volumes equivalent to condiments. *Wise Traditions* magazine probably devotes at least one major scientific article per quarterly issue to the devastating human problems caused by eating soy products the way modern Americans do. Soy products induce infertility, make boys effeminate, cause serious digestive disorders and a host of other maladies. Perhaps one of the best recent books on the subject — and extremely readable, by the way — is *The Vegetarian Myth* by Lierre Keith. Americans owe it to themselves to at least be exposed to the scientific community that discredits virtually everything the USDA and Monsanto spout as gospel. Remember, Monsanto loves it when you eat soy. In China, soybeans historically were grown as a cover crop because it's a legume; not to eat, but to plow down to feed the soil. That's normal. It's food for soil life and animals (and then only as a complement rather than mainstay), not humans.

Even the best vegetable operations inject copious amounts of forage into the system via mulching, fallow years, green manuring, or imported compost. Many organic operations use fish emulsion or dehydrated poultry manure. If you check with your organic vegetable grower, you'll find him using, more often than not, imports of products that originate in concentrated animal feeding operations. Again, cheap grain has skewed the value of manure to such an extent that it's cheaper to buy from an industrial animal factory than it is to grow on-site with integrated smaller-scale symbiotic animal operations. In other words, something that looks more like the regenerative, diversified, balanced farmstead of yesteryear.

Vegetables are heavy feeders. Cultivation exacts a heavy toll. Even Ruth Stout's famous *No-Work Garden Book* that utilized heavy annual mulching rather than tillage required importing lots of forage to the garden beds. Think about it: In nature, no system exists without animals. And by far and away the most productive systems involve herbivores. You can't escape it. You can't wish it away. It just is.

To be clear, I love vegetables as much as anyone. We have a huge garden at Polyface. We love our vegetables, and so should you. As I see it, the advantage of vegetables is that they can be grown in tiny spaces. Highly productive per square foot, they allow us to leverage small areas in proximity to where we live and work. They don't have to be fenced in like animals; they don't make any noise; they don't poop. This makes vegetables the ideal food to grow close to where we spend most of our time. In addition, since vegetables are 95 percent water, and water is heavy, it makes sense that the most water-based food item is most conducive to growing next to our houses and workplaces.

What other food item would be efficient to grow in pots on a patio? Only vegetables. A little area goes a long way with vegetables. We could literally grow all the vegetables we needed in this country simply by using our backyards, road edges, and vacant urban lots. Believe it or not, we really don't need square miles of produce grown in California or pivot-irrigated produce farms in Colorado. Organic or otherwise. We just don't need it. If we returned our close spaces to their historic use as vegetable and herb gardens, the industrial vegetable trade would be unnecessary.

By tucking vegetable production into these currently unused or underutilized spaces, these heavy feeders are also proximate to household dust cleaning, vermicompost from kitchen scraps, or chicken manure from our kitchen chickens. If we took all the biodegradable garbage currently overfilling landfills and sanitation trucks and converted that near where we eat into the fertility for vegetables, the delicious but heavy feeders would be a useful part of our domestic ecology. Using distant animal agriculture to give us healthy bodies so that we have energy to think, tote, and till in our vegetable gardens comes as close as about anything I can think of to historically normal multifaceted symbiotic homesteads.

For a more in-depth analysis of the traditional role that animals have played in cultures, I highly suggest Simon Fairlie's *Meat: A Benign Extravagance*. While I don't agree with everything in the book, it's close enough to be perfect. For a book with lots of figures, it reads like a novel.

Instead of fighting against the animal reality, embrace it for its value. Embrace it for its healing properties. Embrace it for its elegance. In the final analysis, a farm without herbivores just ain't normal.

Here are some gentle reminders from this chapter.

1. Grass is at least as efficient at sequestering carbon as trees.
2. Herbivores are nature's pruners to restart the grass biomass accumulation cycle.
3. Cows can be good or bad, depending on how they are managed.
4. To eat most ecologically, concentrate on grass-fed beef and grass-fed dairy.
5. Normal farms have animals.

Let's Make a Despicable Farm

Modern industrial agriculture touts concentrated animal feeding operations, or CAFOs, as the pinnacle of modern efficiency. A close corollary, of course, is the industrial produce farm or orchard, where large parcels of single-species plants create simple sameness across the landscape. Certainly corn and soybean farms are the plant equivalent of CAFOs. For context, be assured that most of what applies in this chapter to CAFOs also applies to any single-speciated, extremely large-scale farm model.

Confining thousands of animals under one roof certainly is not normal. This modern notion is brand-new in all of history. Never before has this been possible, because a CAFO requires several components.

CAFOs and Cheap Fuel

It requires cheap fuel because it depends on transported feedstuffs, manure, and production (animals, eggs, grain, milk, etc.). Up until recent CAFOs, animals were distributed around the landscape in diversified farms where the feed grew on or near the farm, the manure blessed the adjoining fields with fertility, and production was processed and consumed nearby. As localization gave way to regionalism, then nationalism, then globalism, transportation favored expensive items first. The more value per pound, the more likely its transport will pay for itself. Chicken feathers, for example, will be one of the last things transported. Diamonds will be one of the first.

You can afford to ship coffee, or tea, or spices. But shipping perishable fluid milk or lettuce is extremely expensive. The transportation costs the same per mile regardless of the value of the item being transported. That was the whole Aha! of FedEx, when someone figured out how many ten-dollar packages could go in a plane compared to fifty-dollar people in seats.

Back when transport energy required one-third of a farm's productive capacity, to maintain horses, oxen, or mules, it had to be used sparingly. Imagine every farm devoting one-third of its acreage to producing its energy. Some people think we're heading that way again. If that is true, the abnormality of the CAFO will become immediately apparent.

Bulky feedstuffs like hay or silage (fermented forages) cannot be transported very far because they are cheap per pound. The reason they are cheaper per pound than grain is because they don't pack as much nutritional punch per pound. Grain is much more valuable per pound, and therefore can be transported farther economically. Manure, especially if it is raw and juicy, is too cheap to transport as well. Compost, being much more valuable, can be transported farther economically. Because carbon is bulky and low in value, things like wood chips, sawdust, straw, and peanut hulls can't be economically transported very far. That is why CAFOs do not want to use bedding under the animals. CAFOs prefer slatted floors (the animals live on slats that allow all the manure to fall down into a pit below) or slurry systems (the manure is flushed into a giant lagoon that is periodically pumped onto fields). With all this hauling feed in and hauling manure out, the economics don't allow hauling carbon in too.

Historically, housed animals were always bedded with a carbonaceous diaper like straw or sawdust. The reason is because the manure's nutrients are highly volatile and soluble — if they get wet, they leach into the groundwater and become a toxic pollutant; and if they get dry, they vaporize into the air and are lost, except to our nostrils, which sting at the obnoxious stench. If manure is properly managed, it will never smell.

If you ever smell a stinky farm, be assured that it is wasting its most precious recyclable nutrients and depriving the land of important fertility.

A properly managed farm will be aromatically sensually romantic. If that one rule were applied across the board to America's food system, it would fundamentally change farming to a more normal system. The normal carbonaceous diaper not only soaks up and stabilizes nutrients, it also creates a habitat for healthy microbial activity to keep pathogens at bay. This bedding must be able to deepen in order to create a community with enough mass to maintain a vibrant nematode population to attack pathogens that would hurt the animals. And it takes a lot of carbon, but everything in modern industrial farming is geared toward reducing carbon usage, since it is not economical to haul.

Prior to modern mechanization, slurry systems didn't exist because technology had not invented the types of pumps necessary to load and distribute it. The only way to handle the sloppy bedding was with a manure fork — a special multitined, short-handled pitchfork especially designed for such activity. Raw manure is too sloppy to pick up with a fork, and too inefficient to handle with a shovel. If the animals are walking around in it, they get sick. The only answer, for centuries, was to bed down the animals by adding carbonaceous material to absorb the excrement. Bedding kept the animals healthier, the housing aromatically pleasant, and the cleanout job more efficient.

The most common bedding was straw — the plant part of small grain. In recent times, however, grains like wheat, rye, barley, and oats have been selectively bred to reduce the plant-to-seed ratio. When the combine harvests the grain, it cuts the plant with a knife and sends it through a winnowing mechanism that separates the heavy grain (seed) from the straw (plant material — leaves and stalk). The less straw, the faster the machine can run. Until CAFOs, the straw was nearly as valuable as the grain because it was necessary for bedding livestock, mulching chicken yards, and soaking up pig urine. Raw manure can't be stored, handled, piled, or seasoned without some bulky carbon to give it some body. Otherwise, it all falls through the spade or fork when you try to pick it up. It won't stack because it's too sloppy. And it stinks to high heaven.

I'm sure many old-timers did not realize some of the health benefits of the carbonaceous diaper they were putting down. They just knew you couldn't have healthy animals trudging around in their own feces, and the deeper it was the worse it was. In a day before modern wood chippers and leaf vacuums were developed, straw left over from grain production was the most efficient carbon to bind up this manure and make it healthy and bulky enough to handle.

But once combines came into being, all that changed. The reason they are called combines is because these machines combine the historically separate acts of cutting and threshing. For centuries the mature grain was scythed and later cut (Cyrus McCormick's reaper did away with the scythe) and shocked in the field, where the little teepee-like shocks could dry down and the husks would pull away from the grain, like shells pulling away from nuts when they get dry. A few weeks later, the shocks would be gathered up and run through a threshing machine. The threshing machine had sieves, fans, and shakers that flailed and winnowed the grain (remember the animals treading out the grain in the previous chapter) to separate it from the rest of the plant: husk, leaves, stalk. The plant material residue is all included in the general term "straw."

About the time machinery, and especially the combine, was coming into use, technological advances were cheapening the cost and increasing the quality of concrete. While these might seem like unrelated developments, they actually were symbiotic for developing CAFOs. Combining the acts of cutting and winnowing (threshing), the one-pass mechanical harvester worked much better with less straw. Geneticists worked feverishly to shorten grain stalks so the combine could go faster. Had the demand for straw held apace, farmers would have balked at the new short-stemmed varieties.

But things were changing on the farm. With concrete cheap enough to pour in quantity on farms, scrapable, flushable surfaces had agriculture giddy with the prospects of manure handling without straw. The race was on to get rid of straw. Soon, slurry pumps, augers, and tractor-mounted scraper blades and liquid manure spreaders answered the yearning for a beddingless system. For the first time in human history, animals did not need bedding. They could just poop on concrete and the farmer could hose it down or scrape it down every so often.

Don't ever underestimate the yearning of farmers to be freed from all that manure shoveling. With the advent of raw and liquefied manure handling systems, the need for carbon dropped precipitously. The

whole notion of handling raw manure is brand-new within the last half
century. Until then, all animal housing setups required copious amounts
of carbon. A carbonless manure handling system just ain't normal. In
all fairness, any of us in the same situation would have yearned for a
system that allowed us to escape hand-shoveling manure. Front-end
loaders and efficient mechanical bedding handling systems were developing simultaneously with the slurry technology. Unfortunately, most
farmers opted for the liquid slurry systems, which were the open door to
CAFOs. Farmers who appreciated historical normalcy and understood
the biology of deep bedding systems stayed with them, but handled the
material with front-end loaders.

Even with mechanical handling, the on-farm energy required to
load, haul, and spread carbon-based bedding systems was more than in
a liquid slurry system. The farmer handled all those materials. To most
farmers that looked like way too much effort. Reducing bulk by mini-
mizing material seemed, for most, a more energy- and effort-efficient
option. In a perfect illustration of trade-offs, farmers exchanged their
on-farm materials handling for energy-intensive chemical fertilizers.
Since energy was cheap and the farmer didn't have to expend that energetic effort, that seemed like a great trade-off.

Most farmers opted for moving the energy off the farm. The much
poorer use of their animal manures and the carbon shortfall was not
immediately apparent. All farmers knew was that they had extracted
themselves from the effort of handling carbon with a new system: concentrated chemical-based fertilizers. It was easier on the back, easier on
the pocketbook, and easier on the family. The bottom line is that
CAFOs have taken the carbon out of farming. As a result, on-site-
generated and locally originated carbon has been summarily thrown
into landfills for several decades while energy-intensive chemical-based
fertilizers make up the deficit. Nature can only be tricked for so long,
however, and many of today's problems like plant diseases, erosion,
compaction, and water repulsion indicate that nature will eventually
force a day of reckoning to balance the needs of the soil.

If all the lawn clippings, municipal leaves, and yard wastes generated
in the last seventy years had gone onto farmland instead of into landfills, we would not have needed the chemical-based fertilizers we used,
and that would have kept the soil from being destroyed. If our grain still

had all its stems and leaves, so that when we harvested grain it also generated twice as much carbonaceous straw, the carbon cycle would be in sync. The soil would rejoice.

CAFOs demand long-distance transportation because they are too big to be ecologically appropriate. They take animals, plants, and manure that are supposed to be in a symbiotic dance and separate the partners into toxic antagonists. Instead of the manure being a blessing, it becomes a hazardous waste, especially in fragile riparian (water) areas. Fish kills in North Carolina due to overflowing manure lagoons have occurred numerous times in recent years. Illinois and Iowa both have certainly seen their share of lagoon breakdowns. California mega-dairies have destroyed whole communities. Virtually every state with a CAFO has at least one nightmare story related to these horrible places. None of these nightmares could have happened as recently as a century ago. That many animals could not be concentrated in one place — it was logistically, hygienically, and transportationally impossible.

As this toxicity increases, the transportation necessary to maintain the system increases. Grain must be imported from farther and farther away because it can't be grown in sufficient quantities nearby. The manure must be transported farther and farther away, or burned to power electrical plants (in California). The animals must be imported from farther away because the locality cannot produce enough to feed into the system, and the production must be shipped farther away because it can't be consumed in the bioregion.

While all of this appears to be efficient, it actually is a house of cards that depends on cheap energy. Whenever the industry shows pictures of a CAFO and genuflects at these monuments to the depravity of man, the industrial apologist exclaims, "Look how much food we're producing in such a small acreage."

Whenever journalists come to our farm, the single biggest question is, "But is there enough land to produce it this way?" They see our pigs running around on pasture, in the woods. Chickens are out on the pasture. Cows graze contentedly. Yes, at first blush it seems like this takes more land.

But what you don't see when viewing the picture of that CAFO are the square miles of land required to produce the grain, and the square miles of land required to handle the manure generated by that facility.

The CAFO is not a stand-alone structure, rising out of the landscape in some sort of self-contained system. Every day a tractor-trailer drives up with a load of grain from some distant state or even continent and augers it into giant feed bins attached to the CAFO. Absent that intravenous injection nothing in that facility would live for a day. That production unit is completely dependent on huge tracts of land to grow the food and dispose of the manure. You don't see the pumps, augers, pipes, trucks, slurry lagoons, slurry spreaders, and trains bringing material in and hauling material out. That's not in the picture.

Let's assume for just a moment that the pastured livestock on our farm ate the same amount of imported feedstuffs as the same number in a CAFO. If that were the case, it would not take one more square yard of land to produce the feedstuffs for them than it would if they were housed in confinement. The consumption is identical. The only difference is where the animals are housed. But the fact is that our animals are spreading their own manure, displacing tons and tons of grain production, and being processed and consumed nearby.

It would not take one more acre of land to produce all the animals the world currently consumes if they were all raised like ours at Polyface. This system takes the energy out of the equation. When energy prices really spiked a couple of years ago, we performed a cost analysis of gross sales compared to energy used and we were different by a factor of 10. That's not 10 percent. That's 1,000 percent, compared to a typical industrial farm.

In other words, our fuel costs per dollar in gross sales are only 10 percent of an industrial farm's fuel costs as a percentage of gross sales. That's a lot less energy used per dollar in sales.

Make no mistake, the efficiencies ascribed to CAFOs can last only as long as energy is cheap. The day energy costs return to normalcy, CAFOs will no longer enjoy "economies of scale." They will instead be obsolete.

CAFOs and Drugs

CAFOs have only become possible with the advent of vaccines and pharmaceuticals. Prior to the 1940s, nobody could crowd animals into such tight places at such volumes without disease outbreaks. In fact, most disease outbreaks throughout history have been human-created due to the violation of some specific natural rule regarding density, mass, rest, sanitation, or diversity. Even the bubonic plague occurred during a mini–ice age that drove people indoors, an unprecedented commerce between Great Britain and continental Europe, and massive urbanization under extremely unsanitary and unhygienic conditions. That confluence of factors created the conditions pathogens exploited. Ditto for the Spanish flu in post–World War I America.

Industrial food advocates constantly jeer at me, "Look, we don't want to go back to undulant fever in cows, to Newcastle disease in chickens, hog cholera, smallpox, and whooping cough." They accuse me of being a Luddite, wanting us to all crawl back into some cave and die of tuberculosis.

Well, let's take a look at this in historical context. All innovation has a ragged edge. Around 1910, most metropolitan newspapers carried editorials predicting the demise of cities because they were being covered up in horse manure. With urbanization being the tip of that day's cultural innovation, not everything necessary to metabolize this societal sea change from an agrarian to an industrial economy was yet in place.

The medical community was still arguing about whether sterilizing knives between amputations was really essential. Without indoor plumbing, people took baths once or twice a winter. That was okay when you were just a family living out on the farm, but it got downright nasty when people moved to nonfamilial proximity in cities. Electrification was still a decade away. Sperm whale oil had just been replaced with petroleum oil, all of which was coming from western Pennsylvania and some gushers in Texas.

Stainless steel had not yet been invented; lots of sewage ran in open ditches and cows pooped in municipal drinking-water reservoirs. Chlorine hadn't yet been discovered and refrigeration wasn't invented. The point is that cultural innovation at the tip of urbanization preceded all the infrastructure, policy, and knowledge necessary to metabolize the innovation. This is the inherent nature of innovation.

Today, for example, state governments are going apoplectic over e-commerce because people are buying things without going through a retail store cash register. The standard retail transaction, taxed and controlled, is now being circumvented by a brand-new animal nobody knows how to tame. And state tax collectors are desperate to figure out how to tame e-commerce. This is a modern example of the ragged edge of innovation. The things necessary to assimilate the point of innovation lag behind the point — sometimes by decades, as we saw where there was no Manhattan Project for compost.

So placing yourself in 1910, urbanization had a counterpart in the countryside — industrializing farms, manifested primarily in the increased numbers of animals that a farmer could handle due to mechanical efficiencies. But these farms did not have vaccines, drugs, concrete readily available, front-end loaders, electricity, electric fences, or anything most farmers today would consider common. As a result, farmers began pushing the pathogen envelope.

Nice extensive pig lots that worked fine for five sows to run in and raise their piglets suddenly turned into toxic mud holes with twenty sows. The same thing happened with cows. Without refrigeration, breweries needed to locate in urban settings to satisfy a growing demand for beer. Breweries generated a waste product called distiller's grains. This had always been fed to poultry and pigs, and breweries had always been small enough to dispose of it in locally consumable lots. But not now. It was time to bring in the big eaters: cows.

Milk was a natural item to locate in the cities as well, because it was highly perishable like beer. As a result, confinement dairies began locating next to the large breweries as a synergistic way to recycle the distiller's grains. That abnormal feeding regimen created acidosis in the herbivore rumen, setting up the perfect environment for all kinds of maladies transferred through the milk.

The point of all this is that the diseases that wreaked havoc in the developed world during the 1870–1940 period were largely the result of inadequate infrastructure and knowledge, coupled with greed. Once drugs were discovered and manufactured cheaply, the idea of a CAFO could proceed. Much of the alleged pharmacological progress in the early 1900s was to reduce diseases created by an abnormal feeding, housing, and sanitation regimen. Had it not been for these abnormal farming systems, today's second-generation pathogens would not have developed.

And what do I mean by second-generation pathogens? I mean all those Latin squiggly words like *E. coli*, salmonella, campylobacter, and *Listeria*. And I would include things like MRSA and *C. diff.* in hospitals and antibiotic resistance that is becoming more and more rampant. This collateral damage is starting to take a larger toll on the population than ever.

In school we all learned about Louis Pasteur, who looked in a microscope, identified little bugs that he called germs, and decided that we'd all be healthier if these critters were annihilated. A French contemporary of his, who is still obscure to most people, had a different opinion. His name was Antoine Béchamp, and he advanced the terrain theory. He agreed that germs were bad guys, but postulated that what allowed them to advance on our health was the terrain we created in our immune systems. He argued that our immune systems, maintained by stress-free living, getting enough sleep, hygiene (like taking baths), sanitation (like washing dishes and mopping the floor), and diet created an immunological hedge of protection against these bad guys.

Pasteur, however, carried the day in the court of public opinion. He was more handsome, more flamboyant, and gave a better interview. He would have been a big hit on *Good Morning America* or *The Today Show*. Besides, his theory won widespread support because people love to be victims. We're hardwired to blame somebody or something else for our deficiencies. It's natural to focus on germs instead of immune systems.

Our culture still worships at the altar of the germ theory. I can prove it because we're much more interested in figuring out how to give free heavy metal–laden swine flu vaccinations to our little kiddos instead of ripping out high-fructose corn syrup vending machines from all the schools. Sugar is a significant contributor to immune dysfunction, but we don't hear much about that on the news. Building immune systems requires personal responsibility, and that's much harder than blaming germs. Besides, it's much more fun to kill than to heal. So the germ theory appeals to our morbidity.

Of course, germ theory gradually morphed into the whole cut-and-burn medical mentality. The terrain theory was more consistent with ancient healing arts like acupuncture, chiropractic, naturopathy, homeopathy, and all the rest of alleged medical quackery... that works. Germ theory works great in trauma, where you're dealing with a tsunami of enemy forces. But in a day-to-day wellness maintenance regimen, the terrain is the way to go. Interestingly, in one of the most famous death-bed recantations in all of history, folklore has it that Pasteur endorsed Béchamp moments before he died.

Let's imagine that we wanted to create a pathogen-friendly farm. Think with me: How could we make a really sick farm? We want sick animals, high vet bills, rampant pathogens. Okay, first we'd raise only one species of something. After all, we don't want any confused pathogens trying to figure out who the host is. And we certainly don't want any species unfriendly to the pathogen. Yes, monospeciation is the way to go. That means our farmers would be known as dairy farmers, beef farmers, chicken farmers, orchardists, vineyardists, vegetable growers. Yes, one species it shall be.

Second, let's crowd this one species together. We don't want those pathogens to expend any energy trying to find a great host habitat. After all, we wouldn't want these bugs to work for a living. Crowd up the hosts to make it as easy as possible for the pathogens to live and prolifer-ate. After all, the best way to combat an outbreak of flu in an elemen-tary school is to herd all the kids into the gymnasium and confine them there until the epidemic passes, right? We wouldn't want to call off school and have them all stay at home apart from each other. Clump them together; that's the way to stop the flu outbreak.

Third, let's make sure the animals don't get any exercise. Everyone knows couch potato humans are the most healthy. Make sure their lives are completely sedentary; the less they move around, the better. We wouldn't want muscle tone or healthy cardiovascular systems. Keep them flabby.

Fourth, grow them faster than anyone ever thought imaginable. Shoot the carbohydrates in their rations and blimp them up faster than you can say Jack Sprat. After all, fatter, bigger, faster, cheaper is the mantra of America's food system. We all know that machines run their most efficient when the pedal is to the metal and the engine is scream-ing at the highest RPMs possible. Animals are the same way. Wouldn't want them stunted, not realizing their full genetic potential. Rev them up. Varrooooom! Make them grow so fast they have heart attacks as juveniles. Make them grow so fast their livers swell to double normal size due to abscesses as the filter of the body works overtime to handle toxicity. Make them produce so much milk or lay so many eggs that they cannibalize the calcium right out of the skeleton trying to keep up with production. Leave them with no immune system left.

Fifth, deny them fresh air and sunshine, nature's number one sanitizers. Nothing breaks down pathogenicity like a good airing out in the sun, so we won't abide anything like that on this pathogen-friendly farm. Let's make sure not a ray of sunshine dapples their existence. And make sure the air they breathe is laden with fecal particulate that abrades their tender mucous membranes, creating lesions that allow this fecal particulate to pass right into the bloodstream and override respiratory filters. That way pathogens can fill and consume the inside of the animals in addition to the outside. Wow, we're really getting somewhere. This is fun. Look how easy this is.

Sixth, let's dope them up with drugs to override their immune systems. That will create lethargic immune systems more susceptible to pathogens when they arise.

Seventh, we'll feed them junk food. Sure, unnatural food like dead cows, chicken manure, dead chickens, and grain to herbivores. We'll feed industrial grease residue to chickens. And let's feed pastry wastes to pigs. And the grains we feed, let them be grown with artificial chemical fertilizers so the plants are deficient in vital enzymes and nutrients. Feed only the bare minimum minerals instead of the maximum — always feed to the minimum, not the maximum.

Okay, folks, what have we just described? Modern American CAFOs. And folks, I've got news for you, this ain't normal. Nothing about it is normal. It's not normal for the animals, not normal throughout civilized history, it's not normal for ecology, energy flows, or carbon cycling and sequestration.

In my half century of farming, I have personally experienced three disease outbreaks on our farm, and each time it was my fault. Let me describe each one of them. The first one was around 1990 with broilers. We began having a serious problem with toes curling up at about a week of age. The chicks quickly became immobile, their paralyzed legs hopelessly weak.

Unable to figure out the problem, I took a couple of the chicks to the state laboratory for diagnosis and learned that it was curly toe syndrome and the only solution was to feed antibiotics. The state lab gave me a printout of all the antibiotics useful to combat this inflammation of the nerve sheath and half of them were already useless: The staph infection had built up an immunity to those antibiotics. The chicks were growing too fast for the slower-growing nerve sheaths to keep up with the fast-growing skeleton and muscle tissue. This friction created a staph infection that resulted in the paralysis and eventual death.

Not ready to concede defeat, I looked in my human health and wellness books for what was necessary to maintain nerve health. Vitamin B. What contains large amounts of Vitamin B? Organ meats and greens. Ah, this explained why once I got the birds out on pasture, the problem subsided fairly quickly and the birds were fine. I went to the freezer, grabbed some beef liver, and fed it to the chicks. I had already begun isolating the birds that came down with the malady in a type of hospital pen. They attacked the thawing liver, pecking away at it until even the paper wrap was consumed. The next day, miraculously, several of them were up and walking around.

I kept the liver going to them. Sure enough, virtually all the chicks were up and ambulatory in the next couple of days. Now folks, don't miss a couple of key lessons to this story. First, realize that at this point, I was dealing not only with a nerve problem created by a vitamin deficiency, but also a violent true-blue staph infection. Not only did the liver deal with the nerve issue, it also wiped out the staph infection. Remember that the best taxpayer-funded medical advice was to feed antibiotics as the only remedy even though this disease was already immune to more than half of the potential antibiotics. Yeah, right. How long do you think we can continue trying to outsmart nature? Hmmmmm?

What had caused this problem? We didn't have enough vitamins in their ration. Genetically, the birds were growing faster than the octane of our fuel. At about that time, we discovered Fertrell in Bainbridge, Pennsylvania, and began using their organic premixes of minerals and vitamins in our ration: end of problem to this day. Ultimately, this curly toe malady was my fault, not the birds' fault.

Story number two. Around 1998 we had a lady contact us to raise five hundred ready-to-lay pullets for her. She wanted to start an egg laying operation but didn't want to raise the chicks up to laying age, a period of five months. She knew we had brooding capacity and asked if we'd raise them for her. We said we'd only raise them to about ten weeks because we didn't have enough capacity to go the whole five months. At least by ten weeks they would be old enough to go to her farm without need of supplemental heat from the brooders.

All sounded fine. At ten weeks, we called her to come and get them and she informed us that she had changed her mind after all and didn't want them. This was also the year we labeled "The Year Without a Summer." It was damp and cold all spring. We received double our normal rainfall. We couldn't find anyone else who wanted those five hundred pullets, and we weren't about to destroy them, so we kept them in the crowded brooder. We didn't have anyplace else to put them. The birds were too crowded, but the weather was so bad we dared not put them out to pasture yet.

Soon we noticed some start getting thin, then dying. A couple a day, then several a day. We knew they were too crowded. We couldn't wait any longer. They needed room. So we took them out to pasture with a portable shelter and prayed that the weather would moderate and we'd get some warm days. It did not. Now the birds had plenty of room, but they were exposed, and in their weakened condition, they were even more susceptible to whatever was killing them. I looked in my poultry disease books and found the culprit: Marek's disease. Dead ringer.

Cause: unhygienic conditions. Cure: vaccination. Once they have it, there is really no cure; it just has to run its course, and the veterinary books say you can lose up to 90 percent of the flock. We lost about 60 percent until it quit, but the birds were never strong after that. The next year, we vaccinated. We repeated that for a couple more years and finally quit once we felt like the danger of residues reinfecting birds was past.

Again, the thing to remember about this was that it was totally our fault. Oh, we could blame the lady who reneged on her deal, but that didn't change the fact that it was absolutely and completely our management that created a terrain that allowed this opportunistic pathogen to rear its ugly head. By the way, our farm had raised chickens continually for nearly forty years without ever seeing this. But this particular year, our management deficit had broken down the immunological hedge of protection.

Story number three. We had rented a new farm in the area, and like most farms we rent, it had not received extremely good management prior to our arrival. On this one the pastures were covered with out-of-control blackberry canes. I mean, this was the mother lode. The canes were twelve feet tall with spines that jumped out on you as you walked by. If I'm lying I'm dying. They would shoot out their stickers, embed them in your fingers, ears, and knees. They were alive, these brambles. Horrible.

We took over a herd of two hundred stocker calves, about five or six hundred pounds average, to begin grazing the place. To encourage the calves to stomp out the blackberries and begin the healing process, we placed the mineral box (a two-foot-square wooden trough that holds supplemental salt, seaweed, vitamins and minerals) in the middle of these patches. Some patches covered an acre (about the size of a football field), but most of them were only a few yards in diameter. We would stomp out a little path to the mineral box so the calves could find it, then leave them to do their best.

After a week, we lost a calf. One of the nicest ones. The next day, we lost another one. The next day, two. Now folks, it's one thing to lose a chicken, but quite another to lose a calf. Everyone that has animals loses one from time to time, but calves are worth a lot more than chickens. I called the vet to get a diagnosis. He cut into the hind leg muscle of one that had just died and it was black: blackleg. It's a protozoan that lives in the soil.

The cure: antibiotics. The veterinary books were full of dire forebodings about this disease, a scourge to American cattle producers, who all generally vaccinate for it. Except us. I remember losing a calf or two to blackleg back in the 1960s, but we culled the cow that had the calf that had blackleg and never had any more problems with it. We figure all things being equal, if one calf gets sick and the rest stay healthy, that cow is responsible for that calf. Period. And if she can't put enough will to live, immunity, or healthy vigor into that calf to keep it alive, then she needs to be put in the freezer.

Well, here we were, four dead calves, two sick ones, and a herd of two hundred — er, 196 — looking at us wanting answers. Now, I'm a bit of a lunatic, but not totally foolish, so we took the vet's advice, bought $200 worth of antibiotics, got the whole herd into the corral the next morning, and doped them. Like I said, I may be weird, but I'm not foolhardy — or at least not that foolhardy. Yes, we injected the whole herd with a dose of antibiotics, and we didn't lose another single one. Stopped it cold turkey.

But why? Why there? Although I was glad we stopped it, I wanted to know more. I never wanted this to happen again. So I began searching in all my beef books. I looked up blackleg in every book I have, and my library is fairly extensive. I was down to the last book, and in despair. Every single one said the only cure was vaccination (that's why America's farmers vaccinate for it). Dead ones needed to be burned or buried covered in lime. We had let nature's buzzards take care of the dead ones. That seems more natural to me, and besides, the buzzards are critters that need to eat too. If it weren't for them, this old world would be a pretty smelly place. Thank God for the salvage recyclers.

Anyway, in the last book in my library, in the last paragraph, I read this astounding sentence: "Protozoa live in the soil and gain access to the body through anaerobic puncture wounds, often caused by brambles." Eureka! Indeed, in our effort to stomp out those gargantuan blackberries, we had turned these calves into veritable pincushions. No wonder they got blackleg.

We immediately declared jihad on the brambles and mowed them down with our heavy-duty rotary mower/brush cutter. What a job that was. Even standing on top of the tractor, those canes would dangle over and scratch my head as I drove through. The rabbits and groundhogs that came out of those thickets were legion. But I was on a mission to prepare a healthy landscape for these calves. I'm sure the foxes had some easy pickin's after that job, but we never had another incidence of blackleg, all the way to today. And we created a terrain that maintained the healthy skin on those calves so their immune systems would not be overwhelmed.

I think it's actually much more beneficial to take responsibility for the problem. The learning that happens when we look at a mess and assume it's our fault enables us to grow as individuals, to listen to what life is trying to teach us. To assume these animals are getting sick because some disease fairies sprinkled foo-foo dust on them may sound nice for a while, but ultimately we don't become better people with that attitude. Instruction comes when we humbly ask, "What did I do to make this happen?" At that point, our eyes and ears — indeed, our minds — open and we can hear things others may not hear, and see things others may not see. The others are too busy blaming something or picking up something in a bottle to remedy the problem.

To reiterate, CAFOs have only been possible in the age of pharmaceuticals. As large as the drug industry is in America, it should give us pause that we are ingesting far more drugs secondhand through animals that we eat than we are taking directly via pills and injections. As the surviving viral or bacterial diseases adapt with increased virility, CAFOs are betting that new concoctions from the pharmaceutical industry can stay at least a few days ahead of the mutants. Are we as a culture really willing to bet on that?

Wired for CAFOs

CAFOs required sophisticated infrastructure that wasn't available before the 1940s. The myriad electric motors required to move feedstuffs from storage bins, whether they be silos or grain hoppers, couldn't be used until rural electrification was complete. Rabun Gap, Georgia, did not receive rural electrification until 1965. Our area, just three hours from Washington, D.C., did not receive it until the late 1940s. It wasn't just electricity that enabled CAFOs to come into existence. It was also farm-affordable concrete, rebar, and specific metal castings to make grates and augers. Flexible augers and feed chains, with technologically advanced designs that enabled these devices to go around corners, was part and parcel of this development.

Indeed, today, poultry factories have sophisticated monitoring devices to measure temperature, air flow, and water consumption. Even drip medicators are on monitors so that if anything moves outside a set of standards, a pager goes off on a manager's belt to alert him about the problem. These managers cannot go to church or family socials without being wired to their CAFO monitors. The whole system, for all its seeming strength and power, is actually incredibly fragile.

On our farm, if the electricity goes off, the pastured poultry just go right along about their business. Although weather fluctuations carry their own set of stockmanship requirements, our awareness is plugged into the observable climatic and macroenvironmental conditions, not some R2D2 device purring away on the wall hooked into a pager on our belts.

The whole rationale behind CAFOs is to increase output per person, to make everything run with minimal human input. After all, CAFOs are not enjoyable places to be due to the stench and stressed animals, so who wants to work there? If you drive up to the average CAFO, you won't see anybody. It's a monolithic structure dominating the landscape, without human presence. The CAFO goes against everything a farm should be. A farm should be a place where the human presence cares and nurtures, where human presence drives the design and activities. A personless farm seems like an oxymoron. A personless farm? Doesn't everyone who visits a farm want to meet the farmer? What's a farm without the farmer?

Historically, the farmer was a dominant presence on the farm, not the buildings and machinery. It was the relationship the farmer had with his plants and animals that filled storybooks and attracted visitors. Now we have farms that are unfeeling, clanking piles of machinery chugging along without visible human presence. The nostalgic farm family has been replaced with concrete, wires, and steel. The bond between farmer as caretaker and the biology under his direct stewardship no longer exists. The farmer merely checks computer printouts and whirring machinery.

Again, the CAFO apologists would like you to believe the farmer actually does all of this. But like the cell phone commercial where a parade of technicians follows the guy asking, "Can you hear me now?" these buildings require a huge off-farm team of technical support. When industry representatives effuse to me, "Look how much one farmer can produce," I like to add, "Yes, the farmer plus a host of technicians, mechanics, field reps, drug companies, construction crews, pollution abatement workers, and logistics managers." These are not stand-alone self-contained farm operations. They are monstrosities with a host of personnel behind the scenes making sure things function.

It's unfair to hang all this production on the farmer, as the CAFO apologists do. "Look how many people he's feeding!" they gush. The bottom line is that while it may look like the industrial farm runs on its own, it doesn't. The perception that all this production occurs with very little labor is actually a charade. Also, let's not forget the doctors treating people with foodborne illnesses because of these CAFOs, or the people suffering with *C. diff.* and MRSA, the nursing staff and medical staff taking care of them because of drugged dinners due to animals needing pharmaceuticals to stay alive in these unhealthy conditions. If you took all the personnel and collateral damage associated with this efficiency, it would not look efficient at all. Oh, you can include in that the military personnel stationed around the world to make sure oil stays cheap in order to operate these CAFOs. Add that in, and suddenly this stalwart of American efficiency crumbles like a house of cards.

There you have it, folks. I hope you can now see that when we force habitats that aren't normal on animals and plants, we're going to reap some evil compensation. CAFOs are not normal in any way, shape, or form. They hurt the animals. They assault the landscape. They disrespect the carbon cycle. They guzzle energy. They displace the human element. Folks, CAFOs just ain't normal.

Here are some points to ponder.

1. Examine the terrain of your life, emotionally, spiritually, physically, mentally, vocationally, relationally — is it healthy?
2. If something is out of whack, ask, "What can I do to heal it?"
3. Get together with others in your community and write a local ordinance banning CAFOs in your jurisdiction.
4. Patronize non-CAFO meat, dairy, and poultry products.
5. Remember the carbonaceous diaper — it doesn't even stink.

Scientific Mythology: Centaurs and Mermaids Now in Supermarkets

Corporations owning life. Scientists taking DNA out of plants and putting it into animals, or vice versa. Shooting electron cannons into genes to split off or insert strange chromosomes. Pigs without stress genes. Pollen wafting across fields, sterilizing neighbors' crops. Folks, this ain't normal.

Transgenic modification, commonly known as genetically modified organisms (GMOs) or genetic engineering, is certainly the most abnormal thing being done today and perhaps the most scary. Proponents hold it up as the answer to all of the world's problems. Opponents see it as the most sinister and potentially damaging invention humankind has ever developed. I tend to be in the latter group, in case you're wondering.

First, let's deal with the common retort: "Oh come on, this is just selecting things like people have been doing since the dawn of civilization. This is just an extension of Mendel's peas, an extension of hybridization, just good breeding management. Every farmer does this when he selects one bull over another."

That is exactly why I prefer the term "transgenic" rather than simply "genetic modification." Through selective breeding, in the technical sense of the term, humans have been practicing genetic modification.

When the industry picked up this term as its preferred description, it used clever wordsmithing. Make no mistake, the industry hires the best of the best in order to derail opposition before it starts.

The truth is that this process of genetic manipulation is nothing like selective breeding or hybridization. It is different in many ways, and to help accentuate the differences, I will use the term "transgenec" throughout this discussion. Refusing to let the opposition determine the lingo is one of the strongest ways to maintain clarity.

Historically, genetic selection did not cross-speciate, except perhaps for the mule (a donkey crossed with a horse), but that was still close enough for natural mating. No DNA was bombarded with cannons to force extremely alien material into the genetic structure. If the service couldn't happen with normal male and female organs, it didn't happen. That means the organs had to work together. The plumbing had to match up. Do I need more graphic language here?

In all historic selective breeding programs, the penetrating male and the hollow female sex organs had to fit, to embrace, to connect. That a human was outside the breeding chamber selecting which pairs to mate did not override this compatible plumbing requirement. You could spend a lifetime putting a corn plant and a moth in the same room, but they just won't get it together. You could play soft music, light some candles, add some incense, deliver pizza, wash dishes, give diamond rings, go to Vegas — whatever. You could do that all day, every day, for a million years, and I guarantee you that the corn and moth would not get it on. It just wouldn't happen.

Mood has nothing to do with it. Timing has nothing to do with it. Size of the sex organs has nothing to do with it. I remember well watching a little Scottish Highlander bull service some long-legged Holstein dairy cows on a farm in Minnesota. The cows would go in and out of a barn to be milked, and right at the door, the barn was about eighteen inches above the ground. The bull would wait right inside the door, and when a receptive cow brushed by him, he'd leap on her as she stepped off that eighteen inches, and it was just enough for him to do the job. Quite entertaining. He didn't get every one, but he sure didn't miss much. He had it timed to the inch and the fraction of a second. Bam! Fortunately, it was a small herd of cows so he only had to do about one a week. Any more frequently and he probably would have hurt himself.

Folks, a corn plant mating with a moth just ain't normal. And nature protects its species distinctiveness by creating all sorts of plumbing permutations. The sex organs of flowers are way different than those of whales. Then you have the honeybees, where mating always results in the drone's death, but that one mating is good for thousands and thousands of eggs. Let's be frank. If you and I walked into a garden and saw a tomato getting it on with a pig, we'd freak out. We would immediately wonder what trickery, what video tomfoolery was being played on us.

I'm belaboring the point to help us all understand that nature protects itself from the very things transgenic modification says are perfectly normal. Transgenic manipulation requires an unprecedented hubris, and for that reason alone we should approach it cautiously. If nature seems to have an antipathy for certain procedures, you would think we humans would assume these incompatible plumbing fixtures are for a reason. Maybe a reason we can't yet comprehend, but a reason nonetheless.

The terms "biomimicry" and "biometrics" describe sciences in which biological patterns are assumed to be important. We don't just wade into biological patterns and assume they are dysfunctional. The fact that an herbivore doesn't eat carrion should make us assume that herbivores eating carrion has dangers. And yet for several decades, the USDA and its British counterparts encouraged farmers to feed carrion to herbivores — i.e., dead cows to cows. In fact, the USDA continues to encourage the practice with dead chickens fed to cows. This is being done right here in my neighborhood, and that meat goes right into America's supposedly safe food supply. Aren't you glad your beef is from an animal that was eating dead chickens and chicken manure? Yum. And the USDA wants you and me to think it is the repository of food safety.

For decades, the USDA taught and encouraged farmers like me to feed dead cows to cows as a cheaper way to feed them. Our family, and a handful of other farmers like us, did not buy into this junk science. We didn't buy into it because try as we might, we could not find a single pattern in nature that supported herbivores eating carrion. Cows eating dead cows violated every natural principle we could find. Yet the USDA touted this as scientific, progressive, and state-of-the-art. And we want to put these folks at the helm of food safety regulations? Give me a break.

While land grant universities were cranking out research projects and master's theses and papering the media with reports of this scientific breakthrough, the owner of the small neighborhood abattoir I use to process our beeves and hogs quit buying cattle that had been fed chicken manure and dead cows. He said the meat stunk. He said he got tired of his chill room reeking of chicken manure stench. This type of feeding is still being done throughout the industry. The FDA and USDA think this is great science-based progressive production. I call it sinful, evil, and a violation of nature's rules. And these government agencies are in charge of food safety. Don't you feel secure?

How have we arrived at this kind of thinking? It's because in our Greco-Roman Western compartmentalized systematized fragmented individualized disconnected parts-oriented worldview, our culture views life as fundamentally mechanical. It is interchangeable parts. It is a rearrangement of protons, electrons, and neutrons. It's a huge Tinkertoy set, or a big box of Legos. It contains no mystery. No ethics. No morality. Respect is not necessary.

In the movie *Jurassic Park*, the euphoric scientist, ecstatic over his cloned raptors and other dinosaurs, completely fails to grasp their destructive capabilities even while they eat people, crush cars, and destroy civilization. Although he sees mayhem, he's drunk with achievement rather than remorse. And so the journalist confronts him with the central question of the movie: "But sir, just because we can, should we?" That pregnant question is worth asking every day, for many things.

This is why for much of my life now I've been trying to undo my westernized damaged brain by tempering it with some Eastern holistic community-based, we're-all-relatives connected kind of thinking. A culture that views animals and plants as inanimate piles of protoplasmic structure to be manipulated however cleverly hubris can imagine to manipulate it will view its citizens the same way. And other cultures the same way. Our respecting and honoring the pigness of the pig, therefore, creates the ethical and moral framework upon which we respect and honor the Maryness of Mary and Tomness of Tom.

It is how we respect and honor the least of these that determines how we honor and respect the greatest of these. As a culture, as a nation, we cannot occupy a respected place in the world unless and until we restore sacredness to life. You and I are much more than a dissected pile of organs, blood, bone, and flesh. Life is more than just pieces and parts; it is breath, interaction, spontaneity. Gifts and talents, creativity and intuition, entrepreneurship and work ethic — these define the individual as much as hair color, skin color, and language.

Indeed, our Western accounting methods do not even measure the most valuable things in life. Can you imagine going into a bank for a loan and presenting your business plan to the loan executive, who after studying it rears back in his posh swivel chair and beams: "Why, my lad, this is the best business plan I've ever seen. You're going to be a millionaire within a year. You are a genius."

Then the officer leans forward, suddenly changing expression, elbows on desk, earnest concern knitting his brow: "*But*, what will this do to your marriage? To your children? To the earthworms in your community?" Have you ever heard of such a thing? Of course not. And yet what millionaire successful businessman, losing his marriage, disrespected by his children, wouldn't give it all up to have the adoration of his wife and honor of his children? Where is that value in the business plan? How about the value of clean air, soil, and water? Where is that on the IRS statement? Intuitively, we all know that these things are far more valuable than Wall Street, and yet we skip nonchalantly along as if these things don't matter. And eventually, when they begin catching up to us, we wonder how we ended up here.

Like bovine spongiform encephalopathy, commonly known as mad cow disease. All those nice scientists from 1970 to 2000 sitting in their Presbyterian and Lutheran church pews on Sunday telling the world that feeding dead cows to cows was a wonderful way to feed everyone because their parts-and-pieces worldview said so. Eventually, they were jolted out of their self-assured righteousness when mad cow raised its ugly head. But they didn't repent in sackcloth and ashes, like they should have. Oh no, they went about their Western thought processes with nary a break in stride.

The new thing was transgenetic modification. Why didn't all those scientists hold a nationwide, yea, a worldwide week of mortification, fasting, and humble repentance for foisting mad cow upon the world? Why? Because by the time mad cow arrived on the balance sheet, they'd already moved on to researching how to extract the porcine stress gene, thereby rendering pigs numb to further factory farming abuses. If they could figure out how to eliminate stress from pigs, more could be crammed into tighter stalls, fed poorer feed, and disrespected more profoundly, but at least pigs wouldn't worry about it anymore. Folks, this is being done right now at land grant universities with our tax dollars. Is this the kind of despicable world you want to live in?

Why do chickens have beaks? So they can be cut off, of course. Why do we have to cut them off? So they don't cannibalize each other in their cell, where each bird does not even have enough space to lie down at the same time. If this incredible lack of respect defines our current modern culture's attitude toward our animals, then how much respect can we have for our neighbors?

Monsanto, arguably the world leader in transgenic modification, has sued when a neighbor's crops have been affected by seed from patented Monsanto crops. Let's get this straight: Monsanto creates brand-new life forms that could never occur with historically respectful mating procedures. Because the powers that be, both Republican and Democrat, worship at the altar of conquistador hubris and Western parts-oriented thinking, Monsanto can patent these life forms.

Monsanto or its duplicitous and complicit farmers plant these new life forms. These new life forms contain seed and secrete an orgy of sexual material called pollen, which drifts on the air currents. This seed contaminates, or maybe the pollen impregnates, a neighbor's old life forms, normal life forms, historically respectable life forms, bio-mimicked life forms. Are you with me here? Isn't this kind of like your neighbor coming over and spray-painting your house? Wouldn't you think Monsanto would be liable for its out-of-control seed or encroaching on the neighbor's plants? I mean, the neighbor may be expecting his plants to grow like the seeds he planted. But no, now suddenly those plants are adulterated. Wouldn't you think the owner of those new life forms would be responsible for keeping them home, to ensure that they can't just run rampant, inflicting their odd protein and Frankenstein DNA structure on the neighborhood?

What if someone's dog ran loose breeding with everyone else's pooches? Wouldn't an animal control officer show up, badge and gun in intimidating display, to tell the offending dog owner, "Listen, buddy, you'd better keep your dog at home."

But Monsanto enjoys a special dispensation — indeed, a brand-new interpretation of personal property and responsibility. In fact, a brand-new interpretation of the Golden Rule. In this hubris, according to Monsanto, it's "Do unto others whatever you want with blatant disregard for their well-being, their security, or their desires." Because, dear people — are you sitting down? The courts of our culture have ruled that the poor abused neighbor, the one with the new life forms that came in from Monsanto's plants, is liable for this unsolicited orgy in his fields.

In other words, the neighbor whose plants were contaminated by Monsanto's adventurous and predatory life forms is liable for patent infringement. Jeffrey Smith in *Seeds of Deception* and Marie-Monique Robin in *The World According to Monsanto: Pollution, Corruption, and the Control of Our Food Supply* have done a masterful job of exposing this malevolent, despicable batch of evil humans we call Monsanto. And what's most amazing, President Barack Obama, supposed friend of the common man, has put Monsanto's own vice president, GMO shepherd Michael Taylor, in charge of food safety. It's hard to comprehend a more obvious example of intellectual schizophrenia. It makes you wonder who really is running the country.

President's Obama's secretary of agriculture, Tom Vilsack, was voted Governor of the Year by the transgenic-loving industrial agriculture sector when he was governor of Iowa. Is it any wonder he would approve transgenic alfalfa, more corn, and sugar beets? As of April 1, 2011, eighty-one transgenic crops have been approved by the USDA, and not one single request has been denied. Who in their right mind thinks these people should be in charge of food safety?

With all the press devoted to organics, local foods, and farmers' markets in the last couple of years, proponents of these trends too often think we've won the day. This is a huge mistake. In early 2011, the official organic market share was 3 percent of food consumed. Local is under 2 percent. Even if there were no overlap, this heritage-based type of food is still less than 5 percent of America's food system. Sometimes I have to check my euphoria about the new interest in these issues with the stark truth that every day, Washington, D.C., consumes five tractor-trailer loads of french fries. Wrap your head around that one time.

The local, ecological, normal food system receives an inordinate amount of press for a couple of reasons. First, it's new. New always excites journalists. Second, this awareness is a direct extension of the environmental movement, which has been owned by the more liberal political side. Journalists by their own admission tend to lean about 80 percent liberal. In general, journalists love environmentalist farmers. But don't be naïve. When the doors close on the politicians, they know more Americans drink Mountain Dew and believe Monsanto than drink raw milk and believe Alice Waters. Sorry, Alice.

Part of English jurisprudence is the sacred notion of property. Your house is your castle. Even the Pentateuch uses property and animals as an extension of self. The kind of attitude, both corporately and cultur- ally, that says I must pay Monsanto for life forms that trespassed from their garden into my garden is indescribably preposterous. It's the kind of thing that makes us stutter. How do you find words to describe this travesty of justice? This travesty against everything that is reasonable? Folks, this ain't normal. Our culture has lost its collective mind.

Take a stiff drink and sit down for this. Our culture now believes that if your open-pollinated heirloom tomato plant, that you've lovingly planted, weeded, watered, and nurtured, gets impregnated by the neighbor's Monsanto transgenic Frankenstein tomato, *you* must pay Monsanto royalty fees for using their prostitutes. That's what this is. It's prostitution food. All of life can be owned by the highest bidder. And if you think people are promiscuous, check out the plants. Their orgasm of pollen just drifts along on the wind, where any partner will do.

When they first began working on transgenic life forms, scien- tists said that the pollen would stay at home. After all, they knew pol- len doesn't travel very far. Kind of like the arrogance with which Dr. Francis Collins and the Human Genome Project began mapping human DNA, assuring everyone that they would find at least 100,000 pairs due to the statistical probability analysis carefully docu- mented on computer spreadsheets, based on known genetic variability. Ahem. The reason the project finished a year ahead of schedule was not because the scientists were efficient, but because they only found 25,000.

Their conclusion, in a rare form of scientific humility, was, "There must be a lot of hanky-panky going on up and down the DNA to account for the variations, and we don't know how that happens." Well,

I'll be. You mean you're willing to admit that something is still mysterious? Quick, call the *New York Times*, get this on the front page: "Science Admits Mystery."

Yet Monsanto goes wading into this field like a swashbuckling pirate, with peg leg and patch, shooting at random, exploding genetic havoc into our gardens and animals. If for no other reason than these life forms cannot be kept home, transgenic manipulation should be terminated. That alone is enough reason to pull the plug. Can you imagine if I created a huge vehicle that could start itself, steer itself, and that I couldn't turn off, and I released it on a community? Everyone would be outraged. They'd demand that I stop construction until I could prove that it wouldn't run over somebody's child or through their living room.

Monsanto does the equivalent and the culture puts its attorneys in charge of food safety. This type of inconsistency between thought and practice is more typical than most of us are willing to admit. In fact, all of us have our inconsistencies, even though they are a lot easier to spot in others than in ourselves.

Ultimately, my respect toward the pigness of the pig is grounded in design. For me, it's a benevolent Creator's design. For others, it's evolutionary design by functionality. To others who follow the Gaia theory, Mother Earth invented the pig. In any case, to view DNA as no more special or sacred than a piece of plastic or extruded copper fitting is to approach all of life as a simple mechanical function. Biology is more than mechanics.

As John Ikerd, regenerative agriculture evangelist and professor emeritus of agriculture economics at the University of Missouri, says, the pillars of industrialism are simplification, specialization, routinization, and mechanization. That is not biology. I suggest that biological systems, in direct opposition, are complex, diversified, spontaneous, and dynamic. This is the great epiphany that awaits scientists who view life through a mechanical worldview.

This is what Sir Albert Howard, godfather of scientific aerobic composting, said in his foundational book *An Agricultural Testament*: "Artificial manures lead inevitably to artificial nutrition, artificial food, artificial animals, and finally to artificial men and women." By every measure vegetables grown today with artificial fertilizers contain less nutrition than those grown in compost. The nutrient profile of meat, poultry, dairy, and eggs grown on pasture versus factory-grown is as different as night and day.

You can't just take apart a grain of wheat, analyze its components, then fabricate them in a laboratory and recreate the same nutrition. The whole is worth more than the sum of the parts, and though that is a very Eastern concept and finds no quarters in our enlightened Western heads, it is nonetheless true. This is the theme of Michael Pollan's fabulous examination of modern nutrition science in his book *In Defense of Food.* Transgenic modification is the same worldview, the same mechanical mindset, used by food fabricators as they create amalgamated, reconstituted, extruded, genetically prostituted pseudo-food.

I am not a scientist. And neither are most people. I learned long ago to lead with the heart rather than the head because, ultimately, all of us make choices based on emotion. We really aren't rational beings. But we know what we know. We know what we've seen. Our perceptions are a collection of experiences and exposures.

I learned long ago at farmers' markets that most people can't handle science. I would crack out one of our eggs in a saucer and one from the supermarket in a saucer, displaying them prominently at the front of our market table. Women would come by, children in tow, and ask what I was demonstrating. I started out with vitamin B and polyunsatured fat, and by the tenth word the child was pulling on Mommy's arm, pleading, "Mommy, can we go now? This guy is boring."

After this happened a couple of times, I decided to switch to the Socratic method (I pride myself in being a fast learner when it comes to communication). To the query, "What are you showing here?" I responded in like manner: "What do you see?"

She'd stop and say, "Well, this one has rich color and the other one is kind of pale."

I'd reply, "What's the first thing you notice in your children when they aren't feeling well?"

Now folks, a word to the wise on this one: Don't try this with men. It doesn't work. I've never met a man yet who saw discolored cheeks in his kiddos. Only women can see this. Fortunately, all the shoppers are women, so you're pretty safe duplicating this line of questioning.

To which she would answer, "Oh, their cheeks get pale, off color."

Then, after a moment's hesitation, the Aha! moment: "Oh, healthy eggs, sick eggs."

"Bingo! You got it. You are so clever and observant and a wonderful mother. Our world would be so much better if we had more tuned-in mothers like you. Congratulations." By this time, beaming Mom is totally captivated by my song and dance.

"What else do you see?" I press.

She looks again, eager for another home run in this Socratic test. "Well, this one stands high up and the other one is kind of spread out."

"Have you ever heard of muscle tone?" You have to be very discreet on this question. Never ask the more obvious corollary, "Have you ever heard of middle-aged spread?" No, my friends, that won't get the job done. Phrase it as muscle tone and you'll have them eating out of your hand.

"Why yes. So this one is flabby and lacks exercise."

"Bingo! Right again. My, my, you are the best mom in the world."

"I'll take two dozen."

"You've just acquired for your home the world's best egg, guaranteed to cure everything that ails your little ones. Make sure they get all they want."

I realize this may seem like cheap gamesmanship to some, but it works every time. Why? Because we intuit things. Even scientists intuit things. Like how many genetic pairs occupy human DNA. And these moms out shopping for their family's sustenance can intuit truth like this in a few seconds of conversation that is just as accurate as all the empirical data you can imagine.

To be sure, if everyone jumped ship to real food, Monsanto would be in a world of hurt. And Tyson and lots of others. These outfits cannot afford to have people embrace the truth. It's too devastating to their businesses and so the need to disparage people like me as insufferable Henny Pennys, paranoid fearmonger antiscience Luddites, is driven by the very real understanding that if my thinking became normal, it would invert the entire food system. That is why I've focused in this chapter on the philosophy, the ethics of transgenic modification. Anyone interested in the topic, anyone willing to see the data impugning this evil science, can find it readily in countless research venues.

Scientists always have a conniption when I say this, but I'll say it anyway (I like watching people have conniptions): Science is not objective. I know, in the theoretical sense science is objective. You run the experiment, measure the results, record the data, and analyze it with no bias. The problem is, we are biased beings. Every one of us. We come to every situation with predetermined ideas. How many times have people looked at the same data and come away with two completely different interpretations?

How many times do scientists set up experiments within the framework of their own predilections? An old saying goes something like this: It's hard to get people to see things that might jeopardize their paycheck. Scientific inquiry starts with basic assumptions, like creationism or evolution; mechanical life or biological life; spiritual world or no spiritual world; God or no God. These basic biases affect how we set up experiments, how we see the data, and how we interpret the results.

The scientists I like prove, beyond a shadow of a doubt in my mind, that transgenic modification is horrible, that compost is better than chemical fertilizer, and that grass-fed beeves are better than grain-fed. For every scientist I like, I can find at least one that takes the opposing view. How do we account for such heated debate if science really is objective? The reason is that it's not and neither are we. We are emotional, subjective, biased beings and that is why our philosophy, or value system, is the key to how we interpret data, how we set up experiments, and what we ultimately believe.

This is why I've moved to the philosophical part of the transgenic discussion. In 2010 some sixty-seven scientific studies, from different parts of the world, impugned transgenic modification. Some showed the yields were less than traditional crops. Some showed more disease vulnerability. Others showed mutant weeds and other biological anomalies. But believe me, if I brought these up in a debate with a Monsanto scientist, she would have a cogent, scientific, hard data–supported analysis to shoot me down, point by point. This can be maddening, unless you realize that science is an extension of the human psyche, and the human psyche ultimately operates in a biased state.

In fact, I would suggest that our philosophical or spiritual bias must trump science to keep us from becoming too clever for our own good. We are smart people. We can invent things that we cannot emotionally, spiritually, mentally, or physically metabolize. My dad used to call this "overrunning your headlights." Too often we don't realize what we're doing until the car crashes into something we couldn't see or avoid.

Our culture worships science as if it is the answer, the arbiter of disagreement. Many people think that if we could just set up the right experiment, collect the right data, and get the right interpretation, the irrefutable empirical evidence would convince even the staunchest detractor. Not so. Ultimately, we measure data against what we intuit, what we believe to be so. For the record, I'm a strict creationist — I mean six days and the whole "God spoke" thing. Every time I see scientific data about life, it substantiates my creationist view. I think this transgenic debate is a little like that. You either get it because of how you see life or you don't.

Part of this debate centers around the differences between the question "How?" and the question "Why?" As a culture, we've become adept at technical things, the how. I submit we are woefully ignorant of the why. Until we can answer why, the how is not important. Philosophy protects us from scientific machinations. If we can't first handle the philosophical ramifications of our science, maybe we'd better put the experiments on hold until we deal with the question, "How then shall we live?"

The very real ramifications of patenting life, owning life forms, cross-pollination, and other issues are absolutely more important than whether these transgenic life forms can grow bigger plants or fatter animals. And yet so intoxicated are we with the how to grow them fatter or bigger or faster or cheaper, we aren't asking why. Why do we need these things? I would argue that we need these things because we've failed to fully leverage nature's productive expressions, and now we're grasping at dubious technical solutions to make up for the shortfall. We don't need them because they are necessary; we need them because as a culture we've wasted our energy, our resources, and our innovation on things that assault natural templates rather than massaging them with human cleverness.

Lest anyone think I'm refusing to address the alleged benefits of transgenic manipulation, let me just say that I don't see any of these developments as necessary. When somebody says, "The only way to fix this is…" I immediately tune him out. Almost nothing can be fixed only one way. To assume that transgenics are the only solution to disease or production is simply myopic and simplistic. This includes many of the supposedly excellent things that transgenic manipulation promises. Paul Stamets, unquestionably the world leader in harnessing fungi, has illustrated time and time again the remedial wonders of simple fungi, from oil spill cleanup to toxic waste sanitation. May his mycelium increase. May it all increase.

As for feeding the world, I think I've dealt with that adequately in other sections of this book. Problems created by technology generally don't have technological solutions. Einstein said you cannot solve a problem with the same thinking that created it. Solving factory-farm-caused and megaprocessing-facility-induced pathogen-laden food with mandatory irradiation, for example, is not the answer. Neither is solving weeds with Roundup Ready soybeans. Already, a new generation of superweeds is invading fields as unintended genetic consequences weave their sinister web.

High-tech, capital-intensive, nontransparent, corporate-controlled solutions will not, in the end, make life better for the peasants. Never has and never will. At our farm, we have a 24/7/365 open-door policy for visitors. Anyone may come unannounced anytime to see anything. That's our level of open sourcing. Our farm freely shares techniques, rations, everything. In the big scheme of things, we don't even own the land; we're just custodians for a few years. When nature's final balance sheet is tallied, I believe the principles that have guarded genetic integrity for millenia will outlast those developed by corporatists seeking patents and profits without regard to ethical, moral, or biological ramifications.

The world of transgenic manipulation is full of intrigue, secrecy, backroom deals, and evil intent. To even conceive of a plan to patent wild seeds and then charge groups of indigenous people royalties to harvest them is evil. This is not competition in the marketplace. This is not normal business. The devil incarnate could not be more conniving or sinister. Those are strong words. But I am tired of these mega-outfits, with evil agendas, wining and dining our elected officials, revolving in and out of regulatory agencies, receiving accolades for their United Way contributions, and parking their recruitment trailers on college campuses to snatch the best and brightest of our young people to become their next storm troopers. Folks, this ain't normal.

What can we do about this transgenic fixation in our culture?

1. Don't buy food with transgenics in it. That means buy organic, buy local, buy unprocessed, and know your farmer.
2. Develop a study group in your place of worship to examine what the apologists for transgenics say against the tenets of your faith tradition.
3. As a culture, we should admit our error in patenting life, and criminalize this insidious slavery in which one being owns another.
4. Look in the mirror and decide once and for all: Am I biological or mechanical? Is my deepest essence a machine or not?

You Get What You Pay For

The percentage of American per capita income spent on food is the lowest of any country in the world. This historic low just ain't normal.

Never has a society spent less of its disposable income on food, as a percentage of all expenditures. Another interesting downtrend is the portion of the retail dollar that goes into the farmer's pocket. Just forty years ago, that was nearly fifty cents on the dollar. Today it averages only eight cents, and it's continuing to trend downward.

Much of that decrease is due to the consumer buying highly processed food. Obviously, off-farm processing and value adding is compensated at the retail level but does not change the raw commodity value at the farm gate. In true Hegelian fashion, two simultaneous kitchen trends are occurring today. One is the eating nook, in which kitchens are smaller than entertainment rooms. These are designed specifically for people who assume food preparation occurs outside the home. The other is the ultimate gourmet foodie kitchen. For the most part, however, these are not being used to cook much food. As a percentage of total per capita income, Americans spend less on food today than they did in 1960. When you figure in the value of all that processing, it's an amazing statistic.

With so much food prepared outside the home, how could the price have dropped like this? The answer: Commodity prices have fallen. In most commodities, the price has steadily dropped over the past fifty years. To keep up with inflation, wages, energy, and machinery costs, major commodities would need to be three times what they are. To keep up with land costs, they would need to be twenty times what they are. With this abnormal plummeting of farm gate value, our culture has created a bottom-feeder attitude toward farmers.

What happened to Jefferson's intellectual agrarian dream? It's been replaced by a redneck hillbilly D-student trip-over-the-transmission-in-the-backyard tobacco-spittin' stereotypical steward of our most precious resources. Known as rural brain drain, this phenomenon has gradually taken the best and brightest to urban centers and left the underachievers in charge of the landscape.

Is that what we want as a nation? Two couples drove in recently, in their brand-new BMW, to see the farm and buy some pastured meat and poultry. Out for their Saturday afternoon jaunt in the country, they were clearly upper crust. The two immaculately dressed silver-haired stylish country club men in the front seat. The two garden club social-ites with their perfectly coiffed hair and jacket brooches in the backseat.

I was in the sales building with two apprentices when these couples walked in, exuding an air of ownership. We chatted good-naturedly for a couple of minutes, and then one of the ladies, startled, exclaimed, "You gentlemen are really articulate. Why on earth would you want to be farmers?"

You see, dear people, this is a universal mentality in our culture. And it ain't normal. Perhaps we should be reminded that this great nation was started primarily by farmers. Half the signers of the Declaration of Independence were farmers, and these were also the most respected, revered people in the culture. Today, even with all the books I've written and presentations given, I still sense the condescension from talk show hosts and event organizers: "After all, you're just a farmer."

Recently I was passing through immigration in San Francisco after speaking at the University of British Columbia in Vancouver. I handed my passport to the INS agent and he asked me what I was doing in Canada.

"Speaking at UBC in Vancouver."

"What do you do for a living?"

"I'm a farmer."

Those of you who travel know that these are no-nonsense people. You might mess around with your local deputy sheriff, but you don't mess around with INS agents in international airports. He looked at me, dropped the passport, and sternly admonished me, "No joking, what do you do?"

"I'm a full-time farmer."

I thought he was going to pull me out and put me in an interrogation room. As sarcastically as he could, he said, "Since when do farmers go around making speeches?"

"Well, I was talking about sustainable agriculture and local food systems," I responded, as humbly and penitently as I could. You pick your battles.

He stared at me for a long minute and finally, visibly disgusted, stamped the passport and let me through. Folks, I am not making this up.

We had an apprentice fall in love with a Canadian. He lived in Washington State right across the border from British Columbia and they had met at a Christian summer camp in BC. He returned to his family's thirty-acre farm and began farming successfully. When he filled out INS paperwork to get his fiancée and soon-to-be bride across the border to live with him, he put "FARMER" in the blank for "OCCUPATION." The INS denied the request because farming is not a valid occupation.

He had to agree to do something *valid* for five years in order to get her across the border. So he began driving trucks. The prejudice against farming as a valid vocation permeates our entire culture. I will never forget the last time I conferenced with my high school guidance counselor and told her I wanted to be a farmer. I thought she would go into apoplectic seizures. "What a waste of brains. Are you going to throw away your academic ability?"

Even in college, where I excelled in intercollegiate debate, friends and faculty thought I'd failed them by returning to the farm. In fact, when I left my newspaper position on September 24, 1982, to return to the farm full-time, everybody thought I was crazy. After all, everyone knows that there ain't no money in farmin'. For decades we've shipped our best and brightest off to town to become white-collar doctors, lawyers, accountants, and engineers, and reserved food production to society's dolts.

Does that make sense? Do we really want society's bottom feeders to be in charge of our air, soil, and water? Compare that with the culture in Spain that manicures cork forests to grow the world-famous acorn-fattened black-footed hog. In that culture, the man who knows how to prune the cork trees is revered as much as the medical doctor.

Here is a wonderful excerpt from Adam Smith's *An Inquiry in the Nature and Causes of the Wealth of Nations*:

Not only the art of the farmer, the general direction of the operations of husbandry, but many inferior branches of country labour [*sic*] require much more skill and experience than the greater part of mechanical trades. The man who works upon brass and iron, works with instruments, and upon materials of which the temper is always the same, or very nearly the same. But the man who ploughs the ground with a team of horses or oxen, works with instruments of which the health, strength, and temper, are very different upon different occasions. The condition of the materials which he works upon, too is as variable as that of the instruments which he works with, and both require to be managed with much judgment and discretion. The common ploughman, though generally regarded as the pattern of stupidity and ignorance, is seldom defective in this judgment and discretion. He is less accustomed, indeed, to social intercourse, than the mechanic who lives in a town. His voice and language are more uncouth, and more difficult to be understood by those who are not used to them. His understanding, however, being accustomed to consider a greater variety of objects, is generally much superior to that of the other, whose whole attention, from morning till night, is commonly occupied in performing one or two very simple operations. How much the lower ranks of people in the country are really superior to those of the town, is well known to every man whom either business or curiosity has led to converse much with both. In China and Indostan, accordingly, both the rank and the wages of country labourers are said to be superior to those of the greater part of artificers and manufacturers. They would probably be so everywhere, if corporation laws and the corporation spirit did not prevent it.

I find these classic passages captivating not only for the brilliant and flowing prose, but also for the timeless wisdom contained in truth. At the risk of boring you, let me share another of my favorites. In this case, it's Benjamin Franklin, written in 1784 while he was living in Paris:

> Many persons in Europe having directly or by letters, expressed to the writer of this, who is well acquainted with North America, their desire of transporting and establishing themselves in that country; but who appear to him to have formed through ignorance, mistaken ideas and expectations of what is to be obtained there; he thinks it may be useful, and prevent inconvenient, expensive and fruitless removals and voyages of improper persons, if he gives some clearer and truer notions of that part of the world than appear to have hitherto prevailed.
>
> The truth is, that tho [sic] there are in that country few people so miserable as the poor of Europe, there are also very few that in Europe would be called rich. It is rather a general happy mediocrity that prevails. There are few great proprietors of the soil, and few tenants; most people cultivate their own lands, or follow some handicraft or merchandise; very few [are] rich enough to live idly upon their rents or incomes; or to pay the high prices given in Europe, for painting, statues, architecture, and the other works of art that are more curious than useful.

You can certainly get a sense of Franklin's utilitarian values. He sees it as an American virtue that few are wealthy. Compare this to the society aspired to in the classic *Pride and Prejudice*, where the whole goal was to marry into status and not have to work for a living. Franklin, the unequivocal senior statesman compared to the other younger members of the Continental Congress, applauded the universal need to work for a living. This was no welfare state. I love his phrase about financial status: "a general happy mediocrity." If this was normal for the early days of America, we've certainly strayed from it, with our assault on the middle class and the stratification of economic standing wherein the rich are super-rich and the poor are super-poor.

Let's enjoy some more Franklin:

> Hence the natural geniuses that have arisen in America, with such talents, have uniformly quitted that country for Europe, where they can be

more suitably rewarded. It is true that letters and mathematical knowledge are in esteem there, but they are at the same time more common than is apprehended; there being already existing nine colleges, or universities, viz.: four in New England, and one in each of the provinces of New York, New Jersey, Pennsylvania, Maryland, and Virginia, all furnished with learned professors; besides a number of smaller academies. These educate many of their youth in the languages, and those sciences that qualify men for the professions of Divinity, Law, or Physic. Strangers indeed are by no means excluded from exercising those professions; and by the quick increase of inhabitants everywhere gives them a chance of employ, which they have in common with the natives. Of civil offices or employments, there are few; no superfluous ones as in Europe; and it is a rule established in some of the States, that no office should be so profitable as to make it desirable.

These ideas prevailing more or less in all the United States, it can not be worth any man's while, who has a means of living at home, to expatriate himself in hopes of obtaining a profitable civil office in America; as to military offices, they are at an end with the war, the armies being disbanded. Much less is it advisable for a person to go thither who has no other quality to recommend him but his birth. In Europe it has indeed its value; it is a commodity that can not be carried to a worse market than to that of America, where people do not inquire concerning a stranger "What is he?" but "What can he do?" If he has any useful art, he is welcome; and if he exercises it, and behaves well, he will be respected by all that know him; but a mere man of quality, who on that account wants to live upon the public, by some office or salary, will be despised and disregarded.

Franklin is clear that if you think you'll be respected because you come from a name of status, or if you think you'll find a job with the government, forget it. Again, how different we are today. I have quite a few college classes here at the farm for tours, and it never ceases to amaze me how many of them think the only thing they can do is work for the government. These environmental sciences or environmental studies majors, along with political science majors and planning engineer majors, are steered into government jobs. Not only is this abnormal, I'd call it downright un-American. It disrespects Franklin and all the founders, who saw in this great nation an entrepreneurial spirit, where civil appointments and social status favoritism were rare.

Franklin continues:

Land being cheap in that country, from the vast forests still void of inhabitants, and not likely to be occupied in an age to come, insomuch that the propriety of an hundred acres of fertile soil full of wood may be obtained near the frontiers in many places, for eight or ten guineas, hearty young laboring men, who understand the husbandry of corn and cattle, which is nearly the same in that country as in Europe, may easily establish themselves there. A little money saved of the good wages they receive there while they work for others enables them to buy the land and begin their plantation, in which they are assisted by the good will of their neighbors, and some credit. Multitudes of poor people from England, Scotland, and Germany, have by this means in a few years become wealthy farmers, who in their own countries where all the lands are fully occupied, and the wages of labor low, could never have emerged from the mean condition wherein they were born.

This was and still is the land of opportunity. I think it's fascinating how Franklin describes the population density of Europe and the vast numbers of poor. In order for the rich to live as sumptuously as they did, many people were poor. If anyone wondered about the underpinnings of this nation being agrarian, this paragraph dispels the question. This is partly a sales job, to be sure, but I appreciate the attractiveness of the agrarian life that Franklin paints. In other words, it was normal to consider farming a noble, respected vocation. I realize my quotation here is long, but I'll bet many of my readers have never actually read anything that Benjamin Franklin wrote. We read allegations about him, but we don't actually read the living history in the words of his time, unadulterated and unfiltered by modern prejudices. I like to just let the historical figures speak, and in doing so have found them refreshing and profound. When I come across passages like this, I feel like I haven't even studied history. I hope you'll be enlightened along with me.

Franklin continues:

From the salubrity of the air, the healthiness of the climate, the plenty of good provisions, and the encouragement to early marriages, by the certainty of subsistence in cultivating the earth, the increase of inhabitants by natural generation is very rapid in America, and becomes still more so by the accession of strangers; hence there is a continual demand for more artisans of all the necessary and useful kinds, to supply those cultivators of the earth with houses, and with furniture and utensils of the grosser sorts, which can not so well be brought from Europe. Tolerably good workmen in any of those mechanic arts are sure to find employ, and to be well paid for their work, there being no restraints preventing strangers from exercising any art they understand, nor any permission necessary. If they are poor, they begin first as servants or journeymen; and if they are sober, industrious, and frugal, they soon become masters, establish themselves in business, marry, raise families, and become respectable citizens.

Notice that craftsmen don't need any permission to perform their craft. Now that's different. Today you have to get five licenses just to hammer a nail. Artisans supplied the needs of farmers. That's a strange twist. Wouldn't it be something if all the manufacturing in America were seen as a support for farmers? Today, farmers are universally viewed as peasants to produce raw ingredients for manufacturing. In this next section, he calls the "mechanic arts" respectable — this would be equivalent to what we call blue-collar jobs today. The singular emphasis Franklin puts on utilitarian crafts is truly profound. If this was normal at the dawn of our country, we have certainly become abnormal now. I'm waiting for the day when environmental sciences majors realize that the most valuable thing they could do is actually cover their hands in calluses growing ecological food.

Franklin goes on:

Also, persons of moderate fortunes and capitals, who having a number of children to provide for, are desirous of bringing them up to industry, and to secure estates for their posterity, have opportunities of doing it in America; which Europe does not afford. There they may be taught and practice profitable mechanic arts, without incurring disgrace on that account; but on the contrary acquiring respect by such abilities. There small capitals laid out in lands, which daily become more valuable by the increase of people, afford a solid prospect of ample fortunes thereafter for those children. . . .

Several of the Princes of Europe having of late, formed an opinion of advantage to arise by producing all commodities and manufactures within their own dominions, so as to diminish or render useless their importations, have endeavored to entice workmen from other countries, by high salaries, privileges, etc. This however, has rarely been done in America; and when it has been done it has rarely succeeded, so as to encourage private persons to set it up; labor being generally too dear there, and hands difficult to be kept together, every one desiring to be a master, and the cheapness of land inclining many to leave trades for agriculture. Some indeed have met with success, and are carried on to advantage; but they are generally such as require only a few hands, or wherein great part of the work is performed by machines. Great establishments of manufacture require great numbers of poor to do the work for small wages; these poor are to be found in Europe, but will not be found in America, till inlands are all taken up and cultivated, and the excess of people who can not get land, want employment.

Notice the appreciation for entrepreneurship. He chides European businessmen who try to expand and get big by offering high wages. While small businesses are still the backbone of America, I'm chagrined by the number of college students I meet whose ambition is to go work for a huge company. On the other hand, I see a steady stream of late-forties and mid-fifties folks who desperately want to extricate themselves from corporate jobs. They originally took the Dilbert cubicle job because it offered steady pay and, after all, their family and friends told them farming wouldn't pay. At midlife, tired of the corporate cubicle, they're afraid pushing papers around for "the man" will be their legacy. I think Franklin here perfectly describes a normal yearning: Own or work in a small business. A farm certainly qualifies. I can attest to that because my book *You Can Farm: The Entrepreneur's Guide to Start and Succeed in a Farming Business* is still selling thousands of copies a year even though it's a decade old. I'm convinced that thousands of sharp, bright Americans would farm if they actually thought they could make a living at it and be respected by their families.

Franklin finishes:

The almost general mediocrity of fortune that prevails in America obliging its people to follow some business for subsistence, those vices that arise usually from idleness are in a great measure prevented. Industry and constant employment are great preservatives of the morals and virtue of a nation. Hence bad examples to youth are more rare in America, which must be a comfortable consideration to parents. To this may be truly added, that serious religion, under its various denominations, is not only tolerated, but respected and praised. Atheism is unknown there; Infidelity rare and secret; so that persons may live to a great age in that country without having their piety shocked by meeting with either an Atheist or an Infidel. And the Divine Being seems to have manifested his approbation of the mutual forbearance and kindness with which the different sects treat each other, by the remarkable prosperity with which he has been pleased to favor the whole country.

Is that cool, or what? I think this passage shows a lot about the vision for this country. Notice the egalitarian ideas, the agrarian vision. I had to let it run to the virtues at the end just for fun. I think the last paragraph about morals and divinity are especially interesting in the light of modern revisionists who paint Franklin as a loose-living playboy. Although Franklin was not a farmer, he understood its importance as the foundation of a culture and the initial resource developer of a landscape.

Until we attract the best and brightest to be our landscape stewards, we will suffer a lack of ingenuity and business acumen that would keep farmers from doing many of the things they do, such as signing up for feudalism, otherwise known as becoming a contract grower for Tyson or some other conglomerate. Such as planting Monsanto transgenic seed that precludes me from planting other kinds.

How will we know that this dumb farmer prejudice is gone? You'll know when the next time you go to a soccer game and all the soccer moms are sticking out their chests strutting the accomplishments of their little prodigies in a prodigious praise parade, one of the moms has the audacity to belt out, "Well my little Johnny (or Mary) is going to be a farmer." If all the other moms suddenly stop in silent reverence and exclaim, "Cool! Awesome! Far out!" you'll know we're making progress as a culture.

I have a question for you greenie foodies: How would you feel tomorrow if your farmer rolled into town driving a new BMW? Be honest now, what would you think? If it's anything less than, "Well, it's about time. I'm sure he deserves it," then you aren't getting the point of this message. Why shouldn't good farmers who know how to grow food of sufficient quality to keep us out of the hospital be treated and rewarded like the heart surgeon who fixes the problems caused by cheap food?

We will only have the best and brightest farmers when eaters realize that excellent farmers deserve white-collar salaries, and when eaters demand their abilities in the marketplace. Frankly, I am tired every time the USDA issues a press release lauding the fact that Americans pay less per capita on food, as a percentage of income, than any other country in the world. No government agency has been more successful at annihilating its constituency than the USDA. I call it the U.S. duh.

Of all the governmental agencies, the USDA has been the most aggressive at creating and perpetuating this cheap food policy. Don't people understand that a cheap food policy will create a cheap farmer policy? And a cheap farmer policy will create a cheap landscape policy? And a cheap landscape policy will create a cheap soil policy? No civilization can be any healthier environmentally or economically than its soil. No health care system and no bank bailout program can compensate for a bankrupt soil policy, which is exactly what a cheap food policy creates.

This of course leads directly to a discussion about elitism. The most frequently asked question I receive in all my presentations is this one: "But can a local ecologically regenerative pasture-based food system feed the world?" I already dealt with that. The second most frequently asked question is this: "Isn't this local ecological food movement really a niche for the elite?" The corollary is this: "How do we get this kind of food into urban food deserts, and to the poor?"

Let's deal with this head-on.

1. This is better food. It tastes better. It's nutritionally superior based on mountains of empirical tests. It's safer from pathogens. We say, "You get what you pay for" when talking about vacations, clothing, houses, and automobiles, but somehow this is not supposed to hold true when it comes to food.

The poultry industry and its collusion fraternity at the Food Safety and Inspection Service (FSIS) allow water chill tank agitators to insoak several percentage points, by weight, of water into chickens. Lots of water gets sold to unsuspecting Americans this way. Because the tissue of factory birds is soft rather than firm, it is extremely absorptive. The tissue is actually spongy due to lack of exercise and lack of a chicken-friendly habitat. As a result, the carcasses soak up lots of water chilling down in tanks of cold water. That water is sold to you at whatever the price per pound is for chicken. Do you want nutrition or water?

The very clear vitamin and mineral point differences between ecologically grown foods versus chemically grown is well documented. When A. P. Thomson, founder of Golden Acres Orchard in Front Royal, Virginia, sent his biologically grown apples to the state lab for sugar and nutrient testing the first time, the lab asked for a second sample, assuming something was wrong with the calibration on their equipment. The readings were off the charts. Thomson sent a second sample. Same problem. The lab technicians could not believe their instruments; they'd never seen anything like it.

Acres USA magazine reprinted a study by Doctor's Data laboratories originally published in the *Journal of Applied Nutrition* in 1993, and the differences were astounding. Here is a listing of the percentage increase of the biologically grown product over the chemically grown:

PERCENT INCREASE					
ELEMENT	APPLE	POTATO	PEAR	SWEET CORN	WHEAT	AVG.
Boron	60	110	110	10	0	70
Calcium	40	50	40	1800	120	63
Iron	30	−20	240	160	75	59
Magnesium	40	50	30	300	430	138
Manganese	50	0	120	1,600	540	178
Selenium	0	220	40	300	1,300	390

Now can you see why the lab techs thought their machinery was loused up? This data has been out there for a long time. In spite of studies like this, the chemical cartel continues to pooh-pooh the data and say there is no difference. Anybody who has tasted a compost-grown carrot or tomato compared to a chemically grown one can tell the difference.

Our farm has paid for some studies over the years. I'll share some highlights. One of our customers had a friend at the National Institutes of Health who ran a fatty acid profile. The critical one is f22:6n3 due to omega-6 to omega-3 ratios. Our f22:6n3 average was 552.5 and the factory egg was 185.4. The other critical one is f18:3n3. There our eggs averaged 252.6 and the factory eggs 87.3. These essential fatty acids feed the brain. They turn genes on and off. This is important stuff, folks. And yet the industry routinely pontificates that an egg is an egg is an egg.

We had a fat profile run at the Virginia Tech Human Nutrition lab comparing our pastured chicken fat to Tyson chicken fat. The professor in charge of the lab didn't want to do it, insisting that we were just wasting our money since chicken is chicken. A few hundred dollars later he ran the test. When he handed it back, he said, "See, I told you there was no difference."

No difference? I'm looking at the computer printout right in front of me. Our birds averaged .54 percent fat and the Tyson birds averaged 2 percent. When measuring that fat profile, the polyunsaturated fat (the really good stuff) was 23.3 percent compared to only 19.5 percent in the factory birds. If a licensed dietician is reading this, you know these numbers are huge. In fact, a dietician working in our community hospital at the time was so impressed by the comparisons she saw in her own lab that she began prescribing our birds to heart patients when they were discharged. Is this food worth more? You bet it is.

Are you ready for another one? Two senior biology majors at one of our local universities ran a bacteria test on our chickens compared to the USDA federally inspected birds in the supermarket. They ran a swab test on the ready-to-eat carcass and cultured the bacteria, measuring in colony-forming units per milliliter. The commercially processed birds from Holly Farms, complete with official federal inspection stamps, averaged...drum roll, please...3,600 CFU/mL. Polyface pastured birds averaged 133. I don't know if you're quick with percent-ages, but that's a 2,500 percent difference. If you were concerned about your health, which one would you buy? Is it worth more? Yes.

I won't bore you with tests on grass-fed beef compared to grain-finished — but again the differences are 300 percent in B vitamins, huge differences in conjugated linoleic acid. The differences are noth-ing short of astounding, and they're worth more at the cash register.

Perhaps in few things are the differences more apparent than in a pastured egg compared to an industrial battery egg. Keeping, handling, beating, taste — everything is far superior to the industrial counterpart. A couple of years ago *Mother Earth News* paid for a study pitting twelve pastured egg producers against the USDA standard nutritional egg pro-file. We sent samples to a lab and the Polyface results are below. Yes, they are astounding indeed.

	USDA	POLYFACE FARM
Vitamin E	0.97 mg	7.37 mg
Vitamin A	487 IU	763 IU
Beta-carotene	10 mcg	76.2 mcg
Folate	47 mcg	10,200 mcg
Omega-3s	0.033 g	0.71 g
Cholesterol	423 mg	292 mg
Saturated Fat	3.1 g	2.31 g

This food is worth more because it's better by any measurement.

2. Economies of scale favor the industrial sector. It takes a while for a new paradigm to evolve to the same point of efficiency as the one it's replacing. Right now, the fledgling local foods movement, or should I say the normal foods movement, is pegged at anywhere from 1.8 to 1.9 percent of all food consumed. I am not including organic apples shipped in from China. I call that industrial organic.

Interestingly, I was in a meeting with organic Chinese farmers, and they decried the compromise and adulteration of American organics. "Ours is much more stringent and trustworthy," they said. Anytime I'm around American certified organic growers, they say the Chinese sys-tem is flawed and untrustworthy. Dear people, this is why local trumps organic. And it has to be transparent local. I heard a farmers' market vendor speaking at a conference recently tell consumers, "If you want to know who to patronize, shop at a market stall for three weeks in a row. Any farmer who has not invited you to his farm by your third purchase does not deserve your patronage." Well said, my friend.

The intricate collaborations that drive the industrial food system have been developing for decades. The distribution networking to go loaded and come loaded takes scheduling finesse and lots of players with shared interests. If you have a vehicle making deliveries, you never want it to run empty. Ideally, you try to haul something both ways. This local food movement, in its infancy right now, is not yet sophisticated enough to have enough players with shared interests to create these economies of scale. As it regains market share, however, these relationships will develop just as surely as they have in today's industrial food system. As that happens, prices will come down.

3. Buying unprocessed and preparing food at home is perhaps the best way to combat high food prices. Potato chips sell for eight dollars a pound. I don't know any local artisanal vegetable grower, organic or otherwise, that sells potatoes for eight dollars a pound. But with your handy-dandy kitchen techno-gadgetry, you can buy the most expensive potatoes, put a bit of sweat equity into the kitchen, and have to-die-for potato chips cheaper than any at the supermarket.

Bagged, shredded cheddar cheese is as expensive as unshredded better cheese. How hard is it to grate cheese? Boneless skinless chicken breasts are several times more expensive than whole broilers. You can bone out a breast in about thirty seconds. Any processed potatoes or carrots are incredibly expensive. Buy them whole and raw, then do to them whatever you want to do to them: sliced, diced, whatever. Frozen whole dinners triple the cost of the ingredients. Probably the worst is breakfast cereal. Talk about a lot of money for a little bit of nothing.

Teresa has made our own granola for thirty years. She purchases the raw ingredients: oats, sunflower seeds, coconut, and wheat germ primarily. She puts it in a shallow pan and bakes it in the oven. It's fabulous, healthy, and cheap. Just add whole raw milk and enjoy.

Processed food is expensive. Even fast food is expensive. To get the same nutrition out of one pound of primo Polyface salad bar ground beef, you would need several Big Macs, and they would cost way more than $4.50. Although I have never seen a study to this effect, I'm sure that if you took the average shopper's grocery cart, piled up all the processed food and its cost, then made those same items in your kitchen out of unprocessed ingredients, you could buy the best of the best and still save money.

College students notoriously complain about time and money when I start saying things like this. Recently a global food issues professor asked me to come and lecture to her students. She wanted to do something different, so I decided to cook omelets for them. I asked the professor to go down to a local shop and pick up local salsa and some artisanal cheese from a local dairy. I brought our pastured eggs and cold-pressed apple juice from Golden Acres Orchard, where we buy all of our apple juice.

This wonderful cold-pressed juice has an inch of sediment in the bottom of the jug and feels like eating fresh apples when you drink it. In fact, you have to pace yourself or before you know it you can drink the equivalent of eating six apples and it will take you twenty-four hours to, shall we say, metabolize the juice. This can create an event in your composting toilet.

I showed up with eggs, juice, skillets, and butter to the classroom in this prestigious all-girls' college. The professor had secured a room with a four-burner range, and while she laid out the salsa and cheese, I cracked and beat up the eggs and began heating skillets. In no time, we were in full swing, cranking out these sixty-second omelets as fast as the students could line up to get them. We filled them with salsa and cheese and everyone had a glass of apple juice.

At the end of the exercise, we figured that this meal cost about $1.50 and took about three minutes per cover to prepare, start to finish, including cleanup. Everyone loved the food — it was outrageously good. So I asked for a show of hands: "How many of you have watched a movie this week?" Every hand went up. That's ninety minutes — enough time to prepare thirty of these meals.

I plunged forward: "How many of you have bought a soda out of a vending machine this week?" Every hand went up. "Two?" Every hand was still up. We'd already passed the $1.50 mark, so there was no need to belabor the issue. Then I moved in for the kill: "Now, who wants to tell me they don't have time or money for this?" Not a hand went up.

Their embarrassed expressions showed we had indeed created an Aha! moment. I savored the epiphany for a moment, letting the students squirm.

Then I said this: "Don't ever let yourself be a victim. Our culture thrives on victimhood. We love to invoke 'I can't' and make excuses. The truth is we tend to make time and have money for what we think is important. It's okay to eat junk, but be honest and admit that it's because you don't care enough or you're lazy, or whatever. You and I can't change everyone else, but we can sure change the one looking at us in the mirror. Resolve to do that, and you'll lead by example and find the world lining up to follow. Be the change you want to see and refuse to blame others or circumstances."

Whew! How's that for a pep talk? When somebody says they don't have time or money for food preparation, I want to visit their house and look for a TV, a frozen pizza, and canned spaghetti. All of that wastes time and money.

I was speaking at the University of Guelph in Ontario many years ago and the town hall format included three of us on a panel. One of the other panelists was a high-powered attorney living in a fifth-floor condominium in Toronto. Here is my paraphrase of her opening five-minute monologue.

She and her husband had a baby. When her baby was born, she realized she was responsible for the health and well-being of this little life. She decided to breast-feed to take over autonomy in that department. Then she and her husband decided to take all the time and money they would spend over the next year on recreation and entertainment and go on a local-food treasure hunt, with the goal being that at the end of the year there would be no bar codes in their pantry. And as she stood there, young mom with a successful career, she beamed: "We did it."

They found farmers with grain that they could buy a bushel at a time. Do you know how much flour you can mill, with a little kitchen mill, out of a five-dollar bushel of wheat? At least a hundred dollars' worth. They found their dairy, their beef guy, their vegetable producer. They even found herb growers, molasses, and honey. They decided to shut off the TV, forgo the vacation, and enjoy finding their local-food treasures. Isn't that a great story?

I'm not saying you're in sin unless you do this, but I'm holding it up as an example of one family's determination to not be victims. I agree that this is a challenging bar, to be placed so high. Most of us won't jump that high. But are we even willing to jump half that high?

4. Nonscalable government regulations inordinately discriminate against smaller processing businesses (abattoirs, kitchens, canneries). Subsequent chapters will go into this in great detail.

If the food police, building inspectors, zoning administrators, and other public servants (said tongue in cheek, of course) would not place inordinate hurdles in front of wannabe entrepreneurs, we would see a proliferation of bootstrap businesses like we haven't seen for decades. Without question, a person working in their own kitchen can procure and prepare nutrient-dense soups and stocks as cheaply as the industrial sector. Inner-city gardens in vacant lots are incredibly productive.

Ecologically friendly food can be grown on your house lot, in the community, at a price competitive with anything in the monocrop industrial system from far away. The problem is not production; the problem is processing. Most of the price discrimination on local food is not so much in the growing; it's in the preparing. Production is not very regulated by the food and building police; processing is. Therein lies the problem. That brings us back to the earlier discussion about buying unprocessed. Unfortunately, most people aren't going to buy unprocessed.

If we're going to get affordable market penetration, especially in urban areas, we need to free up cottage industry to use already owned domestic culinary infrastructure and leverage it in the community. How many church kitchens sit idle during the week? How many people who love to prepare food would do so for their neighbors, their urban community, if they could stay home and do it as a business?

Every week I travel around the country meeting thousands of urban consumers, and hundreds of farmers. The farmers are ready to grow. The eaters are ready to buy. But between them is this chasm that is daunting and, for most, insurmountable. We need a tsunami of public awareness that the biggest impediment to affordable local food, even in the most urban areas, is the labyrinth of regulations that stifle entrepreneurial creativity.

Teresa and I co-own a community federally inspected abattoir called T&E Meats in Harrisonburg, about twenty-five miles away from the farm. Because we use legal labor, and craftsmanship, and cross-train so people don't get repetitive-motion disorder, it costs us three hundred dollars to process a steer commensurate to what Iowa Beef Processors (IBP) does for fifty dollars. This has nothing to do with cost of production; it has everything to do with nonscalable regulatory overheads. Inspector overtime, practically daily inspection changes from the food police, infrastructure requirements that must include a separate bathroom and office for the inspector — these are all prejudicial against smaller operations.

Here's another economic reality. As recently as fifteen years ago, hides were still tanned in America. No more. It's all done in China. That means the hide purchasers that used to go around to all these community abattoirs don't exist anymore. As recently as 1995, T&E Meats received nearly sixty dollars per beef hide. Today, it's fifty cents. Why? Because with the consolidation in the meatpacking industry and the loss of domestic tanning, the hide market all runs in container loads.

A huge plant processing five thousand beef animals (beeves) a day — do you realize what that is? That's one hundred tractor-trailer loads of beeves a day. Think of the stench, the blood, the guts, the hooves, the hides. Yes, the hides go directly into a shipping container trucked directly to a dock and loaded onto a vessel heading to China. For our little plant, where we generate perhaps twenty to forty hides per week, there is no point of entry anymore. We've been shut out of the market. That amounts to $50,000 per year loss to our little community abattoir, enough to pay for a new furnace, a new roof, upgraded electrical or a walk-in cooler, or even a raise for everyone who works hard to make sure our local farmers can access restaurants, schools, and families in our community. The consolidated megasize of everything sucks the income right out of the community.

Look, folks, if we want to talk about elitists, I think the real elitists are the people in this country who want to deny you and me the freedom to buy the food of our choice. The food police who raid food clubs and farms. The consumer advocates who want government inspection on every morsel of food consumed. True elitism is some bureaucrat standing up on his hind legs saying consumers are too stupid to find a clean farmer. The real elitists are those who say farmers are dirty and want to hurt their customers. I don't understand why I'm called an elitist for wanting to eat what my grandmother grew up on. Real elitists are the ones who deny me that privilege, and erect a host of barriers to protect global industrialists from peasants with pitchforks...like me.

5. Diversified farms like ours do not receive government subsidies. The farmers growing non-transgenic grains for our farm omnivores (poultry and pigs) do not receive subsidies. Our processor, T&E Meats, does not receive subsidies. In fact, if we get busy enough to need a second shift, we have to prove need in order to get an inspector.

If the government doesn't want to send our puny little plant an inspector, the FSIS just rules that no insurmountable need has been shown. One of the dirty little secrets in the processing industry is that even if a facility complies with everything the food police require to be licensed as a safe food business, an inspector is not guaranteed. Without an inspector, you can't run the plant. And since bigger plants have more prestige than small ones, the food police have a prejudicial attitude toward community-based abattoirs. If a small plant decides to add a second shift, it must submit a request and the government food police get to be judge and jury, deciding if the need merits an inspector. If not, it's tough cookies for the little abattoir. Sorry, end of discussion. Subsidies and corporate welfare are for the big guys, not the little guys.

Let's think about an analogy. Suppose the nation had five auto manufacturers and the government decided to subsidize four of them to the tune of $5,000 per automobile. Would it be fair to scream at the fifth one about their high prices? Of course not. And yet that is exactly what people do when they accuse the local, ecologically based food system of high prices.

We're charging the true cost of goods and labor, not some artificial one. The truth is that the cash register price for regular industrial food at the supermarket — processed or not — is a lie. It does not represent the subsidies. The biggest subsidies are not direct payments to farmers, they are the tab society picks up for externalized costs. The costs of 500,000 cases of foodborne bacterial diarrhea that Americans will get this year from dirty food. What's the price on a case of diarrhea? I don't know, but I guarantee you if those were added to the supermarket cash register, food wouldn't be as cheap as it is.

Here at Polyface and the farms like ours, all the costs are figured in.

We're not creating a Rhode Island–sized dead zone in the Gulf of Mexico. We're not making three-legged salamanders and infertile frogs. We're not killing earthworms; we're growing them. We're not destroying the soil; we're building it. We're not increasing atmospheric carbon; we're sequestering it in the soil where it belongs.

The collateral damage from concentrated animal feeding operations, pesticides, herbicides, and toxic manure lagoons has not even begun to be tabulated. It may be decades if not centuries before the true cost of this abnormal food system gets tallied. I tell people our Polyface food is the cheapest food on the planet, because all the costs are figured in. It's not a price charade.

6. Plenty of money exists in the system to pay for good food. Can you think of anything people buy that they don't need? Let's see, we need to think real hard here. I'm not talking about you, I'm talking about that guy sitting next to you on the airplane or in the subway. That person. I know you wouldn't buy anything that's unnecessary. How about Starbucks? Soda? Tobacco? Flat-screen TV? How about hundred-dollar designer jeans with holes already in the knees? Body piercings? Tattoos? Movies? Disney vacations? Snazzy cars, designer clothes? McDonald's or KFC? *People* magazine? The trip to Las Vegas? Fund-raisers for Democrats? Fund-raisers for Republicans? McMansions? Jewelry? The steeple on the church?

You see, when you come right down to it, the system has plenty of wealth for all of us to be elitists and eat like kings. Really. It's just a matter of priorities.

Recently a Permaculture group asked me to speak at a fund-raiser. The fund-raiser was not for them; it was to purchase Community Supported Agriculture (CSA) shares for needy families in their community. CSA farms sell shares of their production and disseminate it throughout the season to their shareholders. In Europe, they are called box schemes. The event packed out a large city auditorium, and at the end of the night, after paying all expenses, had enough left over to buy CSA shares of local fresh produce for thirty-five four-person families.

See, that's refusing to be a victim. That's real, honest-to-goodness charity, which always starts on my doorstep, not someone else's doorstep. If that model were duplicated throughout the nation, thousands upon thousands of families could join the ranks of local greenie foodies.

We can all do better. If we can find money for movies, ski trips, and recreational cruises, surely we can find the money to purchase integrity food. The fact is that most of us scrounge together enough pennies to fund the passion of our hearts. If we would cultivate a passion for normal food and normal living like we've cultivated it for clothes, cars, and entertainment, perhaps we would ultimately live healthier, happier lives.

We started this chapter talking about cheap food policies and disrespected farmers. I would suggest that the real elitists in our culture are those who would deny the first-line stewards of our nutrition and our landscape their rightful place in society. I'm all about restoring the Jeffersonian intellectual agrarian. Every one of us — farmers, urbanites, condo dwellers — can join this great return to Jeffersonian normalcy by elevating the place of food in our lives to its rightful altar. That can be one giant step toward restoring normalcy.

How about some practical ideas?

1. Complain to your farmer that he isn't charging enough.
2. Display good stickers on your refrigerator or car bumper: "Know your farmer"–type language.
3. Do some price comparisons between processed and unprocessed foods.
4. Look at your expenditures and see what is unnecessary. Add that amount to your food budget. Do that for three months and then tell me you don't have enough money for good food.
5. Before saying anyone can't afford good food, make sure their house contains no alcohol, coffee, tobacco, soda, frozen dinners, flat-screen TVs, iPods, tattoos, or unsingable music.

Get Your Grubby Hands

Throughout history, civilizations have encouraged successional, multi-generational land control. People universally assume that it's good policy to maintain uninterrupted land management and/or ownership to ensure continuity and stability. Most people think it's pretty cool when a business has been in the same family for several generations. That our culture has declared war on generational wealth transfer just ain't normal.

And just what would such a war look like? Inheritance taxes. Farmers are notorious for being unable to agree on things. The corn growers have a different interest than the hog growers. The vegetable growers have a different interest than the sugarcane growers. The sugarcane growers want to keep subsidies. The vegetable growers don't get subsidies so they'd like them terminated. But on one thing I have found absolute and universal agreement: Inheritance taxes are evil.

In general, what I will say in this chapter applies across the board to any family business, but I think it's most acute in farming because farmers are notoriously land-rich and cash-poor. Their assets are the least liquid and their value least negotiable. In a family business, two assessors might ascribe a very different value for goodwill, for example. But land is a more standard science and not as subject to interpretation. The market is what it is, without a lot of wiggle room.

The biggest issue for farms is that the value has no relation to its productive capacity. Stay with me on this. If you have a landscape business, for example, the lawnmowers, shovels, chippers, and weed whackers have a value directly related to their ability to generate income. It's a close relationship. If lawnmowing suddenly became extremely lucrative, the machinery to do the work would rise in price. If lawnmowing took a nosedive, the machinery would drop similarly.

Most businesses have this kind of tight, responsive dance between productive value and infrastructure value. But since the 1970s, land prices have spiked without any correlation to productive capacity. For the first time in our country's history, land value has no relationship to its production value. If farmland doubles in price in a decade, no more sunlight hits that land at the end of the decade than hit it at the beginning.

Farmers generally have all their equity tied up in their land. While others put money in stocks and bonds, treasury bills, IRAs, gold, silver, or other investments, farmers plow everything back into the farm. The farmland represents the farmer's investment portfolio. It is his equity, his retirement, his savings — everything. It is for him what all these other investments are to the 99 percent of us who are not farmers. As we begin this discussion, then, everyone needs to understand that whatever attitude you take toward a farmer's land, that same attitude should be taken toward your investment portfolio.

I can hear the breath sucking in. Many of you never thought about it that way, did you? When people cavalierly talk about what a farmer should or should not be able to do with his land, how it should be valued or not valued, just imagine those same attitudes toward your stock portfolio. How would you like a decision by the zoning board to suddenly change the value of your investment portfolio? How would you feel if tomorrow over a cup of coffee a friend who owns the same $100,000 stock value in the same company told you that a local government agency just changed his valuation and quadrupled his value. It didn't extend to you.

That is what happens when farms suddenly get rezoned commercial or residential, or the government decides to run public water and sewer lines out into farmland. Of course, the opposite happens as well. By down-zoning, value is taken away. This is what happened to friends of ours when the board of supervisors arbitrarily and suddenly down-zoned their land from agriculture to exclusive agriculture. Suddenly, many things that could be done on the property under the old agriculture zone could no longer be done under the more stringent zoning; hence their property value dropped precipitously. Across the road, where the zone remained agriculture, land value held constant.

Historically, whether it was primogeniture (eldest gets the inheritance), patriarchal blessing, or deeded land patents, societies have always protected land succession. When land can't be bequeathed, it upsets the entire society. At the far end of this discussion, of course, is war, which is always about who controls what territory. Clearly, land control is a hot issue.

May I be frank? Our 550-acre farm right now is valued at $1.5 million. Mom and Dad bought this farm in 1961 for $49,000. Not one more ray of sunshine falls on this farm now than it did in 1961. And although we have certainly increased its productive capacity, thirtyfold would be a stretch. By a long shot. Even if we've increased its productive capacity by five times, that's a far cry from thirty times.

With President Obama's new legislation in December 2010, our culture unilaterally decided that for me to inherit this farm, I should pay the government 35 percent of its value. That's a little more than half a million dollars. Would you stop reading and contemplate that for a minute? Can you think of any reason why I should pay the government more than half a million dollars to keep this farm?

Come on, all you liberal Democrats who think we need to tax the wealthy. I'm one of those supposed wealthy people. One of our neighbors just had to pay $300,000 inheritance taxes just to keep owning his farm. It wiped out his entire life's savings. Fortunately, he was not a farmer, so he had some savings from a life of what people around here call "public works." That's any off-farm job. This story could be repeated thousands of times. In the name of anything that makes sense, why in the world would a culture make it practically impossible for its farm businesses to pass to the next generation? This is not only unreasonable, it's downright malicious. There is not a valid reason on God's green earth why a farmer should have to pay hundreds of thousands of dollars to the government in order to stay on his own farm.

Succession is hard enough as it is, without throwing this inheritance monkey wrench into the mix. The biggest reason farm succession planning is difficult is because most of the time, not all the children have an interest in the farm. In fact, many, many times none of the children has an interest in farming. Tragically, many farmers encourage their children not to farm, so the children dutifully leave and head to town for a real job. A job that gives paid vacations and medical insurance. A job that offers societal recognition. A job that lets you live where you can get cable television and pizza delivered to your front door. And when the farm transfers, there's no one to transfer it to because they've all gone to town. I actually receive letters from elderly farmers who ask me if I can find a young person willing to inherit their farm.

These elderly farmers love their land, and they don't want to give it to their children because they know their children will sell it to the highest bidder in a heartbeat. They love it too much to do that. The thought of McMansions sprouting up on their beloved pastures and woods breaks their heart. In fact, my heart breaks for them. I realize that some have been curmudgeons whose "never good enough" or ultra-patriarchal demeanor chased the kids away. That happens more than you can imagine. But to age on the farm with no youthful zest to enthuse your heart with freshness is beyond depressing. Of all the farming accomplishments for which I've received awards, the one that means the most is not a plaque on the wall. The best one is that we have four generations living on this farm. And every day I am surrounded by youthful enthusiasm, both from children and grandchildren. The intern and apprentice contingent adds to this mix, as do subcontractors and our whole radiant team. The Polyface team is absolutely the most energetic, enthusiastic, passionate, and capable bunch of people you could ever want to meet. That's the best succession plan.

But we've still got this land thing. What happens next? I don't have half a million dollars sitting in the bank to give the government when Mom passes. And, for crying out loud, why should I have to? That's the question begging to be answered. Even if it were possible to amass that kind of cash in preparation for inheriting the farm, why should that be a requirement? I look at these bright-eyed, bushy-tailed young people, excited about taking this farm into the future. That half-a-million-dollar bill hangs in front of me like a huge weight. Mom, please stay alive.

I know some of you estate planners are out there saying, "Well, fool, get your ducks in a row. Set up a trust. Start a buyout plan. Get with it to prepare." Yes, I assure you we are doing all of that, but it's complicated. It takes a lot of time and money to pay for the attorneys. I'm belaboring the raw money because I think it's important to understand the bare-bones result of this inheritance tax policy. Of course we can try to avoid it, and I certainly don't intend to lose this farm. But when I could be doing so many other more productive things, to be saddled with the time and money to figure out how to escape this inheritance penalty is plain wrong. It's probably worse than that, but the alternatives aren't civil enough for this conversation.

I want to build a Ferris wheel sprouter. I have an idea for a rotary cylindrical rabbitmobile. How about vermicomposting? A moldering toilet. I have a ton of things that would heal the land and make our production models even better. Why should I have to take time and creative energy to figure out how to escape half a million dollars to the government just to stay on this farm?

So back to the siblings who don't want the farm. In many cases, one child does stay and run the farm. The others go to town and have their careers. That's fine. One child spends his career on the farm. Mom and Dad are now in their eighties. This farmer child is in his late fifties or early sixties. All Mom and Dad's equity is in the farm. What do the other two siblings get? If the farm is left in three equal portions with an undivided interest, what do the nonfarming siblings want out of it? Do they want to sell? Do they want the farmer sibling to rent it from them?

You see, if the farmer sibling had not stayed and worked the farm, it would have collapsed long ago when Dad and Mom got too old to operate it. The farming son held it together, fixed the fences, kept things up. And now suddenly he's faced with a three-way equal split that gives him no more than the other siblings because Mom and Dad associated equal inheritance with equal love. But it's not equal inheritance. The farmer child put his life into that farm. If we're talking about fair, why should either of the other siblings get anything? It seems to me that fairness would dictate that the farming child get the whole thing.

The child who has distinguished himself as a farm lover and developed a track record for success on the farm should not be saddled with a payout to the siblings who left as soon as they could. This scenario happens thousands and thousands of times a year and it will continue to be a dilemma because the average American farmer is now nearly sixty years old. In the next twenty years some 40 percent of America's farmland will pass to the next generation. Succession planning, with the dynamics described here, the family emotions — it's hard enough as it is. To then throw in half a million dollars of inheritance taxes is just adding insult to injury.

Unfortunately, land preservationsts tend to view conservation easements and similar instruments as ways to ameliorate these issues. But what good is preserving land if we don't preserve farmers? What do people like about farmland? The bucolic pastoral landscape does not happen by itself. It takes farmers to handle the livestock, repair the fences, clean up dead and downed trees, and paint the buildings. Without farmers, all you have is abandoned dilapidation and wilderness. That's not what soothes the human spirit.

Pastoral pictures on the wall have a soothing effect on the soul. I think it's mainly because it signifies order. I appreciate wildness, yes I do. But a neat farmscape, a pastoral setting, indicates a caretaking that wildness does not evoke. It expresses stewardship, home, and hearth. That is what draws us in.

Unless and until land preservation groups wrestle with this successional issue, as far as I'm concerned they are just spitting in the wind. If all the effort to create land conservation easements had gone into eliminating, once and for all, inheritance taxes, it probably would have done more to ensure that farms stay as farms than any other single instrument. When problem-solving, we need to go to the heart of the matter, not skip lightly over symptoms.

As fewer people have any link to a parcel of land, the land ethic in this nation is eroding dramatically. One elderly farmer friend recently explained it this way: "Everything is about recreation. America is one big playground. Your farm and my farm, they're just a big playground." I daresay he is right. The boldness exhibited by some groups to either take private land or narrowly define its use would make the founders of this nation start the revolution all over.

A farmer friend in California wanted to return to his family ranch. His grandfather had put the ranch together and his father had moved into the ranch dwelling after the grandfather died. The father worked in town but enjoyed the ranch, running a small horse boarding business as a small side income. The mom operated a dog grooming business at the ranch. The son, now in his early twenties, decided to return to the ranch with his wife. The ranch only had Grandpa's original ranch house on it. The problem? In an effort to preserve open space, the greenies had pushed through legislation that precluded a second home being built on their ranch — their ranch! What was this young ranch-loving couple supposed to do? I suppose the greenies would want them to go live in town and commute out to the farm. That makes a lot of sense from a carbon footprint standpoint. Besides, commuting is expensive, and in this case, any reasonable person can see that it's nonsensical.

They looked at numerous alternatives. Every door closed. In desperation, they ordered a yurt from Pacific Yurts. These structures are not considered buildings. I think they are one of the best loopholes going right now. They are not a recreational vehicle, so you can't "park" them illegally. But they aren't a building, so you can't build them illegally. There's no law that says you can't camp on your own property. They built the yurt. If you haven't been in one, they are chic. Very cool.

Soon, a baby required more room. So they put in a second one, connected by a breezeway. A third one now complements the whole compound, and ten years later they are making do in their tri-yurt. Would they like a house? Absolutely. Would life be easier in a house? Probably.

Now let me ask you: If a law passed suddenly that said you could not access your investment portfolio — could not buy or sell for, say, five years, and the reason was because the politicians just wanted to keep things the way they are — what would you think? Yes, I thought so. You'd say it's outrageous. You'd stomp and fume and shake your fist and say, "It's not fair. This is my money. These are my stocks and bonds. I should be able to do with them what I want."

Oh really? Gentle people, that is all a farmer is asking to do. In our environmentalist land-planning focus groups we don't think about these kinds of ramifications, do we? The law of unintended consequences is very real. We are facing these same problems on our own farm. We are desperate to erect apprentice housing, and even housing for managers, gardeners, orchardists. Goodness, on 550 acres we have plenty of nooks and crannies to tuck little earth-sheltered solar-operated hoophouse-roofed domiciles around where nobody would see anybody else. But we're in an agricultural zone.

The farmland preservationists have decreed that houses and farmland do not go together. Now, I realize we're an unusual farm. The rule was instituted to stop random development. But when the land use plan came out, farmers who happened to own land close to town, who had their farms suddenly zoned commercial, received a windfall. Their land suddenly jumped from $5,000 an acre to $30,000 an acre. Overnight, with the stroke of a pen. The day the politicians ratified the zoning was the day the land values changed.

Farms drawn outside that arbitrary line couldn't even build a house for a farm manager or sell off one lot to a friend. Often these zoning lines are drawn by planning experts, brought in from faraway places. They fly in, look at maps, and start drawing lines. That these lines arbitrarily and overnight create millionaires and paupers never enters their minds because they are doing a good thing: land use planning. Their noble land use planning ministry overrides any unfairness, any capricious occurrences, because this is important work. Again, imagine if that kind of capricious external control were applied to your investment portfolio.

I have a friend who wanted a woodworking shop next to his house. He happened to be located in an agricultural zone. No can do. Oh, he could build the woodworking shop, and he did. He can do tremendous work. He can fix chairs, build furniture. Nice work. He just can't sell anything or charge for his services, because that's a business, and we wouldn't want a business on agricultural land.

A dear farmer friend is the fourth-generation farmer on his land. Her dad is my age and the land was annexed by the city about twenty years ago in an acrimonious, drawn-out legal battle between the city and county. The city won and this farm, a beautiful rambling complex of pasture, farmsteads, and barns covering some twelve hundred acres and operated by three family members, was suddenly faced with city taxes. Suddenly their $15,000 property tax went to $60,000. No more sunlight. No more grass. Nothing changed except a governmental paper designation. The market value for this land, of course, went through the roof.

Some people would say, "Well, what are they complaining about? They got a bonanza, a veritable windfall. They should be grateful, the ungracious dolts."

You're missing the point. My farmer friend, the daughter in this case, grew up there. Her family has owned that place for going on four generations. To be summarily thrown off your land by political machinations is un-American. The city says this developable land is costing them tax revenue. By the city raising the taxes like this, the family must leave the farm. Meanwhile, the city has hundreds of vacant houses, vacant commercial buildings, vacant storefronts. The city's economic woes certainly have nothing to do with the unknown development potential of these twelve hundred acres.

Our country has become a theocracy. It worships money. Money makes anything right. Eminent domain is overused to condemn land or buildings to make way for shopping malls and condominiums. Our county came very close to taking three farms to bring in a subsidized Toyota plant. I used to think eminent domain was necessary. Now, in most cases, I know it's not. Perhaps if eminent domain didn't exist, it would force the powers that be to become more creative in their answers.

Instead of running sewer lines, maybe we need to encourage composting toilets. Maybe instead of running water lines, we need to encourage cisterns. Maybe instead of running roads, we need to cluster houses within walking distance so they aren't spread out all over the land. I don't know what all the answers are, but I've seen some extremely creative ways to house people and integrate communities without eating away at so much land.

I've heard that once land is developed, it's gone forever. Don't believe it. Where are the ruins of ancient civilizations? If everybody vacated New York City today, within three years you would see trees sprouting through sidewalk cracks. Within a decade you would see vines growing up the sides of the skyscrapers. And within a hundred years it would be a forest. In truth, I have no desire for that to happen, but I'm using perhaps the most extreme development example to debunk the notion that development destroys land forever. It does not. All those suburbs can just as easily become farms again.

I was setting up an electric fence down by the creek in the meadow in front of our house. The public dirt road runs adjacent to that creek. We have a simple electric fence running along the creek to keep the livestock out of it, allowing the edges to grow up in brush and trees. I was on the meadow side of the creek, hidden from the road.

Suddenly, I heard a gunshot. It came from the road, about fifty feet away from me. I ran down to the bridge and doubled back up the road to a pickup. Sitting in the cab was a young man in full hunting array. I startled him — probably not as much as he startled me — and asked him what he was doing.

"I shot at a deer standing right yonder," he said.

"That's my field, and I was standing right there," I yelled. I had brought a rebar electric fence stake with me, just in case, and brandished it menacingly, calling him by his license number.

"I didn't know you wuz thar," he drawled, trying to move his chaw of tobacco to one side of his mouth to gain better verbal clarity. He needed more than that with me, let me tell you.

"This is private land. What gives you the right to drive down this road and shoot into my field?" I pressed.

"I didn't see a 'No Tresspassing' sign."

"So if you go to Wal-Mart and you don't see a 'No Stealing' sign, does that mean you figure whatever you see on the shelves is fair game?" Good pun, huh?

"Well, no, I don't reckon."

Just so we're all on the up-and-up here, I'm presenting this to you in the printable version. I'd been minding my business, quietly setting up an electric fence, when Pow! That high-powered rifle within a few feet, on an otherwise quiet and bucolic afternoon — you'd better believe I was ready to wrap that rebar stake around his little neck and squeeze that chaw right out of his mouth.

What do you think he'd been taught? Where do you think he got the notion that wildlife and land are there for the public's taking? Where do you think he got the notion that he could go anywhere at any time as long as specific "No Trespassing" signs did not bar his entrance? Dear people, this abnormally cavalier approach to private property has been fostered by sincere-minded people who think they know a lot more about land use than those of us out here chopping the thistles, moving the cows, and keeping the roof on the barn.

I know plenty of people are sputtering right now, "But, but, but, what about all the farmers who pollute? What about concentrated animal feeding operations and manure spills? What would you do if a neighbor upriver sent pollution down your stream? What if somebody built a feedlot next to you?"

First, I am not opposed to community-wide land use decisions. If a community wants to bar CAFOs, that suits me fine. That affects everyone equally — nobody can have a CAFO. My problem is the unfairness of an urban planner sitting in his office and arbitrarily drawing a line on a map that keeps my own son from joining me on the farm but makes a guy half a mile away a multi-multimillionaire overnight. If all developers had to bear the entire weight of their projects, without a single concession on taxes, infrastructure development, or anything else, the projects would be built more slowly.

A Target Distribution Center came into our county onto prime farmland. It cost that forty-acre building less to hook up to the county water and sewer system than it does a single-family residence. That is the kind of thing that drives development. If development had to truly bear all of its costs, it would occur more slowly, and more organically.

Second, while I lean libertarian, the trade-off is that I am extremely big on personal responsibility. If someone sent pollution down my stream, I would fight to make sure that person cleans it up. Completely and entirely. Right now. Not a decade from now. If it bankrupts the operation, that's fine. If that rule were applied around the country, many of our Fortune 500 businesses would not exist today. I don't think that would necessarily be a bad thing.

Again, I'm not opposed to business, or even big business. But I am vehemently opposed to businesses that dump, businesses that punch their neighbors in the face. With regulatory bureaucracies enforcing fairness instead of courts, bigger businesses purchase concessions like Superfund status instead of being held personally liable for their misdeeds. This is a fundamental difference between socialism and the rule of law. Nobody should need an Environmental Protection Agency to say that polluting the river is bad. If polluting the river is wrong, let the perpetrators be brought before a jury of their neighbors (peers) to assess a penalty. That keeps the politicians out of it. It also keeps the bureaucracies out of it, which is a good thing because the regulating agencies are governed by a revolving door with the industries they regulate.

What we need is for businesses — and anyone else for that matter — to be scared to death to hurt a neighbor. That should include the military, the president — anybody. If some big daddies get a spanking, maybe they won't get so big for their britches.

Third, no paradise exists this side of eternity. No policy is all positive without any negatives. The trade-off to food that heals the land and heals the people is that it is more expensive at the cash register. The advantage is you don't go to the hospital as much.

Well then, maybe we don't need as many hospitals. Oh no, Humana stock falls. But instead, cottage industry thrives. Some nurses and doctors could open mini-practices in their neighborhoods and garden on the side. I'm trying to help us all understand that everything relates to everything. You can't have a change in policy without creating a domino effect.

When the Obama administration put in the Cash for Clunkers program — remember that? — it was intended to stimulate the economy. What it did was deny thousands and thousands of first-time or impoverished car owners the opportunity to own a car. Many of the clunkers were not clunkers at all, but excellent lower-valued used cars. These are the cars that less affluent people like me buy routinely. I've never bought a new car. By ordering these cars crushed and not recycled into the used car market, this program denied cars to people least able to afford a new one. It was one of the most elitist things I've ever seen. Unbelievable.

When the help for the mortgage crisis went into effect, if people defaulted on their mortgages, they could refinance at extremely low rates. Why in the world were these supposedly smart politicians surprised when people just quit paying their mortgages so they could go into default and get the new lower rates? The experts who designed the program for President Obama were blindsided and aghast that people would do such a thing. Duh?

The chairman of the Federal Reserve claimed the bank crises that eventuated the Bush and Obama bailout plan could not have been predicted and blindsided him. Oh really? Nongovernment investment counselors told clients all about the impending day of reckoning. You can't mandate banks to give people loans who would never qualify in a normal market without jeopardizing the mortgage industry. Policy has consequences. It never ceases to amaze me how the people supposedly in the know can miss major ramifications of their policy. That's what they're doing with farm inheritance taxes.

When you tax inheritance, you destroy farms. It's plain and simple. I can't think of any culture, at any time in history, that actually discouraged land transferring between generations. Usually people go to war over such things. It's sacred even in primitive tribal cultures. Even in slash-and-burn tribal cultures in the heart of Indonesia, the fields are allocated by tribal leaders based on historic use by those families. My brother lived in Indonesia for fifteen years, and he knows about such things.

Has our culture become too sophisticated to put value on things as mundane as land transfer between generations? If we are going to preserve the culture of agri-culture, it starts by revering those who have poured their lives into a piece of land. Enough pressure exists on agri-culture to create ownership changes anyway. Land will continue to change hands, just like it has for centuries. But making it difficult to transfer from one generation to the next with inheritance taxes is both aberrant and immoral.

From a policy standpoint then, here are some options.

1. Eliminate all inheritance taxes. Period. Death should not be a taxable event. This will make farmland transfer easier and take a huge incentive to development out of the system.
2. Vigorously prosecute those who pollute, or whose actions penetrate another's property. The old adage, "Your freedoms end at my nose," is probably appropriate here. Anybody who pollutes should clean it up, and bear all the cost of the cleanup. We don't need a bunch of environmental regulations to make this happen. It's simple: Is toxicity running down the creek? If it is, find out where it's coming from and go after the perpetrators.

   In the world of industrial agriculture, all sorts of protections exist to make sure polluters never pay for any cleanup — or never even get fingered. Again, the industrial ag sector cozies up to the regulatory people and they solve their issues over games of golf. If there were no regulators, and private citizens forced redress through the sheriff or state police, then the public-private fraternization would be less likely to occur. Today, the Internet has democratized information and can be a huge lever to activate boycotts and public knowledge.

I don't think any of these egregious perpetrations are beyond the ability of people to respond by refusing to buy. For example, right now, a CAFO egg factory receiving a USDA inspection label has much more credibility than a pastured operation without all the infrastructure required for the inspection label. If there were no inspection label, it would be us little pasture-based farms against the factory. As it is, it's us against the USDA, the insurance companies, the land grant universities, the scientific community, the industry.

Want another example? Every year, we harvest several deer from our farm and take the boneless trim plus some pork fat up to a family near Harrisonburg that turns it into wonderful bologna. We'll get a hundred pounds or more and eat it ourselves, give some away, and share it with apprentices and interns. It's a perfect quick and filling lunch. But we can't take beef to this same shop because food safety regulations preclude it. This bologna tastes better, is more nutritious, and is far safer than anything with a USDA label on it at the supermarket. But the whole system decrees that ours isn't as good, and many people believe it, just because it doesn't carry the USDA approval. If there were no USDA requirements for bologna, our product would speak for itself in both subjective and empirical ways, but we can't even have that discussion due to the regulations.

Perhaps one more example. What we call our salad bar beef is completely grass-fed, without any grain, on land that has received compost and biomimicry grazing for decades. We can't call it organic, though, because the government owns the word. Rumors are circulating that in the future we may even have to get a license to use the word "grass-fed." But right now, most organic beef in America is grown in feedlots, where the nutritional profile is the same as any regular industrial feedlot beef. The fact that grass-fed may be far superior never gets a hearing because the environmentalist, foodie, and government are gaga over organic, and that's the licensed term.

3. Eminent domain should be allowed only for things that, if not done, would threaten life and limb. Not security. That word has now been trivialized to the point of meaninglessness. I think "threaten life and limb" might work. If not taking the land won't endanger life and limb, then it should be left alone.

4. All land preservation groups should devote themselves to figuring out the impediments to profitable farm businesses. Once they figure that out, they should throw all their lobbying clout into solving those problems. I think what they'll find are that the impediments to profitable farming are actually many of the things they voted for, like more food police, more green space restrictions, more worker protection.

   Anyone who thinks the only way to ensure worker protection is with a regulatory bureaucracy is just not being creative. Worker protection can be forced through the marketplace, through independent certifications, through public awareness. If there is enough public pressure to create a regulatory bureaucracy, why not just use that lobbying clout to force integrity in the marketplace?

5. Allow agricultural land to be used broadly. If a farmer wants a commune on his farm, what's wrong with that? If he wants a nursing home, restaurant, soup kitchen, farm store, day camp, what's wrong with these uses? The truth is that profitable farming is no more static than the culture. What was profitable thirty years ago is not necessarily what is profitable today. To freeze what farms looked like thirty years ago is both unrealistic and anachronistic. Farms need to flex with the times.

   Now that our culture has nearly twice as many people incarcerated in prisons as we have living on farms, we have a new set of business realities, new pressures, and new opportunities. These farms must be able to adapt to this new climate. To freeze them in yesteryear is to condemn them to failure. And folks, that ain't normal.

Sterile Poop and Other Unsavory Cultural Objectives

What in bygone eras used to be a fairly simple transaction between producer and buyer, generally with a middleperson thrown in somewhere, has in recent days become a labyrinth of logistical and protocol nightmares. You would think that a supermarket located ten miles from our farm, for example, could stock our eggs or chicken or hot dogs. You would think that a university just twenty miles away could access our farm's bounty just by calling us and placing an order. You would think that a restaurant that wants our sausage could get it fairly easily.

Never in the history of civilization have the current number of hurdles between local food systems and food needs been erected. People constantly ask me, "Why can't we buy your stuff at the supermarket? Why can't we get it in our university dining services?" I'll answer those questions with some real-life stories. These are not embellished or strained.

Several years ago a local university's board of trustees adopted a local food sourcing pledge. They hired a new chef for their dining services and he immediately contacted our farm to begin getting pastured chicken, beef, and pork. We were ecstatic and assured him we'd be glad to oblige. We didn't hear back for a couple of weeks so I called him. He answered the phone and immediately asked if he could call me back in a few minutes. Fine.

The phone rang a few minutes later. He had gone out to his car and left campus to talk to me on his cell phone. He said he needed to get to a private place where no one could overhear the conversation. As is often the case, the university had contracted out its dining services to a specialty company like Aramark or Marriott. The noncompete clause of the contracts prohibited any food from coming onto campus that wasn't a registered vendor to that company. He was frustrated with this new hurdle and said that his superiors had decided to just buy chicken from Tyson since they had a processing facility in the town — and they would call that chicken local.

What do we mean by the word "local"? Perhaps no one has better defined this than Michael Shuman, founder of BALLE (Business Alliance for Local Living Economies) and author of *The Small-Mart Revolution*. He uses the acronym LOIS to stand for "locally owned and import substitution" as the descriptive term for businesses that qualify for local. The idea is that the people responsible for decision-making — the top people in the organization — must live in the same community as the lowest people in the organization. They attend the same churches and have children on the same soccer team.

By that definition, of course, the Tyson processing plant, just because it's located in the same town as the university, is certainly not a local business. The CEO does not live there; none of the board members live there. And yet this is the kind of cleverspeak people use to talk the talk instead of walk the walk.

Another chef contacted us from another nearby university and began buying product...for only a month until Aramark found out. We ran into the same noncompete clause as before, except with a new wrinkle. Aramark had the dining service contract, but subbed out the food acquisition portion to Sysco.

I talked to the regional director of Aramark and asked him why he couldn't okay shipments of Polyface products into the university — in this case, the University of Virginia in Charlottesville. The students were begging for our product; the chefs wanted it. We were in more than twenty upscale restaurants within blocks of the university. It wasn't a matter of legality; only an internal protocol forcing them to use Sysco vendors.

In our conversations, he kept saying that his priority was to protect the health of the UVA students. I asked him why he couldn't personally come out, check us out, and sign off on the product. Evidently he felt much safer dealing with meats from concentrated animal feeding operations located in China, as long as they had paperwork behind them, than dealing with a farm located a few miles away where any student could come and self-inspect anytime.

About the same time, we had a restaurant call and ask for fifteen hundred pounds of sausage a week. That's significant, but the twist was that the product must be delivered on a Sysco truck so that it arrived with everything else. I've often wondered about the propriety of toilet paper, shrimp, and eggs coming in the same truck. But that's the new model.

I called Sysco and decided to see what it would take to become a vendor. I'm thinking, if you can't fight them, join them. Remember, for both UVA and the restaurant, our delivery bus went by both their front doors every week anyway. It wasn't like adding these clients would have been difficult for our distribution. The stops would have been easy.

The only thing Sysco wanted was a $3 million product liability policy and hold harmless agreement. I certainly didn't have any trouble signing a hold harmless agreement, but at the time we only had $1 million in product liability insurance. I have never been fond of liability insurance, partly because I think our culture has too many bloodsucking lawyers and partly because your risk of being sued is in direct proportion to the amount of insurance you have. Insurance provides a bigger pot to go after.

But because I like challenges and enjoy breaking down arbitrary hurdles, I decided to pursue getting the $3 million coverage to see if we could actually become a Sysco vendor. After many phone calls, I was told such an option did not exist for us. Nobody would write that kind of protection for a farm, end of story. I kept seeking, though, even mentioning it in my public presentations as I traveled: "Does anyone know where such coverage exists?"

Finally an insurance agent in South Carolina came up to me after a speech and said he'd like to work on it. A year later, after many interviews and signed forms, we had the coverage as an umbrella under ANPAC (American National Property and Casualty Company). We changed all our farm insurance, homeowner's, automobiles, everything.

Another driving force on this was workmen's compensation. Because we had hired a couple of employees, by law we had to join the mandated workmen's compensation program through a licensed underwriter in the state of Virginia. Our local agent recommended Liberty Mutual, a national company, and that was a nightmare. For example, our delivery driver had to be classified as a live animal hauler — an extremely risky position.

Because we were a farm, their rules precluded our having a delivery driver who handled dead product. After all, we all know that farms don't handle meat. They handle live commodities. No farmer in his right mind would want to dress his own chickens. No way. He wants to borrow $500,000 to build a confinement house so he can sign a contract with Tyson to grow chickens for a few cents apiece. It's the new voluntary feudalism agreement. I become your slave and you become my master. The master can terminate the contract at any time. I'm completely dependent on the good graces of Tyson. Sounds like a good deal for any farmer, doesn't it?

But a farmer that actually processes his own chickens and peddles them to neighbors? No, we can't have any of that. Ridiculous. So the only delivery driver a farm can have is a live animal hauler, period. As a result of the high risk in that job description, which is certainly very real, we paid several thousand dollars extra for a position we didn't even have. And that's just the delivery.

You should have seen the auditor (yes, we were red-flagged and got kicked into audit within thirty days of our first premium check) when he found out we had workers who handled both cows and chickens. No, that would never do. You see, every worker must be classified as a poultry worker or a beef cow worker. Fortunately, cattle workers could also work with hogs, but they were not supposed to work with poultry. The whole system was set up for industrialized monospeciated farms. The fact that at our farm we all work with all the animals was way outside the box.

Not only that, but these exposure rates are based on confinement systems, where fecal dust, lots of electric motors, concrete, and stressed animals live. At our farm, the animals gambol in fields, in the fresh air, and are blissfully content. No concessions are given for such a bucolic production practice. Farms like ours aren't supposed to be big enough to have workers. Farmers who do what we do are supposed to be limited to hobbyists. No credible farmer would eschew animal factories.

It seemed like every couple of months we received a new amended bill in the mail until we were paying upwards of $12,000 a year for our little crew. It was outrageous. By this time, Teresa and I had purchased half ownership in the federally inspected abattoir we used, and even with nineteen full-time employees the workmen's comp bill there was way less than we were paying for our little crew here on the farm. And it was primarily because our farm was not considered normal. Let me tell you what ain't normal: It's saddling a little farm like ours with this capricious and asinine bureaucratic mumbo-jumbo that saps all of our creative energy and time. What happened to the good old days when if someone wanted to work and someone wanted to hire, they just shook hands and went about their business?

The best thing to come of our product liability search was that ANPAC took over our workmen's compensation policy and saved us nearly $10,000 a year in premiums just by filling out the paperwork differently. In a small business, that's a lot of money. Few things have made me happier in recent years than to tell Liberty Mutual to take a hike. Good riddance.

With the $3 million liability umbrella under our belt, I called my Sysco lady back to get signed up and rolling. I was excited. She answered the phone and then hesitated: "Things have changed since March 2010. Sysco has put in some protocols."

My heart sank. I'd been working for two years to punch through this insurance thing, and now I was literally a couple of months behind a new protocol. I asked her to go ahead and send me the requirements and we'd talk later.

I printed off the protocol: seventeen pages. I stared at the stack of papers. Outside, cows needed to be moved and chickens watered. I had Post-it notes hanging all over the computer from serious institutional wanna-buys. I'd spent two years trying to punch through the insurance problem; now this. I wanted to cry. Do you understand this? I have cows to move, chickens to water, acorn finishing glens to set up for pigs, fences to mend, and a host of other things to do, and I'm staring at seventeen pages of fine print that reads like a science experiment:

Grinder establishments have demonstrated programs in place to assure they only purchase domestic beef or veal for grinding from slaughter suppliers who can affirm the following:

*3A1 Validated HACCP Plan — with at least 2 post evisceration interventions that reduce E. coli 0157:H7 to below detectable levels.

*3A2 A scientifically based plan that identifies unusual event periods and includes corrective actions which may include customer notification.

*3A3 A protocol for verification of E. coli 0157:H7 trim testing at a minimum frequency of Quarterly via a valid method.

*3A4 A system including COAs showing all source material lots intended for grinding were sampled via robust N60 protocol and tested negative for E. coli 0157:H7 using lab methods as sensitive as FSIS and/ or approved by CFIA....

Annual Independent Third Party Audit Including a specific E. coli 0157:H7 Addendum for Grinders.... Auditing agencies must be approved by Corporate QA....

Grinders and Processor shall perform "Mock Recalls" on a routine basis... to measure trace back to suppliers and trace forward to customers. Mock Recalls include an assessment of the records associated with HACCP, SSOP and Prerequisite Food Safety Programs.

Establishments shall have contingency plans providing the capability to perform recalls or market withdrawals at all times.

Grinders shall document the effectiveness of the mock recalls....

All ground products must be conveyed through a working metal detector at least capable of detecting and rejecting product with stainless, non-ferrous and ferrous metal standards....

Suppliers shall have demonstrated programs for controlling wood pieces and nails from damaged raw material pallets....

Ground products shall be manufactured with grinders equipped with functional bone chip (hard and soft) removal systems in the final grinding process.

Folks, this ain't normal. First of all, we're not buying material from anyone else: It's our animals, raised in our pastures. Can you imagine our farm trying to fill out this paperwork? It would be like trying to explain that our workers actually handle chickens, pigs, and cows on the same day in the same pasture. We might as well be from Pluto. The whole protocol is set up for megaprocessing facilities buying foreign and domestic product by the tractor-trailer load. The undefined abbreviations are some kind of industrial code — it would take a day just to find out what all the abbreviations mean.

Notice that nowhere, in any of this, is anyone concerned about feedlot growing conditions, exposure to chemicals, soil development, nutrient profiles, saturated fat, or anything remotely resembling ecological management. This is all part of a totally abnormal feeding and production protocol. The reason that in the last thirty years all those squiggly italicized Latin words like *E. coli*, campylobacter, *Listeria*, and salmonella have become part of our everyday lexicon is because, for the first time in history, we are housing and feeding animals in a completely abnormal way. It is nature's language begging, pleading, "Enough!" We have abused, mishandled, disrespected long enough. And all of this, dear people, has come at the encouragement of the great U.S. Department of Agriculture.

The pervasiveness of these strange ills bespeaks a disregard for everything that is natural and normal. It is not normal for cows to eat cows. It is not normal for chickens to be confined by the multi-thousands in football field–sized houses breathing fecal particulate so toxic that it rubs lesions into the tender mucous membranes of the respiratory tract and opens the blood's hemoglobin to direct fecal particulate contamination. This is how salmonella, for example, gets into the bloodstream of animals. Folks, this ain't normal.

As I see it, the food safety requirements assume unimaginable pathogenicity coming from the farm. Whether it's milk, beef, poultry, pork, or vegetables, the pathogen-friendly production environment is a template that cannot be changed. After all, changing it would be inefficient. What this means is that food safety becomes an after-the-fact sterilizing objective. Those of us who produce in a nonpathogenic way do not receive any concessions from the overburdensome protocols put in place by paranoid food service professionals. This is the number one hurdle denying local farmers access to local markets.

It certainly isn't normal for a restaurant up the road to be unable to procure meat or poultry from a nearby pasture without it going through the kind of testing and infrastructure demanded by seventeen pages of protocol. Did you catch the requirement for routine mock recalls? Put yourself in my shoes. I'm a small farmer. Right, I'm going to conduct mock recalls. I don't know how to do one. I don't know what these people are looking for. Who am I supposed to call? This one item would take a week for me to ascertain what is acceptable.

Did you catch the sophisticated metal and wood detector? These things aren't cheap. These protocols are written for the plants that you see on television, or in *Food, Inc.*, where miles of shackles, hundreds of workers, and thousands of carcasses dangle through a labyrinth of nuts, bolts, and conveyors. At our little plant, we do everything by hand.

We kill each animal one at a time. There is no chain conveyor system. You can eat off the floor it's so clean. We spray it down between each animal. We debone by hand. In the big processing facilities, they dump bones and carcasses into huge stiff spinning rubber-fingered vats that shred off ligaments and every vestige of tissue from the bones. In this setting, of course, the potential for debris and chips is huge. When you do this work by hand, the risk is exponentially less.

I called the Sysco lady back and said, "It would take a dozen industry experts working full-time to comply with this."

She quickly responded, "Oh yes, I know, and that is what's frustrating. My phone rings every day with requests for local product, but with these requirements, no local company can comply with the mandated paperwork and expensive equipment."

The one-size-fits all mentality is not just in the government's food police bureaucracy; it's also in the industry. This creates a fraternity, a country club if you will, that is practically impossible to crack. It acts as a firewall to competition. Indeed, it effectively eliminates the antidote to all the problems these protocols are trying to address. Forcing farms like us through the same sieve as Iowa Beef Processors is not only ridiculous, it's actually malicious.

The big corporate food system makes statements about safe food and quality assurance, but in the end, it's all about the good ol' boy network, protecting the industrial machine. Nobody is asking about happy cows, happy pigs, or happy chickens. The whole system is predicated on raising them in despicable, totally abnormal conditions, and then trying to rectify the damage with infrastructure, irradiation, technology, and paperwork. Why not just raise them clean to begin with?

I find no small satisfaction in knowing that at least the poop I'm eating has been sterilized by chlorine and irradiation. Why not raise them clean enough and process them slow enough that poop doesn't adhere to the carcass?

When the animals come in covered in manure from filthy growing conditions, and the insides are toxic from filthy air, of course it's going to take a heavy-handed approach to compensate for the pathogens. But if we raise them in a sanitary animal-friendly way to begin with, these procedures are unnecessary.

Lest anyone reading this think the whole issue is uniquely animal-based, similar protocols are being developed in plant farming. And they have the same result: draconian measures that effectively prevent local and small operators from accessing the market.

According to a July 13, 2009, *San Francisco Chronicle* article by Carolyn Lochhead, organic farmers must insure sterility around their fields by tearing out hedge habitat for beneficial insects. Even a squirrel trespass is cause for scorched-earth destruction, all in the name of sterility. Antiseptic procedures to sanitize food production are directly opposed to the biological systems encouraged by organic farming.

This is all done, according to the credentialed food safety experts, to rid the food system of deadly, mutated, new bacterial strains. The killer bacteria live in the guts of feedlot and confined grain-fed dairy cattle. The killer bacteria does not live in the guts of pastured and forage-based cattle. That the scientists won't even discuss this reality shows their agenda to maintain and protect something that ain't normal.

According to the article, corporate food businesses would much rather have a "dead pond" than a "dead child." In a strange twist, according to the industry, lettuce trucked two thousand miles from sterilized fields in California would be considered safer than the lettuce grown locally by an Amish farmer in the Midwest who cultivates his fields with horses. After all, horses are dirty and machines are clean.

Do you see the parallels between Sysco demanding metal detectors on conveyors and import-tracking paperwork for my locally processed and hand-cut beef? They consider fecal feedlot beef trucked two thousand miles and covered with chlorine and official paperwork cleaner than my pastured beef from just down the road.

The sterility demands on lettuce growers even requires the farmers to deny access to any children younger than five years old in order to guarantee that no diapers will enter the farm gate. Indeed, truth is stranger than fiction. I wish I were making this up, but it's straight out of the news report.

What does it say about a food system when children cannot walk through the fields? Folks, this ain't normal. Nuclear reactors, I can see. Even junkyards, maybe. But gardens? Farms? Children not allowed to visit? What have we created here?

"It's all based on panic and fear, and the science is not there," says Dr. Andy Gordus, an environmental scientist with the California Department of Fish and Game. He adds that "frogs are unrelated to *E. coli*, but their remains in bags of mechanically harvested greens are unsightly, so the industry has been using food safety as a premise to eliminate frogs."

Did you catch that? Frog remains in bags of lettuce? Folks, this ain't normal. Let me ask you a question: Have you ever accidentally put a frog in your lettuce bag when you went out to the garden to harvest your greens? No? Oh, come on, surely this has happened at least a couple of times. No self-respecting gardener, working with efficiency in mind, could possibly miss every frog in the lettuce patch. Surely you'd get one once in a while. Come on, tell the truth. I know there's a frog in that bag somewhere. See, dear people, when Baltimore and Philadelphia demand lettuce from California, a tender, tiny, fragile, mostly water crop, this is the inevitable result. You can't blame the industry for trying to fill a demand. What we need to do is realize it's our collective responsibility to stop this insane demand and grow the lettuce in our own backyards, under cold frames, on our rooftops, or buy it from local farmers. Period. You cannot have sanity in the food system with this abnormal demand for convenience.

How long can this craziness continue? I'm still waiting for the day when even 10 percent of the population wants to return to normalcy, where cows eat grass, chickens chase bugs around pastures, lettuce grows in local gardens, vegetables grow in a rotated sequence, and neighbors can do business with each other.

Interestingly, I recently spoke at a conference along with a huge specialty vegetable grower. He said the California *E. coli* spinach problem mentioned in the above article was a result of pure greed. The white-hot demand for the product moved production and processing into overdrive. The processors cut huge corners. For example, the lettuce is not supposed to sit in the harvest wagons waiting to be processed for more than an hour or so. Instead, they were backed up for several hours. The bagging speeds were running two or three times faster than acceptable, which meant workers could not look at the lettuce as well.

Since this is a huge processor, of course, you never heard the business impugned by government agents. Instead, the food police scratched their heads and hem-hawed around, kicking at the dust and gee-whizzing into futility. The truth is that the violations of safe food handling protocols were flagrant and purposeful. If those corporate executives had faced punishment in a court instead of being protected by their food police cronies, perhaps these kinds of shortcuts would not occur as often.

Two years ago our farm had extra eggs in the spring so I called the local Kroger and Martins supermarkets to see what it would take for them to accept our eggs. These places donate to the United Way and tout themselves as interested in the community. But that's sure not what you get when you ask them to stock local food products. I never even got to the price discussion. After numerous calls, I finally got to the manager, who couldn't do anything but refer me to corporate headquarters. I called there and could never get past the robot.

Again, the firewalls against penetration are severe. I could never talk to a person. What does it say about a food system in which the manager of a local store cannot even make a decision about handling a local product? And then won't even shepherd the local producer through the process to see if someone higher up is interested? If the local managers were interested in local food, at least they could move the request on up the corporate chain. But in my experience, they want to get you off the phone as quickly as possible. After all, they have Twinkies to shelve.

Our farm lasted at Whole Foods for about three months. The Charlottesville store contacted me and wanted to carry our eggs. I warned them that our plain pulp cartons were not up to the high-petroleum plastic four-color flashy cartons I was used to seeing there. They said no problem. My intuition thought better, but I didn't say anything.

We started selling eggs at Whole Foods, and within six weeks, their marketing people called: "We need to do something about these plain egg cartons."

I was ready. We had already gotten tired of making five calls a week to get their order. Every week we were supposed to talk to someone different. What a pain. I've got better things to do than sit on the phone chasing around Bob, Henry, Megan, Charlie, and finally Betsy this week in order to get the order. And next week it's Pat, Bill, Zoe, Clyde, and finally Michael. I responded, "Look, if you need sexy egg cartons to sell our eggs, then you need to educate your customers. We don't intend to patronize big oil just so we can sell eggs at Whole Foods." We quit doing business with them a few weeks later.

A year later, Whole Foods courted us again for beef, pork, and chicken. One stipulation: Our animals had to be killed by gassing. Now folks, that ain't normal. Gassing shuts the nervous system down and doesn't let much of the blood pump out. That is why in both halal and kosher abattoirs, the animals cannot be gassed. Furthermore, it's inexact and doesn't actually kill some of them. We prefer the simple throat slice — basically halal and kosher — to let the autonomic nervous system continue to function and pump the blood out of the body.

That black you see around the bones of supermarket chicken is because the birds are electrocuted and don't bleed out very well. We took some birds to a small federal plant one year in order to sell them across state lines at a farmers' market, and the birds were killed by electrocution. The blood buckets contained half the blood we see on the same number of birds we do under our ancient methods here at the farm. These methods, by the way, are historically normal. The reality struck me that Whole Foods thinks all kosher and halal slaughter techniques qualify as animal abuse.

Oh boy, I thought, wait until all the Jews and Muslims hear about that. They'll sure enjoy shopping at Whole Foods. As a result, we refuse to have our meats at Whole Foods. In addition to being a bad technique, gassing is dangerous for workers and requires huge infrastructure that smaller abattoirs can't afford. Just to make sure nobody is missing the point here, we're talking about hurdles that keep local foods from institutional markets. These are the reasons why you can't buy our stuff at these locations.

As I've articulated in this chapter, the impediments change from market venue to market venue. It might be insurance. It might be mock recalls. It might be infrastructure. It might even be packaging. From a small farmer's perspective, they are myriad and maddening.

Some chains are requiring compliance with new best agricultural practice (BAP) standards in order to sell there. These BAPs, of course, are created by agricultural universities in collusion with the food industry. They all play golf together, lick the turf chemicals off the balls, and then come up with BAPs. For manure management, the BAP is a manure lagoon, not compost. A lagoon is as unnatural as it gets. Show me a manure lagoon in nature. The whole point is to keep the manure out of the water, not put it in water. Lagoons have all sorts of problems compared to compost, not only from a nutrient profile, but also from an infrastructure standpoint. It's a big swimming pool for poop. It's dangerous for people, requires capital-intensive single-use machinery, and stinks to high heaven.

How about animal veterinary care? BAP says everything should be vaccinated. And routine medication is a great thing. And confinement housing is wonderful. And pastured poultry are pathogen vectors. That's the government-industrial BAP. As these proliferate, they will shut more doors on ecologically based, historically normal production practices from ever getting onto a grocery shelf.

Perhaps one of the most interesting hurdles we've encountered occurred at one of our white-tablecloth country club restaurants several years ago when someone discovered that our eggs did not have a USDA-inspected label on them. Again, the threat of litigation scared the country club's board members to death and they swooped down on the artisanal chef, demanding why he would get eggs without a USDA stamp. "Because they are better. They are the best anywhere around," he said.

The important thing to remember is that on eggs, that stamp has nothing to do with testing for things that people fear. With eggs, the big fear is salmonella. But the USDA-inspected stamp does not check for salmonella. It only certifies that if you say the eggs are grade A, the air cell is a certain size and the viscosity of the albumen is a certain thickness. That has absolutely nothing to do with bacteria.

It also certifies that the shell is not cracked and that if you say it's a large, it actually is a large egg, not a medium or jumbo size. It simply means that your scales are accurate. Again, this has nothing to do with pathogens. People, please understand that most USDA-inspected stamps have nothing to do with actual pathogenicity. They are stamps about size, color, fat covering, skin tears, and the like. A grade A broiler has nothing to do with pathogenicity. It has to do with size, skin tears, and fleshiness.

Should I scream here, "The emperor has no clothes?" Americans have been totally snookered into believing that all this regulatory elitism actually protects them, and the ugly truth is that it generally does not test for anything that can actually hurt you. So eggs coming out of a factory house from debeaked chickens crammed nine to a sixteen-by-twenty-two-inch cage can be plunged into a fecal chlorine bath and sold with a USDA-inspected stamp on them. But eggs from a home-based pastured operation are extremely difficult to get licensed.

I hope I've given an answer to the question, "Why can't I get your stuff at the store?" For all the problems, plenty of alternative marketing venues exist, and people who want our kind of food need to patronize and encourage those venues.

From Community Supported Agriculture to farmers' markets, to direct-from-the-farmer schemes like our Metropolitan Buying Clubs, to small retail boutiques, to the occasional sympathetic grocery manager, plenty of venues exist to provide all the product Americans need without going to supermarkets. When foodies say, "Demand this food at your supermarket," I want to respond, "Quit going to the supermarket. Go find your farmer instead. Thousands and thousands of farmers are out there ready to serve you. Shut off the TV, skip the party, and go find your farmer. We're here and we're ready to serve you outside this abnormal system."

And folks, once you start dealing with your local farmers, you will reenter the world of normalcy. And it will feel great. You'll feel good physically, spiritually, and emotionally. Believe me, you'll know deep down that this is the right thing. Who needs supermarkets? We lived without them for centuries. Their intransigence and bureaucracy render them stodgy and negative. Get jazzed up. Be hip. Start dancing with your farmer, and your chickens will turn into chic-ens.

Here are some action steps you can take.

1. Buy local — really local. Locally owned, operated, and marketed.
2. Don't demand government stamps of approval for anything. In fact, look for the nonapproved item.
3. Patronize plain packaging. Pay for the product, not the packaging.

I Hereby Release You from Being Responsible for Me

Lawyer jokes. I love 'em. The one thing I dislike almost as much as dealing with government bureaucrats is dealing with liability insurance. I think my negative perceptions of liability insurance really nosedived thirty years ago in 1982 when Teresa and I were just getting started.

Although our farm is 550 acres, 450 acres of it is forested. It's very much a forest farm, with only about 100 acres of open fields. In these parts, that's a fairly large tract of forested land. And this forested acreage is surrounded by public land, owned by the Virginia State Commission of Game and Inland Fisheries, called the Little North Mountain Wildlife Management Area. This public land is really a subsidy for below-cost timber sales to the forestry industry and a taxpayer-subsidized playground for recreational hunting.

Our private forestland extends into this surrounding public land like a deep peninsula. Of course, on our acreage, we're building ponds, developing springs, putting in pig pastures, and acorn-finishing pigs. Simple one-strand electric fence designates three- to five-acre tracts that we run pigs through one time per year for about two or three weeks. The pigs root out brush and brambles, eat bugs that would hurt the trees, and stimulate leaf litter decomposition with the gentle stirring. Hogs and forests have gone together symbiotically for centuries. Our diversified management mosaic attracts wildlife from the surrounding static forest and puts inordinate deer pressure on our land. As we began direct-marketing beef and chicken, we had interest from a couple of the customers about hunting.

Never being one to shy away from symbiotic enterprises, I put together a fee hunting program whereby people we had vetted could come and hunt for a day. A detailed map of the farm with large fifty-acre areas, designated by number, allowed hunters to come and be in a protected area without infringing on someone else's spot. Everyone signed in and signed out, dropped their money in a lockbox, and marked on the sign-in sheet where they would be hunting.

Many hunting groups either buy or lease land for their hunting. The problem with the public hunting land is that anyone can go there and it's not very secure. Unfortunately, alcohol, recklessness, and other things sometimes accompany hunting, so the demand is significant for private hunting opportunities. Our per diem flexible system was ideal for people who wanted to get to a secure, private place without all the formality and fraternity of a hunting club.

It worked fine. I always checked the sign-outs about half an hour after dark to make sure everyone had come out. That was a security measure we offered. If someone didn't come out, we would go looking for him. The system was unique and worked very well for the short time it ran. Why short time?

Because it didn't take long for our pastured poultry and direct-marketed beef to attract some attention in the local press. At the time, our farm homeowner's policy was through Farm Bureau Insurance, affiliated with the American Farm Bureau Federation, which is arguably the nation's number one farm lobby. The local insurance agent paid us a visit and said that if we sold one chicken directly to a consumer, Farm Bureau would not insure us for anything — even if our house burned down.

Folks, you need to understand this. Farm Bureau's position was not that it refused to accept product liability. If that were the case, we could have simply removed product liability from the policy. As I mentioned in the previous chapter, since the risk of being sued is in direct proportion to the amount of liability insurance you have, I'd just as soon not carry any liability insurance. That way it would be hard for someone to sue and collect anything.

What Farm Bureau said was that if a neighbor came and bought one dead oven-ready chicken from us, the insurance company would not cover our home, our barn, our animals — nothing. They were perfectly happy with the hunting arrangement. The hunting liability was no problem. But those chickens and that beef, they just couldn't abide that liability. After all, poultry and beef are far more risky than guns.

The hunting deal was small and fledgling. The poultry and beef were our livelihood, so we couldn't afford to quit direct marketing. Again, it wasn't the poultry and beef production that was the problem. It was the fact that we were selling dead animals. You see, farmers are only supposed to sell live animals to processors and marketers who are supposed to make all the money — those notorious middlemen. After all, we couldn't have all that middleman money going to farmers. No, that wouldn't be right. Farmers are supposed to be peasants, serfs, impoverished dolts, remember?

We felt like our only response was to begin searching for an insurance company that didn't fear direct marketing. I certainly learned at that time just how firmly the Farm Bureau Federation is entrenched in the industrial agribusiness paradigm. While it purports to represent farmers, it really represents the corporate agribusiness community. Of course, since most farmers are completely dependent on corporate agribusiness, that suits farmers just fine. In all fairness, this policy may have changed by now, but if it has, Farm Bureau has certainly been a Johnny-come-lately to the local food scene.

We soon found another local insurance underwriter who didn't have any problem with the direct-marketing approach. It was fairly small, innovative, low-risk. No problem. But they did have a huge problem with the fee hunting. No way. Too risky. If we let people come for free, or took down our "Posted: No Hunting" signs and let any riffraff come and hunt, drunk as a skunk or whatever, we had no liability.

Is that crazy, or what? In other words, if a guy comes on our property and shoots someone, as long as we didn't try to exclude him or protect ourselves, we wouldn't be liable. But as soon as we close our boundaries and vet those allowed in, then we're liable for what happens. If someone gets wounded here, he can sue me for letting the other person on the place, but if I take down all my posted signs and let anyone hunt on my land who wants to, then I absolve myself of all liability. Folks, is this normal? This is nuts. I realize that all you attorneys out there understand this perfectly. To me, it's unreasonable, unfair, and nonsense.

In the final analysis, though, you have to pick your battles, and you can't right all the wrongs in a day, no matter how much you'd like to. Since hunting was small and fledgling, we jettisoned that enterprise and went with the new insurance underwriter. Several years later we added product liability when even this underwriter got nervous about our exposure. It was no big deal, though. Cheap and easy, it gave us $300,000 of product liability coverage. At the time, that was the minimum required at most farmers' markets and a generally recognized acceptable level for local community-based direct-marketing farms.

As our farm sales have grown, we've added coverage to keep up with exposure and today carry the $3 million umbrella coverage I discussed in the previous chapter in order to get our farm products into mainline distributors. Even though we've worked hard to secure the coverage, these companies, who run scared from litigation every single day, heap on cover-your-tail procedures that inevitably deny access to smaller outfits like us. We still can't get on a Sysco truck.

This whole litigation climate is destroying innovation because it makes people too afraid to move. If I think you might sue me, I'm going to move much more cautiously in my relationship with you than if I know you won't sue me. Polyface now leases several farms in the area. These are landowners who, for the most part, have approached us and asked us to manage their properties. It allows us to expand to meet our market demand but maintain a decentralized, spread-out production and processing model consistent with our ecological and business values.

Each agreement contains a no-litigation clause. No matter what happens or who is at fault, neither party can sue the other. Instead, we must go to binding arbitration. I have been in courtrooms several times and find them outrageous. I think if we elected non-attorneys as legislators, and selected judges from regular people, including the Supreme Court, we would have more reasonable decisions. The Constitution does not encourage attorneys to be judges. Our cultural assumption that only licensed attorneys are eligible to be judges automatically excludes innovation. It assures a fraternity of like-minded people who will assuredly protect the culture's power brokers.

Wouldn't it be a hoot to put a couple of farmers, a used car salesman, two schoolteachers, a plumber, and construction worker on the Supreme Court? It might just restore sanity to the bench. It would sure make for some interesting reading. Why not put honorable, distinguished businesspeople on some of these benches? Maybe they would not worship the law so much, and start telling the jury the truth: that a jury can throw out a foolish law. Instead, these law-worshipping judges, steeped in conventional fraternization, refuse to tell the jury how much power it has.

I think our culture is paralyzed, again, by constipation of imagination. Is there no recourse for redress other than litigation? Probably the closest thing to a free market that exists in the United States right now is eBay. If I buy a product that doesn't work, I don't need to sue somebody; I just tell people not to patronize that company. If a doctor louses up, why don't the nurses and other staff let people know that the doctor is a bumbling idiot? No, they circle the wagons in their fraternity to protect the professional institution. Teresa's longtime gynecologist recently retired early because he said he got tired of paying $50,000 a month for his medical malpractice insurance.

To my knowledge he's never been sued. He's a pillar of the community and has delivered lots and lots of babies. But $50,000 a month! He said, "I like to talk to my patients, but with this insurance premium, I don't have time. I have to keep that door swinging as fast as possible just to pay the overhead." Our area lost a great doctor when he hung up his stethoscope a couple of years ago. So all you people who think litigation is the way to balance the playing field in our culture, just think about what is *not* being accomplished, and the good that is *not* being done, because of our litigious culture.

Life happens. We make decisions. Sometimes things don't work out like you planned. If somebody's negligence hurts me, the government is supposed to punish the perpetrator of the harm. If you look at the biblical justice system in the Mosaic law, you don't see suits. You see governmental redress. A thief must restore what he stole. If a farmer has an unruly cow and it hurts someone, that farmer can be executed for not dealing with the unruly animal. Now, for goodness' sake, don't let the execution punishment override the point that the judicial model did not depend on the harmed person suing the farmer; it depended on the government bringing the negligent farmer to trial.

Instead of the state dispensing justice, we have litigious vigilantes. When a woman sues McDonald's because her coffee burned her when it spilled in her lap at a stoplight, that's nonsense. These frivolous suits are costing millions of dollars, creating a professional sue-er class. (Yes, the pun is intentional.) Since the government appears uninterested in dispensing justice, which is its obligation, it instead imposes a host of regulations, licenses, and bureaucratic paperwork.

Routinely our pasture-based meats, poultry, and eggs are not served at establishments because they haven't been certified by some agency or organization. It reminds me of a discussion I had with one of our state general assembly delegates, who said one of the biggest problems in the large poultry processing plants is personal hygiene of the workers. He said many of these workers go to the bathroom and don't wash their hands before coming back onto the processing line and handling meat (or vegetables in other areas).

A plant can have all the stainless steel and written sanitation policies in the world, but at the end of the day, if a worker uses the bathroom without washing his hands, the subsequently handled food could be tainted. Therefore, to protect themselves, the industry and food police are trying to require irradiation, chlorine baths, and other highly toxic procedures. Eggs are a perfect example. Industrial eggs are washed in a chlorine bath. Since the shells are permeable, some of that chlorine enters the egg. This is standard food safety protocol. In fact, some health department inspectors believe an egg not washed in chlorine is not fit for human consumption. I have a whole story about this and other related incidents in my book *Everything I Want to Do Is Illegal*.

We don't wash the eggs from our farm in chlorine for a number of reasons. First, eggshells are porous and some of the chlorine leaches into the egg's interior. How much chlorine have you been eating lately? Yum. Secondly, our eggs don't have the pathogens that factory-farmed eggs have. Third, any pathogens our eggs might have are gentle natural pathogens, not mutated superbugs created by bathing the laying hen operation in antibiotics, hormones, artificial feed ingredients, and toxic sanitizers sprayed around the buildings.

In our litigious world, nobody cares about these alternatives that act as their own product liability protection. It's a pass/fail system. You're either in or out. You either follow these accepted procedures or not. As a result, standard operating procedures have become too onerous for small operations. For the record, in principle I don't have any problem submitting our products for testing, but if the tests cost me $500 apiece then I have a problem because I don't have enough pounds or pieces to justify the expense.

One big fear facing the heritage-based food community is the anemic bacterial tolerance of people. Due to the fear of litigation, most food processors confuse safe with sterile. I have news for you: Our bodies do not want sterile food. Plastic is sterile. Glass is sterile. Sterile is not biological. Sterile does not feed our three-trillion-member internal community.

As more and more eaters realize that sterile is not nutritional, they ask for living food. The problem is that if you've been eating sterile for a long time — and in the case of many children today, your whole life — suddenly exposing your body to living food can cause a toxic reaction. This is especially true with raw dairy products. Anyone who begins reading the current literature promoting raw dairy products will quickly find out that bacterially alive food is what this is all about.

A big difference exists between the mutated bacteria found at the end of a factory and the weakened strains found at the end of a pastured livestock operation. The same could be said of raw-milk cheeses. Food police are swooping in and closing down cottage-industry cheesemakers, alleging pathogenicity. The truth is that benign strains of campylobacter, for example, are part of the living food system. Eating some mold is a good thing. These historically normal bacteria help our immune systems. When we sterilize the food, or have a zero tolerance policy, the survivors — and there are always survivors somewhere — mutate to these more toxic strains that our bodies can't handle.

The reason the industrial food system must kill everything through sterilization is because the bugs, to use a vernacular term, are lethal. When you read about new strains of old bugs, designated by new numbers, these are more virulent strains than natural systems produce. Scientists who accuse people like me of being simple-minded and imprecise with our terms often practice the same broad-brush approach when it comes to these bugs.

A great example is E. coli, which has numerous strains. The scientists in the industry scoff at me with the condescending, "Don't you

know that all cows have always had *E. coli*? It's necessary for their digestion." What you might not see on camera is a rolling of the eyes, shaking of the head, when these credentialed experts dismiss the anti–factory
farming crowd as being simpletons. The anti–factory farming crowd,
of course, accuses the industry of encouraging these bad bugs that hurt
people.

Actually, both sides are right . . . or wrong, whichever way you want to
look at it. The *E. coli* strains that have been in the rumen of the herbivore since time immemorial and do play an important role in digestion
enjoy a natural alkaline environment. When raw forages enter the herbivore's alkaline rumen, they are broken down by many types of bacteria that thrive in that environment. The process is akin to fermentation.

But when a cow eats lots of already fermented feedstuffs like silage,
and especially eats grains, it causes the Ph of the rumen to become
more acidic. This creates a condition in the rumen called acidosis. To
digest this new type of feedstuff, the bacteria in the rumen change to
more acid-loving varieties. Over time, new generations emerge that
thrive in a more acid environment.

In normal conditions, the human digestive system is far more acidic
than an herbivore's. I always wondered how a cow could cough up forage already in its first stomach and enjoy the taste. Whenever I cough
up something from my one stomach, it doesn't taste like something I'd
like to chew on contentedly. Yuck. But a cow is not like that. She enjoys
that sweet taste of the nonacidic forage. If a human were to ingest these
natural *E. coli* strains, our acidic digestive juices would kill them
immediately.

This is why, even in extremely unsanitary conditions, Native Americans and pioneers, and modern-day hunters, never suffer from *E. coli*
contamination. When you kill an herbivore in the wild, it's virtually
impossible to sanitize the carcass. I've field dressed these animals, and
even at best, something is going to touch manure — even if it's manure
from another animal.

But these new, virulent acid-tolerant strains of *E. coli* are a different
story. Already acclimated to acidic conditions, instead of our acidic
digestive system killing these bacteria, the mutated strains kill us. Several years ago when Cornell University's research showed that feeding
forage for two weeks prior to slaughter would practically eliminate the

risk of *E. coli* problems, wouldn't you think the industry would have created new protocols for forage-finished feeding?

No, instead the industry vilified Cornell. The industry said the tests were not conducted correctly, yada, yada, yada. Here was a chance to really do something positive, and the industry pooh-poohed the whole thing. The point is that if I, as a beef producer, don't feed grain and silage to my animals, even if your steak has some *E. coli* on it, you won't get sick. For decades on our farm we've treated ourselves to ice cream bars after processing chicken. We've never even washed our hands. Guts to ice cream. Yum. We've never gotten sick.

Why? The reason is because whatever bacteria we have is a gentle strain. Indeed, exposure to these gentle, normal strains are key to stretching and exercising our immune system. Absent these gentle assaults our immune system becomes lethargic. Absent them long enough and our immune system becomes so abnormal that it can't even deal with these gentle bugs anymore. And that, dear people, is a very real issue in the heritage foods movement.

Antimicrobial soaps play right into this sterility fixation. Honestly, I don't want our farm customers using antimicrobials. They assault the healthy bacteria and break down our defenses. While this certainly sounds like heresy to some credentialed health professionals, I assure you that a whole body of information exists to support my position. If you want to eat sterile food and use antimicrobial soap and bathe in chlorine twice a day, have at it. It's a big world. But realize that by doing so if you decide to eat bacteria-rich living food, you may have killed off all of your defenses to handle even slight problems. If you get sick, will you then sue me? Who really is responsible in this situation?

Every day we have people who for years have eaten nothing but sterilized food, coming into our farm store and buying living food. We know our meat, poultry, and eggs contain bacteria. Good cheese should contain bacteria. That's part of the process, but it's a very different bacteria than that created by toxic bacterial annihilation programs and abnormally fed or fertilized animals and plants.

When the food police or the litigation freaks descend on a farm and find bacteria, it may or may not be harmful bacteria. Right now this is a major battle in artisanal cheesemaking. Living cheese has some bacteria in it. To be sure, just because an enterprise is small does not mean it is clean. I've seen some pretty dirty outfits. The problem is when a small outfit buys in product from industrial sources.

Some of the most treacherous ground is when the industrial and artisanal meet. The safe thing is never to let them meet. They are two mutually exclusive universes.

Some raw dairy farms are having their patrons sign indemnification contracts, hold harmless agreements, or liability waivers. That may be the face of local heritage-based food for the foreseeable future. It's tragic that our litigious society makes us producers feel held hostage, and in turn makes all of us want to hold others hostage. I hate living in fear, looking over my shoulder every day wondering who might sue me. In fact, I refuse to live that way. Long ago I came to terms with my living food, and determined to do the best job I could. If somebody sues me and collects, then God must have something better for me to do. Unfortunately, artisan cheesemakers are actually getting out of the business and changing careers due to food sterility requirements.

This convoluted thinking and blatant misunderstanding of life now means that Coca-Cola is safe, but raw milk is not. Food safety is completely subjective. I don't think for a minute that most of what's in the supermarket is safe. But it's been deemed safe because it only kills you slowly. While thousands of people die due to unnatural food and nutrient-deprived food, the food police go after a cottage-industry cheesemaker because two people got diarrhea. If we really want to be safe, we should outlaw swimming pools and automobiles. They kill far more people than raw milk or home-canned produce. How about Type II diabetes, obesity, childhood onset leukemia, and other food-induced maladies?

The only reason foods that cause long-term illness are deemed safe is because our experts are fixated on the lethal dose concept. If it doesn't kill you right now, then it's safe. That's nonsense. Ultimately, food safety is a subjective determination, but our litigious society is trying to confine it within governmental officialdom.

Recently I heard a news story about a fellow who climbed a security fence to rob a filling station. He robbed the station and decided to exit a little easier when he saw a ladder lying by the fence. He put the ladder against the fence to aid his escape, only to break a rotted rung at six feet up. The subsequent crash to the ground broke a leg and he sued the filling station owner for having improper equipment — and collected. Now folks, that ain't normal.

How does someone get a ridiculous award like that? I don't know. But if we did not have this sue-crazy culture, created by an unreasonable award protocol, perhaps people would begin taking more of their own responsibility. My heart goes out to a family, for example, that loses a child who ate a hamburger tainted with virulent *E. coli* in a restaurant. Of course, what happens is that the restaurant immediately says it complied with all government food safety regulations so it's not liable.

The government is immune from liability, so it's not responsible. The restaurant has a government license that indicates it complied with inspection requirements, so it's not liable. The result is that nothing changes and nobody is responsible. If we didn't have the government involved, then the business would be forced to accept liability. As soon as the business is forced to accept liability, it will become much more careful about how it handles things. It may begin snooping around its suppliers, which may mean terminating buying beef from factory feedlots. When people are educated and understand the dangers of industrial feedlot beef, they may begin choosing not to eat it.

When the suppliers are held liable by the restaurant, then the suppliers begin snooping around the processors. And the processors begin snooping around the farms. As it is today, all of these entities buy concessionary passes from their government fraternity buddies by playing a few rounds of golf and then quaffing a few beers together at the country club. Oh yes, they probably invite a few litigators to join them too. Anyone who thinks this is not reality is either incredibly naïve or refuses to see what is really going on.

Meanwhile, all those parties attack their most vulnerable competitors and the ones who can provide an antidote to the problems: local heritage-based food businesses. If you attend any state meeting of ecologically minded direct-marketing farmers, in an hour you will hear a dozen horror stories about litigation and the food police. I don't know which is worse. The industry wants more food police in order to be absolved of liability. The food police want more power just because they are people, and people love power.

So where do we go from here? Let's think a bit about our litigious

society. Is there a remedy, or are we doomed to keep siphoning off innovative energies, alternative products, and precious capital to this societal scourge?

First, I think we need a Japanese loser-pay system for civil suits. In
this model, if I sue you and lose, I have to pay you the amount that I
sued you for. This would do two things very fast. It would ensure that
the person who sues has an extremely good case. Second, it would profoundly reduce the amount of the recoveries.

As it is, many suits, even those without merit, are settled for some
tiny portion of the amount just to get rid of the litigation. I sue you for
$5 million in a completely frivolous suit hoping you'll settle with me for
$50,000. That's legal blackmail and it happens every day in America.
We have to quit assuming that just because someone files a suit, he has
a case.

We're hardwired to believe bad news. That's why we call them stop
lights and not go lights. The human psyche, for whatever reason, thrives
on bad news. If I come up to you with juicy gossip about so-and-so, you
tend to believe it. Without question. I may be making it up, blowing
some tiny thing out of proportion, or whatever. But we love to believe
the negative.

This is why, for many years, our farm did not take female interns. It
wasn't because they couldn't do the work. We knew of instances where
farmers had taken female interns and gotten crossways somehow, then
been sued for sexual harassment or some trumped-up allegation. It
ruined them. If I go to work in the woods all day with a good-looking
co-ed, and three years later she files papers saying that on such-and-
such a day when we were up in the woods together I groped her, what
are you going to believe? Don't sit there self-righteously and say, "I
would wait to hear the facts." Hogwash.

You know, I know, and everybody knows I'm toast. That's the way our
society is; it's the way of human nature. Adding third parties to every
work assignment was far too cumbersome, so we elected to dispense
with any liability by not having females. Eventually, I was getting
beaten up so badly out on the speaking circuit that I pleaded with my
family for mercy. Females could not believe that we would be so prejudicial. Folks, in our view, this was just prudent business. I love women. I
married the greatest one on earth — sorry, all you other guys. But this is

the direct result of a litigious society. This is how opportunity and innovation are destroyed by the current litigious climate.

I begged the family to let us take females. Just to try it. I was being
vilified, crucified by women. It didn't matter how many earthworms we
grew. It didn't matter what I said about ecology. Since we excluded
women from our intern program, I was worse than a sexual predator.
Interestingly, during that time, we received ten female applications to
every male one. Four years ago the family acquiesced and we opened
up internships to women.

Immediately the female applicants dropped to nothing. In four years,
we have not turned away one single woman intern applicant who made
it through our initial questionnaire process. That may change this year,
but so far we've taken every one who came to our mandatory two-day
checkout. We take two per summer. The only reasonable explanation
for the precipitous drop in applicants, in my opinion, is that it is no
longer forbidden fruit. These women didn't actually want to come as
interns. They were just making a point.

To be sure, we are extremely discriminatory in our acceptance standards. We've had fantastic female interns, but we're very careful to send
three people together when the job is several hours and out in the boon-
docks. This is a completely defensive protocol to reduce the possibility
of litigation. It's a shame that this has to occupy our minds every day, in
making work assignments, in creating the farm schedule, but that's life
in litigious America and it has a direct impact on how farmers like me
make everyday decisions. It also affects the decision whether or not to
have interns at all.

Too often people sit around and discuss these issues as if they exist in
some netherland, some fantasy place 'twixt our ears, above the earth
but not in the heavens. Some ephemeral place of cerebral discussion.
Perhaps in college focus groups or bureaucratic committee meetings.
Actually, these cultural norms touch lives. They create or destroy real
dreams, and that is why we should deal with them head-on and not
cavalierly toss our heads and say, "Tort reform? Oh, you want to destroy
the downtrodden? You want to eliminate fairness?"

Talk about constipation of imagination.

Second, we should put a value on human life. What's a life
worth — $100,000, $200,000, $1 million? Just put a value on it. No

matter what happens, if your negligence kills me, then all you can collect is the value of my life. It should be written into legislation and stan-
dardized. Executives. CEOs. Janitors. One and the same. Forget the
haggling. It's not worth the haggling. Just set a figure and be done
with it.

Third, no emotional trauma. You know what? Our litigious society
has caused me emotional trauma. Who do I sue? All of us have emotional trauma. Look at our parents. Look at our kids. Look at our neighbors. Look at our teachers. I've got emotional trauma, you've got
emotional trauma. Forget it. This discussion is giving me emotional
trauma. Emotional trauma makes for great stories, but we all have it. It's
worth diddly-squat.

**Fourth, anyone at any time and anywhere should be able to sign
away their rights.** I should be able to absolve you of liability for anything I choose. Many years ago, our state delegate tried to get a customer waiver for direct marketers. This would be a waiver that would
ensure informed consent:

"I know this food is not government-certified."

"I am buying this food of my own volition, with no coercion from
anyone."

"I have visited the farm and verify that it satisfies my requirements
for food safety."

"I hold the farmer harmless should anything happen to me as a result
of consuming, preparing, or acquiring this food."

"If I get sick, I will not demand treatment from society's equity."

"If I get sick, I will die rather than seek remedies from taxpayers."

"I hold Santa Claus harmless for the Christmas letter that my friend
sent me introducing me to this farm."

You get the picture. The Virginia attorney general told my delegate
that waivers are not worth anything. He said they don't mean anything
because people will always say they didn't know what they were signing
and didn't understand the legal ramifications of said document, yada,
yada, yada.

We live in a strange time when you can't promise not to sue me so
that you can get better food from me for yourself. That's crazy. Who
owns me? Ultimately, that's the question. Who owns my three-trillion-
member internal bacterial community? The government's track record

on deciding what to promote as safe food is abysmal. The government told us to feed dead cows to cows and gave us mad cow disease. The government told us to subsidize corn growers and cheapened unhealthy high-fructose corn syrup.

The government told us to eat trans fats and hydrogenated oils. The government paid for research to irradiate, transgenically modify, and clone. The government paid for manure slurry lagoons instead of compost. Folks, why in the name of common sense would we entrust the government to prescribe what we can and cannot feed our internal community? Have we no liberty, no autonomy?

The food police don't think we should have the freedom to eat something that might hurt us — as if their sanctioned factory-farmed supermarket fare is good. The truth is that if I don't have the freedom to hurt myself, then neither do I have the freedom to help myself with something that is not government-sanctioned. Many issues are like this, from childhood immunization to accepted cancer therapies. A culture that will not allow its citizenry autonomy in matters of personal food intake will certainly destroy other freedoms very quickly. Ultimately, you are not responsible for me. I am responsible for me. If you disagree, that's fine, but at least let me take responsibility for myself. Isn't that the charitable thing to do?

The food police, however, will not let me take responsibility for myself. Whether I like their prescriptions or not, they demand that I swallow their pills. People, that's tyranny of the worst sort. Choosing my food is as personal and sacred as choosing my religion or what to write.

I've listened in dismay, at public hearings, when the food police say I should not be allowed to sell customer-inspected food because I might get sued and lose the farm. If that doesn't show the true reason for food inspections, I don't know what does. I appreciate that these officials don't want me to be sued. But if it doesn't bother me, why should it bother them? They aren't the ones painting the barn, building fences, paying taxes, and stewarding the land. By what authority should they be able to preclude food choice just because they think it's a risky business decision? Folks, King George would blush at the tyranny in our own country.

In other words, the government, in its all-caring wisdom, does not want me as a farmer to be able to jeopardize my farm's future by deciding, for myself, to sell something to a neighbor. Isn't the government nice? What would we do without such caring bureaucrats? I think I need to sit down right now and send them thank-you cards for sparing me the choice to be reckless.

I think I'll sit down and eat their sanctioned Twinkies and Cocoa Puffs, washed down with a half liter of Coke. That will put me in a better frame of mind, don't you think? My, my, I feel better already. How absurd to think my neighbor and I could transact a dead chicken deal or dozen eggs deal without threat of suit. How utterly un-American. I'm so thankful our military might is protecting this great American tradition. All you fine young soldiers in uniform, thank you for sacrificing to keep our government bureaucrats safely ensconced behind their mahogany desks, drawing fat paychecks extracted at gunpoint from my farm, where in their infinite wisdom they've decided I should not be able to sell a chicken to my neighbor, all to protect me, of course. Good grief, Charlie Brown. This ain't normal.

Fifth, elect some officials who aren't attorneys. Let's put some janitors, some businesspeople, some doctors, some schoolteachers in Washington. Goodness, I'd be happy for a couple of rocket scientists. Maybe even a farmer or two. The point is, let's get some diversity in our legislators. Let's quit putting in people whose passion is parsing words rather than trying to discover truth and fairness.

Sixth, patronize the underdog. I don't care who it is or what it is. I don't shop at Wal-Mart as a matter of principle. I'd rather pay an extra 20 percent than shop at Wal-Mart. I love the underdog. It's fun to help the underdog. If we all search for the underdog, we'll float more boats. And the boats will be far more individualistic and exciting.

Whenever I hear an ad touting, "We're the biggest," I automatically decide I won't patronize that outfit. You won't get anywhere with me telling me you're the biggest. And yes, I'm writing this on an Apple computer. Go Apple. Perhaps the biggest reason Apple appealed to me when I decided to buy my first computer was because, at the time, the e-press was predicting the company's demise. The thought of losing choice stirred me to action, and I bought an Apple. Perhaps that sale saved the company. I wonder if anyone else bought an Apple because of that. I didn't know enough about computers to know if Apple was better. I still don't know, but I'm glad all of us still have a choice. Aren't you?

Amazingly, our peer-dependent celebrity culture runs from fad to fad. Why not hang in there with the stodgy tried-and-true? Who needs to run with the pack? Like Robert Frost said, "I chose the road less traveled by, and that has made all the difference." Why do people run to the crowd? I like running away from the crowd. I always tell farmers that if their farming neighbors think their idea is a good one, don't do it. Only the ideas that brand you as a lunatic will be innovative and radical enough to be the answer.

If all of us patronize the underdog, eventually we'll have a lot more dogs in the race. More dogs can't be bad. Can they?

Here are some points to ponder.

1. Who owns me?
2. Who is responsible for me?
3. Who do I trust to provide me the safest food — a neighbor, or the government?
4. Will more food police, enforcing the government's food agenda, help or hurt food diversity and choice?

I'm from the Government, and I'm Here to Help You—Right

What is the responsibility of government? Farming is ultimately about how to grow the food and care for the land. Food is ultimately about how we interact with that land and how we care for our bodies. With government's dominant penetration in food and farming, the question of responsibility is crucial. Government's size and manipulation of our lives today is far greater than anything envisioned by the people who founded this country. I realize this topic is huge and we certainly won't examine all the nuances in one chapter, but I want to touch on it simply because I have experienced some things that may be of interest to you. In my opinion, the government we have today is certainly not normal.

I was in Australia preparing to go on their *Today Show*. The day prior to the live studio appearance, their lieutenant interviewer called to feel me out and select the themes and issues that would be most interesting for the show. After having me explain a little about our farm, she went after the food processors — them, those guys, those dastardly people. "Don't you think the government should forbid them to process food like that?" she queried.

"No," I responded. "Nobody is holding a gun to consumers' heads demanding that they buy frozen DiGiorno's pizza. Nobody is requiring people to buy food with MSG in it. Nobody has to buy Coca-Cola."

"Well, don't you think the government should protect people from these products?" she pursued.

"No. It's a big free country. People are responsible for what they eat. They are the ones who decide what goes into their bodies."

"Oh, we couldn't say that. That would offend our listeners, to be told that they are responsible," retorted the miffed journalist. In fact, my greatly abbreviated perversion of the ten-minute interchange doesn't do justice to her badgering and then horror that I would suggest people are responsible for their food decisions. What made the interchange all the more epiphanal for me was that she purported to be an allegedly objective hard-news journalist, not a commentator and not a lobbyist.

What if we agreed that this was the role of government, to place stipulations on food processing? How many government meetings, how many stacks of paper do you think it would take to create a regulation about processing? All at the taxpayers' expense, of course.

I was incredulous last year when consumer advocates started lobbying for a tax on high-fructose corn (HFC) syrup. Everyone knows it's bad for you. Instituting an HFC beverage tax, according to the rationale, would deter its use, like sin taxes on cigarettes and alcohol. Obviously, those taxes have worked, haven't they?

My response to this idea was simply this: Instead of putting a tax on corn syrup, why not eliminate corn subsidies? If taxpayers did not subsidize corn, it wouldn't be as cheap to produce, corn syrup wouldn't be as cheap to manufacture, and perhaps a candy bar wouldn't be cheaper than a carrot. I hear people wanting to subsidize produce in order to make it price-competitive with sugary foods. Instead, why not take away the subsidies for sugarcane?

Wouldn't you think that with our nation floundering in sugar, we'd quit subsidizing corn and sugarcane? No, that's far too difficult. Instead, we turn health care over to the government too. Is this normal?

Now that we've broached health care, let's talk about that for a minute. Who is responsible for my health? The government? Since when did the government become responsible for my health? I can hear the responses coming back through these pages: "But this is the charitable thing to do. What about people who can't afford it? Even Jesus said to help the needy."

Let's get this straight: Jesus never invoked the government to help anybody. He invoked His followers to be Good Samaritans, and to help the needy, to make room for children. He never encouraged anyone to use the government to those ends. Why? Because forced charity is not charity at all. If the government comes to me with a gun and takes my wealth to give to some charitable cause, regardless of how noble, the forcible removal of my contribution does not make this a charitable act. Since when did violence become charity? If you don't think taxes are violent, just try abstaining from paying them.

Personally, I resent that our culture now thinks that I am responsible for the health of a smoking, drinking, nonexercising, candy-bar diet, junk-food addict couch potato. How in the name of anything close to normal can anyone suggest that I should be forced at gunpoint (taxes) to pay for this joker's medical care? Even Jesus didn't heal everyone. If charity cannot be done charitably, then it's not charity. Charity that requires violent force doesn't sound very charitable to me.

Anyone who thinks the Internal Revenue Service is not a violent force apparently hasn't crossed a government regulatory agency yet. Anyone who thinks government bureaucrats have a better understanding of charity, of who deserves help and who does not, than private citizens and neighbors is living in la-la land.

Thomas Jefferson said, "The two enemies of the people are criminals and government, so let us tie the second down with the chains of the Constitution so the second will not become the legalized version of the first." That's strong language from a reasonable man.

If I'm not responsible for my health and the food I eat, then what else am I not responsible for? My education? My retirement? My income? My children? My job performance? Maintaining my house? Maintaining my automobile? Folks, as you start down this slope, it's a slippery degeneration to a total nanny state.

Think with me. If we want children to grow up to be responsible adults, how do we inculcate responsible decision-making into their psyche? Do we hover over them from dawn to dusk, following like a little puppy dog, keeping them from doing anything risky? Do we make sure they never climb a tree because they might fall? Never go in the swimming pool because they might drown? Never meet another child because that other snot-nosed kid might call them a name and hurt their feelings? Never get them a bicycle because they could wreck it? Never let them go down a set of stairs because they might tumble? Never let them see a book because they might encounter bad language or bad pictures? Never let them see a movie because it might have questionable content? Never let them choose their clothes because the patterns might clash? Never let them play a musical instrument because they might not be musically talented? Never let them perform in a play because they might forget their lines? Never let them visit family members because family members are always weird? Never let them cook because they might burn something? Never take them camping because they might get bit by a tick and get Lyme disease? Never eat because the food might be pathogenic?

Are you with me? Folks, a risk-free life is a life that's not worth living. Everything that makes life worth living is about taking risks. We've become such an abnormal namby-pamby wimp culture that we're scared to do anything. I think part of that is the abnormal assault on our sensibilities in every day's graphic newscasts about atrocities around the world. Whether it's starvation in Africa or bombings in Iraq or drug violence in Mexico, every day we're bombarded with more horror than the human psyche was built to handle.

Our cultural reaction is to batten down the hatches of our own lives. Self-preservation mode expresses itself in different ways. To people prone to a victimhood mentality, it means demanding relief and protection from someone else — usually a government entity. To others, it means taking the reins of their own destiny, becoming self-employed, growing their own food, milking their own cow, buying a piece of land, and developing a food larder and survival skills. Those two reactions illustrate the implications for how we answer the question: Who is responsible for me?

So if we want to raise responsible children, we cannot protect them from every risk. If we do so, we raise floundering, directionless, dependent young people. Smothering parents raise dysfunctional and totally dependent young adults. This is the same process as building immunity. You don't take a newborn infant into situations conducive to communicable diseases, but neither do you isolate a newborn infant from all human contact. Limited exposure creates immune responses, and as the child ages, the exercised immune system can take more and more assaults.

Using this analogy to decision-making, the way to create wise adults is to expose them to decision-making incidents. In other words, assaults on the decision-making immune system, in the form of bad decisions, develop a better immune system, which in this case is a system that makes better decisions.

What do you and I do when faced with a decision that could have serious consequences? We do some research. We consult people who know more about this than we do. We read, search the Internet — we do our research. This is what *Consumer Reports* is all about. This is why eBay has a feedback loop — a rating system that lets customers rate performance. When the results of the decision rest squarely on my shoulders, I get savvy about becoming informed. Once I feel confident enough to make the decision, I make it. It may turn out to be the wrong one, and I may have ended up being hoodwinked, but I'll be more savvy next time in the same situation. That is the way we create responsible decision-makers.

It's the same way we develop savvy food decision-makers. If the only thing I need to know is that the food has been licensed by the government as safe for consumption, then I'm like the parentally smothered child. I don't have any decisions to make. Such a system inevitably moves the population toward ignorance and complacency. And it makes the population more gullible because the discernment radar is not being exercised. If I assume that anything with a USDA stamp of approval is safe to consume, why do any research? Why care about how it was raised, whether it destroys the soil, or if it contains live bugs? The tidal wave of interest in local, artisanal, ecologically enhancing food is precisely because many people are realizing that the USDA stamp does not measure some of the most salient requirements in food.

The reason personal responsibility is culturally important is because it keeps people on their toes. When we remove decision-making responsibility from the populace, the tendency is for everyone to become lazy. If you had no government guarantee of safety, how informed would you become about the source of your food? Yes, that's what I thought. Pretty cotton-pickin', huh?

Ever since the Oscar-nominated documentary *Food, Inc.* came out, I've made a point of asking cabbies, hotel receptionists, airline ticket counter clerks — people I encounter in my normal travels —"Hey, have you ever heard of the documentary *Food, Inc.?*" Not one in a hundred has ever heard of it. Ditto *The Omnivore's Dilemma*, even though it has sold a million copies. In my circles, these, along with Eric Schlosser's *Fast Food Nation*, have achieved iconic status. But we forget that the vast majority of Americans don't read. They attend Hollywood flicks and eat at McDonald's.

When I do a presentation in some city, my reality check is to remind the audience that although it's wonderful to see the venue packed with five hundred people, in the amount of time we've gathered to promote local integrity food, many more than this, within a few miles, have eaten at McDonald's, Burger King, Kentucky Fried Chicken, whatever. While our normal food and living movement may be gaining steam, it's nowhere near a tipping point. We'll know we've achieved a tipping point when McDonald's starts closing restaurants or begins offering locally sourced, seasonal nonindustrial cuisine. But then they would hardly be recognizable as McDonald's, would they?

Here's the point: The way we create popular food literacy is to put people in the driver's seat. Make them responsible. The way to create wellness literacy is to put people in charge of their own health. Every time the government takes away decision-making power and choice risks, it dumbs down the populace in that arena. Do you wonder why people have such an unprecedented demand for sensationalism, for fantasy, for celebrity? It's because life without responsibility is boring.

Personal responsibility is thrilling. Wow, what a ride! Sure, dependency is easier. It feeds my laziness, but it doesn't feed my humanness. Ultimately, this whole discussion boils down to faith. Do I have faith in myself, in my private relationships, or in the government bureaucracy? A population educationally institutionalized all their life has now been acculturated to assume that government agents are more trustworthy than any other people they encounter.

Do you really believe that? Government agents are people just like you and me. Some are great and some are horrendous, and the more government injects itself into our affairs, the more temptation to create cozy public-private deals. While liberals naively call these partnerships, I see them as political bribery, cronyism, and collusion. That such a vast number of people in our culture now look to the government for salvation, as the first answer to any societal problem, does not indicate a new appreciation for the righteousness of government, but rather a profound political devolution into constipation of imagination.

Let's take a case in point and follow it. Let's revisit Upton Sinclair, 1906, and the founding of the Food Safety and Inspection Service (FSIS). Sinclair, a socialist, wrote *The Jungle* to expose atrocious working conditions primarily in the Chicago slaughterhouses and processing plants. Employees would fall into scalding vats, lose life and limb in exposed grinding machines. It was not a pretty picture.

The result was a little surprising to Sinclair. Instead of being incensed about working conditions, people were more outraged that the hamburger they ate might contain some human flesh or other unacceptable adulteration. The filth that made unsafe slippery floors, the manure everywhere — this got America's attention. The immediate result was that sales nationwide plummeted for the big packers of the day. This was 1906, and the nation still had an extremely healthy and vibrant number of community-based butchers and small abattoirs. People began patronizing these and withdrew their food dollars from the big packers.

Depending on what historian you read, the sales dropoff for the big packers was anywhere from 30 to 50 percent. The marketplace spoke. Loud and clear. How long do you think those packers could have stood that market spanking before overhauling their policies? In fact, many of them faced bankruptcy. Remember, this was a boon to local food systems because people went back to their neighborhood butchers instead of buying the prepackaged, canned meat. This was before refrigeration, so almost all the product people stopped buying was the processed, canned meat.

What actually happened differs depending on what historian you read. Some say the public demanded that President Teddy Roosevelt do something. Others say the packers went to Roosevelt on bended knee and begged him to establish federal government inspection to give them credibility with a disenfranchised public. In either case, at that point, federal government food inspection was born.

What if Teddy Roosevelt had decided to honor the Constitution and not enter the food fracas? What if he had respected the Constitution and said, "You guys are despicable and I'm glad you just lost 50 percent of the market. Now get your act together or you'll lose it all. I'm not the one who made you lose faith with the American people, and I'm sure not going to help you get it back. You made your bed, now lie in it, you sleazy, shortsighted corporate giants."

What if he had said that? First, Americans would have unilaterally abandoned the big packers. Most if not all would have gone out of business. Thousands of people would have been out of work, temporarily. But consumers would have moved their dollars to their community abattoirs. Local butchers would have hired additional staff. Local farmers would have enjoyed more income because the price of the meat would not have had to absorb such costly long-distance transportation. It might even have affected ranch overgrazing in the West.

Americans would have begun comparing notes. They would have visited farmers, local packing houses, and become educated about meat. After all, that's what Sinclair did: educate. With all the publicity about America's current deplorable food system, I encounter people every day who, after watching *Food, Inc.* or reading *The Omnivore's Dilemma*, exclaim, "Goodness, I had no idea!" Although I'm glad they are now informed, I can't help but sigh deep down inside: "Where have you been? I've been preaching this for forty years, and my family has been preaching it for eighty years. Where on God's green earth have you been, for crying out loud? How could you possibly be educated, with postgraduate degrees, white-collar careers, and be this ignorant? How can it be?"

I'll tell you how it can be. We didn't have to think about it. It was easy. No risk of wrong decisions. Just accept the government approval and be glad you can now occupy your mind with celebrity news since you don't have to think about which burger to buy. If Roosevelt had stood up to the big packers and refused government intervention, he would have promoted a food-literate populace. I'm well aware that the official news story is how he stood up to them and controlled them with the FSIS. But the real story is generally not the official one. A few days at a news desk will teach you that.

Then the industry and influential private parties would have banded together and developed a private inspection system like Underwriters Laboratory, the American Automobile Association (AAA), or the star-based restaurant and hospitality rating system. Plenty of private rating systems exist. The Weston A. Price Foundation (WAPF) in its

Shopping Guide rates farmers by how closely they adhere to certain WAPF production values. WAPF was founded in the 1990s by Sally Fallon Morell to champion the health benefits of eating traditional (normal) diets. Weston A. Price was a dentist who traveled the world in the early twentieth century to find societies that had not yet been touched by processed Western foods. In each of these cultures, he found no heart attacks, no arthritis, beautiful wide facial structures and teeth. His work now inspires the international WAPF movement, which, as Sally says, challenges the "diet dictocrats." Sounds like my kind of gal, don't you think?

Some of these private inspection options could have been for-profit membership outfits. A group of people would get together, set up a protocol, publish it, and people who wanted their food subjected to this set of criteria could join for a hundred dollars a year and get the inside scoop (or poop) on the businesses. Some could be nonprofit groups. If the FSIS budget stayed in people's pockets instead of being confiscated by the IRS, there would be plenty of money for the private sector to run this service. With private enterprise running it, the possibilities for innovative solutions to new problems would be far more than they are today with the entrenched government bureaucracy.

Could these private organizations themselves be co-opted by the industries they inspected? Of course. But that would leave room for innovative entrepreneurial upstarts to present their case for "ours is better" and the whole process could be reinvented as often as necessary per marketplace demand. Anyone who thinks the current government system has not been co-opted by the industry is living with their head in the sand.

I've participated in too many official public hearings to think the current system is anything but corrupt to the core. When I testified at the congressional hearing on meat safety, it was clear that most of the twelve speakers wanted twenty-four-hour surveillance cameras on every square foot of every abattoir in the nation. It seemed clear to me that these speakers had gone to the same fraternity parties prior to the hearing. The final speaker just happened to be in the video surveillance business.

In fact, he just happened to have a promotional PowerPoint on how his business could eliminate every problem in the meat industry. In clear deference to the bureaucracy, the head of the FSIS spoke first. He had aides handing him slips of paper during the cross-examination. Although twelve of us were scheduled to speak, he took up about a third of the time. When he finished and left the room, I realized how many department people were with him for backup. It seemed like the whole room left.

So we got to the last guy, the video surveillance dude. The congress-people swooned over his technology. I was sitting there thinking, *Wouldn't it be just like these politicians to require these cameras in every abattoir in the country?* They only cost a million dollars, which is bad enough if you're a multimillion-dollar packer. But if you're a little community abattoir, it puts you out of business. Collusion? Yes, I think so.

I've been to Richmond, our Virginia state capital, numerous times to testify at hearings and committee meetings. Up at the front table, sitting with the senators and delegates, is the lobbyist for the Agribusiness Council, the Corn Growers Association, the Farm Bureau Federation, the Virginia Poultry Federation, the veterinarians' association. Me? I get to sit in back with the peasants in the gallery, waiting for my name to be called. After two hours of posturing and political machinations, the chairman then, almost as an afterthought, calls on me, looking at his watch, admonishing, "Mr. Salatin, please be brief. We only have five more minutes." Folks, if you've never been to one of these, they are obscene. Every time I exit these hearings, I feel like I need to go take a shower and wash the filth off.

Why would anyone want these people to have authority over their lives? Truly, we are sheeple. Rather than think for ourselves, we want someone else to do all our thinking for us. Folks, this ain't normal. Read what the common person read leading up to the Revolutionary War, or the Civil War. Goodness, the average college graduate today couldn't make heads or tails of these writings. This is why many parents are opting for a classical education, in which their children become schooled in rhetoric, logic, and classic American texts. I think it's a wonderful renaissance and long overdue.

The bottom line is that if Roosevelt had not created the FSIS, people would not have starved and the world would not have stopped spinning. Adjustments to the new level of information would have cre-ated societal disturbance. What would have come out of that certainly could not have been worse than what we have today in the food police state.

Let me introduce you to an Old Order Mennonite man named Mark Nolt, from Pennsylvania, who voluntarily turned in his raw milk license a couple of years ago since it precluded him from doing anything besides selling milk. He couldn't sell ice cream, kefir, yogurt, or butter, and his customers clamored for all those things. He turned in the license and invoked his rights under "freedom of contract," which dates clear back to ancient English common law.

Essentially, the right of private contract, or treaty, says that if you and I want to strike a deal voluntarily, it's none of the government's business. If you want to buy my used car, and nobody is forcing me to sell or you to buy, then it's buyer beware and the price and stipulations like warranties that we agree to are our own business. If you ask me to make you a chair in my woodworking shop, and I say yes and quote a price, then we have a private contract.

So Mark simply used that old jurisprudence to market his pasture-based dairy products. His thriving business saw people drive a couple of hours one way to his farm to purchase his outlandishly good-tasting and nutritious dairy products, but the Pennsylvania Department of Agriculture couldn't abide this private contract. Nobody was forcing Nolt's customers to buy. Nolt was not forced to sell to anyone. The whole transaction was private and voluntary. But the food police saw it differently.

So they conducted a raid, complete with semiautomatic weapons, flak jackets, and a whole cadre of gun-toting state police. Nolt does not vote and does not pay into Social Security. He has opted out, putting faith in his own Mennonite community rather than the state to care for him in his older years. He doesn't even drive a car. The food police hauled him to the courthouse for processing, like a common criminal. When they offered him a ride home, he refused, and walked the twelve miles back to his farm.

In the raid, the officials confiscated product and equipment worth about $20,000. The next day, he continued milking cows, making kefir, and selling raw dairy products to his patrons, who swarmed around him like protective bees, encouraging him, giving him donations, and even performing fund-raisers on his behalf. Within a few months, the food police returned, again confiscating about $20,000 worth of machinery and product. He was issued a contempt of court judgment.

The next day, he was back milking cows, making ice cream, and servicing his loyal patrons, who again stepped up to the plate and surrounded him with financial and emotional help. Someday I hope to write a book about Nolt, because his story speaks to the heart of tyranny versus freedom. Here's a simple Mennonite man, caring for his farm, serving his patrons, and everyone is happy. Except the food police.

If I may invoke the Bible, Romans 13 in the New Testament gives us a clear reason for government: to be a "terror to evil" and an "encourager of righteousness." This is by far and away the most cited scriptural writing relative to government.

The more you know about the food police treatment toward Mark Nolt, the more you realize that the government has become a terror to righteousness, and an encourager of evil, a position inverted from the Apostle Paul's admonitions in Romans 13.

I wish Nolt's story were an isolated case. It is not. From one end of this great country to another, private food stores, private clubs, and clean farmers are being harassed by overzealous food police. Who gives them this authority? You and I. We have decided that food is a governmental responsibility. Once we make that assumption, it has broad ramifications for how our food is raised, what kind of farmers we have, what kind of food we have, and ultimately what our three-trillion-member internal bacterial community will ingest.

As this so-called governmental safety net widens, it captures an ever-broadening host of individuals. I do not question that most of this is done with good intentions and sincerity. But the road to hell is paved with good intentions. Remember the prohibition.

On this issue, I differ substantially with many of my sustainable agriculture friends who see this as a big food system versus small system battle. I do not. The pressure for more government food police is coming from the consumer advocacy lobby. That is why I'm belaboring the personal responsibility. I'm not afraid of industrial food corporations at all. They can't do anything to me. But the government comes with SWAT teams and guns — they can do something to me. Make no mistake, well-intentioned consumer protectionists are scared to death of industry corner-cutting. So am I, but the answer is not regulations that inevitably put little producers out of business. The answer is to quit buying from the industrial food system.

Several years ago I was doing a marketing seminar in Ohio for about two hundred farmers. The breaking news of the week was Monsanto's introduction of recombinant bovine growth hormone (rBGH) injections to dairy cows to stimulate milk production. The consumer advocates were outraged and spent millions of dollars trying to stop it, but to no avail. The FDA wouldn't even let milk labels carry an "rBGH-free" designation.

I had already done some figuring and realized that in Ohio, on twenty-five acres, a farmer could milk twenty cows. If he sold the milk directly to neighbors, at supermarket prices, he could net $25,000–$30,000 a year. I asked how many farmers in the room would like to do that. Every hand went up. Well, you ask, why didn't they do it? Raw milk is illegal. Even if you wanted to pasteurize and bottle it, the government requirements, including infrastructure, cannot be capitalized on such a small scale.

If all the effort lobbying against rBGH by consumer advocates had instead gone into releasing entrepreneurial community-based micro-dairies on their communities, our side would have buried rBGH milk in the marketplace. Pasture-based milk tastes better, is far more nutrient-dense, and far safer from a pathogen standpoint. Instead of demanding a government fix, why don't we just release entrepreneurism and let that fix the problem?

We hear a lot today about requiring labeling information on packaging, from "Country of Origin," to ingredients, to nutrition labels. That all sounds fine and dandy, until you're faced with the cost of a nutrient analysis that the FDA will accept. These usually run several thousand dollars per item. While it's true that we could just slap a typical USDA nutrient analysis on our eggs or poultry or beef, and the food police would be fine with that, such a label would be untrue.

At Polyface, our nutrient analyses always look like an entirely different product than USDA standards. It would be a lie for us to put one of those generic labels on our products. But to pay for one for every product is prohibitively expensive. I don't know what to do, but I hope you can see the problem. The same thing affects restaurants. Publishing nutrient analysis for McDonald's, which sells millions of the same item every day, is a spit in the ocean. But for a small, independent local restaurant, it can become onerous enough to put the entire business out of business.

This is the ugly underside of this "I'm not responsible, government is the answer" ship of state. Am I an anarchist? Not at all. I believe in personal responsibility. That means corporate polluters who received Superfund dollars to clean up their messes, in my world, would have not only had to pay all the costs of cleanup, but would have been personally punished for their actions. And by the way, my punishment would not include sitting in air-conditioned prisons watching soap operas on wide-screen TVs every day, getting three squares and no leftovers because leftovers have been deemed inhumane.

I wish I had a nickel for every wannabe farmer who has asked me to sign on as an expert to their grant-writing scheme to jump-start their enterprise. Whose pocket are they going to rob so their business can get a jump-start? Whose money is this, anyway? Remember, the government does not get any money that it does not first take from someone, by force. I know the world has needs. I know our neighbors have needs. If the government let us keep some of our own money, we'd have more to give, and it would be responsible, voluntary giving, not mindless giving.

Today Teresa and I received the news that for a number of crazy reasons, we have to pay almost $40,000 in taxes this year. I am being as transparent and honest as I can. We've worked, scraped, and developed this farm together, as a family. I won't bore you with the story of how hard we've worked. I'll leave that to your imagination. By the way, this is an anomaly — this is the first year this has happened. We've had several things contribute to an unusual set of circumstances that added up to a salary anomaly. We've been below the poverty level virtually all of our lives. We had a windfall year. It was a blessing.

Our reward? Forty thousand dollars in taxes. Folks, that's enough to hire another person. It's enough to build several large ponds and help protect the Potomac from floodwaters. We could put it in our local bank, in a CD, and it could be lent to other local businesses to help them get started. We could give it away to our favorite charities. We could give all our staff a huge bonus (we did anyway). Let me ask you something: Do you think the things we could think to do with that

$40,000 are more creative and noble than what the government will do with it? Think hard and be honest. Really, deep down, do you think the government would put this to better use than we would?

Not only is this confiscatory taxation not normal in history, it's outrageous. In the Old Testament story of Joseph, when Egypt's Pharaoh owned all the cattle, all the land, and all the people after the seven-year famine, Joseph let the people keep 90 percent of everything they produced. I say any tax rate more than 10 percent is immoral, indecent, obnoxious, and outrageous. In America, with all of the taxes figured in, it's almost 50 percent. Our civilization cannot survive this confiscatory rate of taxation.

We're just one small business among thousands. Unfortunately, our story is not unique. It happens to every working family in America, every day. For the tax-and-spend crowd to dishonor hardworking Americans like this just ain't normal. America has always honored work. We even have a Labor Day holiday. Thrift, personal responsibility, and industriousness have defined our culture since its inception.

While we're on the subject of money, let me register my decided disagreement with both the Bush and Obama bailout plans, from the automakers to the banking cartel.

The business and economic failures were enormously disturbing. This is the disturbance that's necessary to freshen up the ground. Consider it spading up the backyard to put in a vegetable garden. The Marines say, "Pain is weakness leaving the body." I don't care how you describe it, but fresh ideas and innovation are born out of disturbance, as Einstein said. To artificially prop up inept business or scalawags or worse, and delay the disturbance, is to deny the culture fertile ground for innovation. It's to deny the culture a phoenix. Yes, collapse would have been difficult. I don't like economic downturns any more than anyone else. But the night is always darkest right before dawn.

You can't have the reckless goings-on in banking without a day of reckoning. The government manipulation of the housing market, by demanding that high-risk loans be made to unqualified people in the name of helping them, had an inevitable fallout. I'm not a banker and I don't understand a lot of this, but I know you can't have the level of government manipulation we've had for the past several decades without lousing things up.

Our family used to own a three-apartment complex in town. Dad and Mom used it as an investment after they finished paying for the farm. The regulations about how we could advertise, who we could rent to, how and when we could kick them out — it was endless. Anyone who looks at anything in today's economy and says it's loused up due to free markets apparently doesn't realize the depth of governmental regulatory manipulation of every facet of America's marketplace. We have not had any free markets for a very, very long time. I can't think of any commodity or any product that enjoys a free market today.

A free market would require individual responsibility. It would require us to return to a constitutional form of government, wherein the government's role is minimal and individual responsibility is maximized. That was the reason for the chains Jefferson talked about — to keep the government from becoming criminal. I would suggest that those chains have long since fallen away, and the biggest criminal in our nation is the government. Ask Mark Nolt.

How do we move away from where we are? My detractors will counter that we aren't in an agrarian economy anymore. What was okay two hundred years ago can't be duplicated today. In fact, they would say today is normal for today, and yesterday was normal for yesterday. They would say normal is simply the status quo. Normal is relative, like the Constitution. It's a "living document," they say.

First, I admit I don't have all the answers — by a long shot. I've picked some fairly safe fights in this chapter. For example, I don't know where I fall on protectionism versus free trade. My libertarianism makes me tend toward free trade, but I also know that the founders of our country planned for the federal government to derive its income from import tariffs. Actually, the federal government received money from the states. Now it's reversed, with the states holding their hands out like whining children. Remember, until 1913 the federal income tax did not exist. Neither did the Federal Reserve. Dear President Woodrow Wilson destroyed the country with a double whammy. Of course, my first worst president was Abraham Lincoln, who gave us the USDA. What an idiotic dreamer. He really thought the government could teach people how to farm. And no, this doesn't mean I like slavery.

But in our nation today, we've traded people slavery for life slavery by allowing the patenting of life to corporations. When the Supreme

Court allowed private entities to patent life June 16, 1980, that legalized owning life. Owning life is slavery no matter how you cut it. As a nation we haven't gotten better on the slavery issue; we've gotten worse. For the pro-life community angry about *Roe v. Wade* to accept this moral earthquake with nary a whimper is both hypocritical and shocking. The government's primary responsibility is protecting the right to "life, liberty, and the pursuit of happiness." All of these speak to basic life freedom. To create new life forms, then buy and sell them, and then with the pollen from these life forms to adulterate normal lives in neighbors' fields, is evil. It's not right to life. In my opinion, it's right to kill; right to prostitute; right to enslave.

Does anyone really think farmers would be worse off today if there had been no government help? Really? Why couldn't Lincoln have had faith that farmers would band together and figure it out? Goodness, soil societies and grazing associations abounded. Private trade associations brought all sorts of new ideas to farmers. Today, the USDA not only refuses to accept any of my ideas, but actually labels them reckless and backward. When you see the track record of government agencies, why would anyone put faith in them? I don't get it.

But back to the tariffs question. What would our nation look like today if the federal government were still only financed by import tariffs and monies from the states? Wow. That's one to think about. And as for free trade, the problem is we don't have free trade. For example, our country subsidizes cheap crops that we dump into other countries, dislocating their agrarian base, and they in turn dump their subsidized commodities into our country and dislocate those industries. Honestly, I'm not sure about that one.

I'm also not sure about airwaves and broadcasting. It certainly needs some regulation. I certainly don't agree with any requirements on content — none — but I'm not sure what is right about who gets to put what frequencies out into the universe. Nobody has to turn any of it on, thank goodness. Why do parents need governmental oversight on TV broadcasting? Did you ever hear of the off switch? Why should that be a responsibility of government? A government that controls your TV will also control your access to compost-grown tomatoes and Aunt Matilda's pickles.

Believe it or not, I've talked with politicians at the federal level who actually believe the government should regulate the vegetables you eat out of your own garden. In Virginia, except for some last-minute terrific lobbying, it would have been illegal to drink milk from your own cow a couple of years ago. This law was averted by the slimmest margin. One senator said during the final showdown, "Isn't this like saying you can't watch the sun rise?" How much micromanagement can we afford, pray tell?

Here are some things that I think would get us started down a path of normalcy.

1. Quit asking the government to solve problems. If a societal problem exists, think about how it could be solved privately, without any bureaucracy, any committee meetings, or any regulatory paperwork. Just start doing what is right because it's right and don't wait for the government to credential it. If drinking rBGH milk is wrong, then don't wait for the government to make it wrong; just quit drinking it. If CAFOs are wrong, don't ask the government to outlaw them, just quit patronizing their food. Never underestimate the power of one.

2. Take charge of your own wellness. Don't expect to live like a slob and assume a government health care system will fix you for nothing. Get spiritually, emotionally, mentally, and physically well. Do whatever it takes. If your job gives you headaches, change jobs. Don't look for answers from the pharmacy. Get off your pills and props. One of the fastest-growing medical niches right now is the personal wellness trainer. I think that's super. Go see one. It will be worth every penny.

3. Drop your income. Work for less. You chief executive officers, drop your pay. Who needs to earn more than $200,000? Nobody. Nobody. Want me to say it one more time? Nobody. I'm not saying the government should make this mandatory; I'm saying if we had a couple of high-profile executives do this, it would create a ripple throughout the entire business world. Just quit paying taxes and give the money to people in a lower tax bracket. Since our country believes in redistributing wealth, go ahead and redistribute it now to your employees and they will love you to the ends of the earth. It might help the company, too.

4. Do it yourself. If you want to start a business, go ahead. What are you waiting for? If you have fire in the belly, go for it. Don't waste your passion on the trauma of deciphering government-speak to finance your project. If it's worth doing, it's worth doing without any government participation whatsoever. And if it won't fly without government participation, figure out how to make it fly. It's up to you, not somebody else. And especially not some bureaucrat.

Should I say, "Get back to the Constitution?" If that is normal, it's going to take some radical thinking to get there. I can say with some strong belief that personal responsibility is certainly more normal than running to the government to wipe every nose. Nothing is as liberating as freedom. Any government that gives you something can also take it back. If we view responsibility like a huge pile of stuff — all the responsibility for all the decisions that need to be made — the more responsibility the government takes the less there is for me. The less responsibility, the more ignorant I become and the less freedom I have. I'll take the responsibility, thank you very much.

The Church of Industrial Food's
Unholy Food Inquisition

Surrounding every morsel of food with a government-mandated protocol and infrastructure is unprecedented in human history. If we fear
what we don't know, it's no wonder that most Americans are paranoid
about food. They don't know where it comes from, how it grows, who
handled it, or how to prepare it. As this fear of the unknown grows, we
try to protect ourselves under a phalanx of food regulations. We demand
the government protect us from them, from those people, not realizing
that the government *is* them, and those people. And that in the final
analysis, it's just us.

The rate and severity of foodborne pathogens and recalls is unprecedented. I find it amazing that even as bad as things were in Upton Sinclair's *The Jungle*, published in 1906, nobody was getting sick. Yes,
things were filthy and workers were treated poorly. Maybe more people
were getting sick than our science at the time could discover. But at that
time, even the largest meatpackers in America were relatively small by
today's standards, and the centralization was not nearly as concentrated
as it is today.

Our nation had gotten along for 150 years without any food inspection whatsoever. During most of that time, of course, food was primarily local. "In 1910, 88 percent of America's chickens were in flocks of

less than 80 hens," according to Allan Nation's *The Moving Feast.* People were eating close to the land. Without refrigeration or efficient transportation, people ate regionally, locally, and almost everyone actually grew some portion of what they ate. The rapid urbanization that came with early industrialization created a new demand for industrial-sized processing. It was still tiny compared to today's industrial-scaled processing, but big compared to the embedded butcher, baker, and candlestick maker of that era.

Teddy Roosevelt's federal Food Safety and Inspection Service (FSIS) grew out of food industrialization. It was never needed for local and neighborhood operations. It only came about when scale and a corporate, mercenary mentality invaded the food system. Before then, food production enjoyed direct accountability due to its transparency. You either grew your own food or you knew the person who grew it and how it was handled. This created a tight feedback loop — remember our discussion of the self-policing eBay?

The mega–food processing facility changed all of that. Freed from the drudgery of manure and gardening, more factory workers quit growing anything for themselves. At this disturbing edge of cultural innovation, abuses became easier and the nation responded with a federal agency. I am confident that even Roosevelt never intended these regulations to reach down into little neighborhood abattoirs. And honestly, although I love a free and responsive market, I have made it a point not to debate people who think we at least need governmental oversight for the processing entities hidden from direct customer interaction. If you have a guard gate, security fence, and no trespassing signs around the facility, perhaps government inspection is appropriate.

Let's assume we have a scale from 1 to 10, with 1 being a Happy Meal and 10 being Aunt Matilda's Sunday dinner prepared from her own garden, her own chickens, her own kitchen flour mill, and her own canned pickles. Here's the question: Does the 1 need government oversight? Most people would say yes. Now what about the 10? Would you believe that I've encountered many people who say yes? Is that unbelievable? But that is a sign of our abnormal times. Fortunately, most people still say no to the 10. That's a relief.

By establishing two different food situations with a broad consensus that one needs oversight and the other one doesn't, then the meaningful

exercise is to walk the numbers toward the middle to determine if anything else can be excused from government oversight. Perhaps a 2 is a
frozen dinner. Yes. Perhaps a 9 is Community Supported Agriculture,
in which patrons invest in the farm and share risk with the farmer. Anyone that interested and committed should be able to buy whatever they
want without inspectors snooping around. How about an 8? Perhaps
that's direct farmer-to-consumer trade of any type, including farmers'
markets. Yes or no?

This seems like a reasonable way to arrive at a point, somewhere,
anywhere, that freedom of food choice is still allowed. As I've already
mentioned, however, we've already come, in our state, within a hair's
breadth of outlawing the freedom to drink milk from your own cow.
And I've met plenty of people who think you should not be able to enjoy
Aunt Matilda's meal prepared from her own garden without government intervention. Encouraging this backyard or farmstead food system, however, is the key to innovation in the food system.

What started out as a reaction to industrial food abuses has now
become the de facto firewall that protects corporate food globalists
from innovative entrepreneurial competition. Today, the size is bigger,
the pathogens worse, the abuses more flagrant, and the concentration
greater than it was in 1906. But we thought FSIS was supposed to stop
all of this and make things better.

I know to you liberal Democrats, what I'm about to say will sound
like libertarian nonsense, but I beg you to stay with me as I walk you
through something you may never have thought about before. Innovation requires prototyping. Prototypes by definition must be small.
Because they are trials and high-risk, you want to minimize your exposure to potential losses. If it doesn't work, in other words, you don't want
it to sink the rest of the business.

All innovation requires this initial small-scale prototyping. The more
regulation in any economic sector, the less prototyping is possible. Regulations tend to be nonscalable and therefore are not friendly to innovation. Realize that in about 1915 some fifteen hundred automobile
models were available. Imagine if today's regulations had been in place
at that time. Imagine if you had to be zoned commercial in order to
build a prototype automobile in your backyard machine shop. We

would not have had nearly as many ideas entering the auto-building prototype phase as we did.

We see this principle evident today. Let's take eBay as an example. Let's say that in order to put an item on eBay you had to have a certified computer license. And you had to submit to a government agent a detailed plan about how you were going to store the item, package the item, ship the item, and guarantee its safe arrival. And before you could log on, you needed an establishment number that showed that you had passed the local fire code (we wouldn't want you sitting there with a nonworking fire extinguisher on the wall when the first hot bid came in) and an electrical inspection to verify that your cobweb of wires under the desk met code. And you needed an inspection from the Occupational Safety and Health Administration to make sure that your office area complied with worker safety. After all, we wouldn't want you getting a splinter in your hind end from the makeshift plywood desk when you jumped up after that first hot bid bleeped onto your screen.

Do you see where I'm going with this? If we had such regulations, would eBay exist? No, of course not. I'm not here trying to advertise for eBay — I've never been on it and don't know how to get on it anyway, but I'm aware of what's going on and I know eBay is a big thing. It certainly represents innovation, and some would say wonderful innovation. The point is that it exists because it was developed as a prototype and can be accessed as a prototype from existing, low-investment infrastructure (i.e., your home computer). Wrap a bunch of regulations around it, and it would go away as surely as snow in July.

Now let's go back to food. Let's say I have some chickens in the backyard to eat my kitchen scraps and the damaged vegetables from my garden. I have extra eggs, and I have neighbors who don't have the skill, time, or desire to cook. I'd like to take my extra eggs and some vegetables and make quiche for these neighbors. I've made quiche all my life for myself and my family. Occasionally I make one and give it away to friends when a loved one dies and neighbors bring food. Folks at church say my quiche is to die for.

My neighbors, who hear about this new idea, are delighted and desperate to know when I'll start. They are ready to buy. I'm ready to make quiche. Only one problem: I don't have a freestanding licensed commercial kitchen. Not only that, I'm in a residential zone that prohibits businesses. I would have to be rezoned, then build a $50,000 self-standing commercial kitchen out where my garden is. Well, that would take away from growing space.

And not only that, I would need to submit Hazardous Analysis and Critical Control Point (HACCP) plans to bureaucrats, who would agree or disagree with my protocol. They might tell me I have to wash the eggs in chlorine. My customers don't want chlorine in their eggs. They might tell me I have to wash my vegetables in chlorine. My customers don't want chlorine on their vegetables.

They might tell me I can't use a compost pile for fertilizer because compost piles are not "science-based." Besides, compost piles are dirty, unsterile. It's more science-based and safer to use chemical fertilizers and pesticides. That would be approved, you see. Not this Luddite backwards stuff like compost piles and wood ash powder. Obviously, my fledgling quiche business is not going to get off the ground. Folks, this ain't normal.

No culture has ever put this kind of heavy-handed requirement on food. What started as a regulation to control industry has instead become the tool industry uses to eliminate innovation in the food marketplace. I could keep you up the rest of the day with examples of this, but my book *Everything I Want to Do Is Illegal* is the unabridged version of this chapter. Get it and read it. For the sake of brevity, I'm going to stay with the broader issue here, the abnormality of food police.

The single biggest reason local integrity food does not enjoy a larger share in the modern American marketplace is due to these nonscalable regulations. Farmers are ready and willing to produce for local markets, and they have the knowledge to do it. Consumers (or coproducers, as Carlo Petrini, founder of Slow Food, calls them) are ready and willing to buy. But between these two parties exists a labyrinth of capricious, nonsensical, malicious, ridiculous — let's see how many adjectives I can think of — asinine, unreasonable regulations that preclude commerce.

Make no mistake, these regulations are not about food safety. They are about market access. How else can you justify that all these items are fine to give away? You can give away raw milk, homemade pickles, quiche, whatever. Giving them away to neighbors and friends is considered patriotic and model citizenry, but if any money changes hands, suddenly you're peddling a hazardous substance and intend to kill people with your recklessness.

You can go out on a 70-degree November day and gut-shoot a deer with Creutzfeld-Jakob disease (the deer equivalent of mad cow), gut it out on the ground, and drag it a mile through the squirrel dung, sticks, and rocks, tie it down to the hood of your Land Rover for a hot afternoon showoff romp through town, then pull it up in a backyard tree where it hangs for a week under birds that roost in the branches; then skin it out, cut it up, and feed it to your children and all your children's friends. That's being a great American.

But try dressing a grass-fed beef in the cleanliness of an unlicensed backyard abattoir and sell one T-bone steak to a neighbor who helps you dress it and cut it up, and you're a criminal. With other hazardous or regulated substances, the prohibitions for commerce apply equally on buyer and seller. For example, with both prescription and illicit drugs, prohibitions exist on both buyer and seller. If you could somehow acquire a box full of prescription drugs, you couldn't just use them or give them to friends. Ditto for cocaine. Jeopardy exists to both have it and sell it.

With food, however, the prohibitions are all one-sided. If you can acquire pickles or quiche or raw milk that's fine, and you can even feed it to your children. The prohibitions are only on the seller — that would be the farmer, or in the above case, the quiche maker. The point is that in other potentially hazardous substances, the money transaction has nothing to do with the legality of the substance. It is a controlled substance and exchanging money has no bearing. In food, however, this is not the case. You can donate the quiche to a local fire department potluck, or a fund-raiser, or give it to friends, and that's all perfectly legal — even applauded. But if you take a penny for the quiche, suddenly it's a hazardous substance that needs a plethora of government oversight. Clearly, the food safety laws are not about safety, but about regulating market access. What is it about exchanging money that suddenly makes the food hazardous?

That the food police are not interested in safety could be no better illustrated than the fact that putting "rBGH-free" on milk labels to show that the hormone trademarked Prosilac had not been injected into cows was deemed illegal. A friend of mine operating a CSA had a couple of beeves processed for his shareholders under custom regulations (the butcher is processing my own animal to be returned to me), and the food police swooped down to impound the product. The inspectors accused him of selling illegal meat because it wasn't processed under government inspection. They wouldn't even let him eat the meat or give it to a homeless shelter — he had to throw it in the landfill. This was simply a labeling-procedural technicality. There was absolutely nothing wrong with that meat.

I have a friend in Florida who was raided for selling raw dairy. Mind you, his customers wanted this product, of their own free will. Eventually Florida let him register these products as pet food and he is selling them just fine. Everybody knows they are not going to pets. These raw dairy products are going to people, of course. If it really is a dangerous substance, don't you think the government would stop it? Why was it hazardous when people were buying it outright, but suddenly it's fine in this pet food charade? None of this is about food safety; it's about regulating market access.

Creekstone Farms in Missouri, a small beef processing plant, shipped most of its product to Japan. When Japan closed its door to U.S. beef due to mad cow in this country, Creekstone wanted to test every single animal it processed. Japan said they'd buy them. But the USDA enjoined the universal testing, declaring that it would establish precedent for other processors that would be too hard to meet. In other words, the USDA couldn't afford to have anyone do something innovative. Unbelievable.

One of the restaurants that buys our pastured chicken serves chicken sandwiches at lunch. They cook the chicken and make a salad to put on the bread. A health department official walked in, stuck her thermometer in the salad, and declared it was one degree too warm and had to be discarded on the spot. Now, gentle folks, you know as well as I do that one degree over cold holding temperature for five minutes is not going to create a safety problem. If that were the case, everyone who has ever made chicken salad in their home kitchen would be sick. Welcome to the real world of the food police.

A big issue confronting local school lunch sourcing is seasonal variations and flexible availability. The food police want the menus displayed two months in advance. Schools trying to use local products don't always know what's going to be available two months in advance. If they change the menu, they're written up for noncompliance. An infraction of food police laws. Imagine that.

The reason I don't go to farmers' markets anymore is because I got tired of the food police coming down and poking thermometers in my display eggs. "Two degrees above cold holding temperature. You must discard that dozen."

"Well, actually, ma'am, this is my display carton. I'm pulling my eggs out of this cooler behind me."

"I can't trust you for that. You have to discard this dozen right now, in front of me, while I watch."

"Okay, and see if I come back to farmers' market anymore." And I didn't. Come back, that is.

I have a friend with an abattoir and one day his employee who was supposed to check the carcass chill room temperature every two hours failed to check it at the 2 p.m. time. The paperwork went across the food police desk with that one box not checked. The food police wanted the entire contents of the room discarded — more than $20,000 worth of meat. The temperature was perfect at the noon check and at the 4 p.m. check. It wasn't reasonable to assume there had been a spike at the 2 p.m. time. The intervention of a senator finally halted an otherwise heinous reaction.

I could go on like this for a day. The point is that the food police are naturally prejudiced against small operators. Many people don't realize that in a culture that worships industrial efficiency, the same mentality rules at the food police. The last time I testified at a congressional hearing in Washington, D.C., about food safety, the head of the FSIS was the first of us to testify. It turned my stomach to hear him gloat about how much more efficient his department had become since most of the local and small-scale community abattoirs had been eliminated.

They actually measure their efficiency in pounds of product per inspector-hour. Now folks, if you're trying to decide if something is okay or not, and you measure success in terms of volume per hour, how much inspection do you think is going on? Precious little. It's a factory mentality applied to meat inspection. With that kind of benchmark for success, you can see why FSIS harasses small outfits and gives a pass to the big ones. By their own admission, the food police despise running around to smaller processing plants. They will do all they can to get rid of these pesky, inefficient facilities. This is an embedded prejudice that no legislation can stop.

A friend started a processing facility and was closed down after one week for being too slow. Gentle people, inspection requirements don't say anything about speed. I thought we were interested in clean food. After he put up all his capital, mortgaged his farm, worked twenty-hour days, jumped through every hoop the food police threw at him, they concocted this totally illegal hurdle: You're too slow. This is outrageous.

These small community-based abattoirs are absolutely essential to legally get meat and poultry to local markets. In fact, the one that Teresa and I own with our partner Joe Cloud in Harrisonburg, T&E Meats, was originally owned by an aging couple who had run it for more than forty years and we bought it in 2008. When we took over there were nineteen employees, and twelve were older than seventy.

We formed Salatin&Cloud LLC and kept the name T&E, which stood for Tommy and Erma May, the former owners. We changed it to True and Essential Meats and began the difficult task of changing from the cheapest place in town to the best place in town. We bought it because it was headed out of business. An aging owner, no succession plan, and a geriatric workforce. When your business is handling thousands of pounds of meat, you need people younger than seventy.

My partner Joe became the general manager and we've fortunately steered the company through two years of get-acquainted financial hemorrhaging. Without this plant, Polyface would have had to travel twice as far or more to get animals processed in order to legally sell them. I meet people all over the nation traveling two hundred miles one way just to get animals processed so they can legally sell the meat. This is another permutation of the food police hurdles against local food systems, and the main reason why local meats are much more expensive than their industrial supermarket counterparts.

At T&E Meats, we are desperate to preserve this embedded custom butchering service for our community. Although Polyface is right now the largest customer, we process meat for anybody who wants the service. Our aged plant is in need of massive infrastructure upgrades, but we've finally turned a couple of profitable months and we're optimistic about 2011. If we can hang in there and be profitable, we will have the satisfaction of preserving a seamless abattoir in the Shenandoah Valley.

When I ask Joe, who is there every day and has a better feel for day-to-day operations, what he fears most, it's increasing government regulations that will require infrastructure we can't afford in our little facility. That includes reading directives and handling food police paperwork that for us is the same as it is for a 5,000-head-per-day processor in Nebraska. The only difference is we don't have the volume over which to spread the paperwork overhead. When the food police decide that a $10,000 head gate is necessary, the big outfit installs it with pocket change. For us, that's two months' profit.

Recently our farm took a small boar hog to process for a church picnic barbecue. We had accidentally missed him when the rest received their male alteration procedure (castration). The inspector threw out the hog — I mean, threw it away into the rendering barrel — because our plant did not have a separate boar hog HACCP plan. Joe didn't know we needed one. Nobody bothered to tell him because we don't have full-time employees to read all the fine print. If we'd known, we would have just backyard-dressed that hog here at the farm and used it for the church barbecue. Folks, this stuff will make you crazy.

These food police don't give a hoot whether our plant is profitable or not, but they have complete authority to shut us down in a heartbeat if they see anything they don't like. In our small plant, though, they actually see things. When I was testifying in that congressional hearing, the head of the inspection workers said that the big plants have cameras and walkie-talkies to warn the different parts of the plant of the whereabouts of the inspectors. That way they can hide things. In our plant, we don't have different divisions, walkie-talkies, and cameras.

I was up at the plant the other day talking to Joe about business when two federal inspection agents walked in, unannounced, flashed their badges, and began asking questions:

"Is this plant inspected?"

I could scarcely contain myself. Here Joe and I were engrossed in an important discussion, in our business, and these two yo-yos walk in off the street without even the courtesy to call, asking the stupidest question anybody could ask. Any bozo could look up our establishment number, confirm our status as a federally inspected plant. Am I wrong to be incensed by this harassment? Remember, people, this is the agency that whines about not having enough manpower to do proper inspections. Hogwash. If they have time to send two agents from out of state and ask if T&E is an inspected plant, they have time to go places that really need it. We have an assigned inspector in the plant every day. These guys could have found out who it was. Honestly, I can't find words to describe how ridiculous this is.

Are you ready for the second question? Here you go: "What do you all do? What is your business?"

I couldn't stand it. Joe, bless his heart, kept his composure and patiently answered their questions. I left. They stayed for half an hour, asking the most senseless questions you can imagine. A kindergartner could not be more childish. And these people draw fat government paychecks that you and I pay for with our taxes. I agree with Jefferson: We need a revolution about every fifty years. I think it's long overdue.

Our little abattoir is the link between any farmer and a school cafeteria that wants to be supplied with local beef or pork. The link between farmer and restaurant. The link between farmer and homeowner. Very few patrons want a live pig showing up on their doorstep. They prefer packages of sausage and pork chops, thank you very much, and the place that people in our multicounty area go to for this service is T&E Meats, long may it survive. Bless you, Joe and staff, for making it happen every day. Polyface would be in dire straits without you.

Let's get this straight. Every time the culture decides through popular vote to ask for government penetration into the marketplace, it creates a climate that pushes the biggest players to curry concessionary privileges with the regulators. The little players don't have the clout, manpower, or capital to arm-twist. The big players do. And that is why every time, every time, every time — should I say it once more? — every time the public asks for government oversight, it eventuates in the bigger players getting more power and the smaller players being kicked in the teeth.

Did smaller players become stronger or weaker as a result of the Bush-Obama bank bailout plan? The big players got more powerful, made unprecedented amounts of profit, and smaller banks lost market share. I don't understand how people who disbelieve the Pentagon can suddenly believe what the Environmental Protection Agency says, or the FSIS, or the Treasury Department, or any other bureaucracy. For some reason, a fancy name, like Homeland Security, engenders trust. People want to believe these agencies actually do something positive. In the end, though, the cure is worse than the disease. This is why limited government was the name of the game when the U.S. Constitution was written.

Will the new government-controlled health care plan allow alternative procedures and encourage nonhospital use? Don't believe it. As a culture we have become brainwashed with this notion that the government knows best. Ultimately, the food police idea assumes that the government is more trustworthy than the marketplace or business. What is the first thing said by the CEO of a company embroiled in a nationwide food recall? You know what it is: "We've complied with every government food safety requirement."

The government penetration into this sphere creates a fraternity of shared ideas. The revolving door of people between the industry/regulatory worlds is not only real, but ubiquitous. This explains the very real anti-small and anti-innovation sentiment within the agencies. It also explains why the big players seem to get a free pass.

We have entered an unmistaken Food Inquisition in America. Heritage and traditional food production and processing techniques are coming under fire as jeopardizing so-called scientific procedures.

I've said it before and I'll say it again. We need a food NRA (National Rifle Association). The only reason we don't have a food NRA is because Americans generally feel much more vulnerable when they lose their guns than when they lose their food. The fact is we've lost our homegrown foods, our local canneries, our abattoirs in every community, our cottage-industry bologna and jerky. We've lost our healthy food system, and while we reach for Twinkies and Coca-Cola, we think we're being fed. Folks, this ain't normal.

Think about this: How many times has the official government food pyramid changed in the last couple of decades? Do you agree with it? Probably my favorite credentialed dietician in the country is Joan Gussow, professor emeritus at Columbia University. She's been feeding herself from her own backyard for years and now discards much of the official government nutritional paradigm. She now believes that some of the things she used to teach were incorrect. She's one of the most honest food experts I know. Her books should be read by everyone.

Now think about the farm bill — what Michael Pollan says should be called the food bill. Think about the official government policies, types of food promoted, subsidized, encouraged. Now let me ask you a question: Is this the food you think we should eat? In other words, if the USDA or FDA formulated your meals, would you be happy? Can you imagine anything else you might want to add? Anything you might want to subtract? These are the people who won't allow transgenic modification delineated on a label; won't allow cloning delineated on a label. Do you want your meals picked by these people?

If the answer is no or even a hesitation, remember that the philosophy that gives the government the right to determine what we can and can't ingest in fats, for example, will be the same one that determines what we can and can't ingest in vegetables.

To the consternation of all my religious right friends, I am a staunch defender of legalized drugs. All of them. A government that tells me I can't smoke dope can also tell me I can't eat compost-grown tomatoes. All it takes is someone to be hurt by compost-grown tomatoes and the whole culture demonizes compost-grown tomatoes. In 2001 and 2004 a salmonella outbreak traceable to one 9,000-acre pistachio-almond farm, the biggest in the United States, resulted in the mandatory steam heating, or fumigation with propylene oxide (an EPA-registered carcinogen), of all raw almonds. The almonds are still labeled raw. Independent growers who direct market have been haggling with the food police for years to preserve their freedom to sell real raw almonds.

By the way, foreign growers are exempted from the rule. As a result, domestic growers have lost huge market share to imported almonds. Did somebody say something about free markets? The point is that the largest grower in the country abused nature's parameters, and as a result, every grower is being forced away from raw almonds. Didn't you just love it in school when a student broke a rule and the teacher punished everyone for the infraction? Oh yes, that's my favorite kind of justice.

The independent almond growers finally won a small victory. It's been a long uphill battle, waged by the Cornucopia Institute, a seat-of-the-pants organic watchdog group, but finally a federal district court in

2010 ruled that it was okay for farmers to take the USDA to court over the mandatory almond pasteurizing rule. Remember, the alleged culprit in the case was the largest industrial grower in the United States. Who got hurt? The little guys. Go, Cornucopia.

Fortunately, these days we do in fact have a food NRA, and it's called the Farm-to-Consumer Legal Defense Fund (FTCLD). It is to traditional foods what the Home School Legal Defense Assocation (HSLDA) was to homeschoolers in 1980. One is trying to preserve food choice; the other was about preserving educational choice. The educational choice issue took a decade to win, but it finally did. The food choice issue is in the early stages, and may be just as long a battle, but I'm one guy who intends to win.

I quote from a memo sent by Sally Fallon Morell, founder of the Weston A. Price Foundation:

February 19, 2010 the Farm-to-Consumer Legal Defense Fund filed a lawsuit against the Food and Drug Administration (FDA) and the United States Department of Health and Human Services to challenge federal regulations banning the transport and sale of raw milk across state lines. On April 26, FDA filed its response to the lawsuit, providing a public record of what the agency's views on food freedom of choice really are.

Here are some of FDA's shocking claims:
- "There is no absolute right to consume or feed children any particular food."
- Plaintiffs' assertion of a "fundamental right to their own bodily and physical health, which includes what foods they do and do not choose to consume for themselves and their families" is similarly unavailing because plaintiffs do not have a fundamental right to obtain any food they wish.
- There is no "deeply rooted" historical tradition of unfettered access to foods of all kinds.

In this official, written, legal response, the FDA makes its position about food choice extremely clear. No American has a right to choose what to eat. Does that bother you? Please tell me it does, especially when this agency now has more power than ever due to the recent 2010

Food Safety Modernization Act. According to the government, laid out here in plain English in court documents, I have no right to freedom of food choice. That means the government owns my body. The government has the right to choose what I can and cannot eat.

And what might this be? Pastured poultry? Raw milk? Compost-fertilized vegetables? Raw almonds? Not on your life. You see, dear people, we must be very careful what stirs us to righteous indignation. In my opinion, probably the single biggest blow to America's food system came with Prohibition, because it forever gave the government control over what we could and could not consume. In that action, the die was cast.

Until then, freedom of food choice was a foregone conclusion in our culture. But once well-intentioned, righteously indignant people decided it was okay for the bureaucrats to crawl between my lips and my throat, criminalizing any other substance du jour was acceptable. This conditioned the nation to accept more and more restrictions until today you can hardly spit without a license.

Be assured that the values on which food police will base their regulations will not be local-friendly, ecology-friendly, or nutrition-friendly. Their paradigm will be based on germ theory. It will be based on the notion that the laboratory knows much better than traditional wisdom. That manipulation of DNA is far superior to respecting the traditional wisdom contained in the native DNA. After all, President Obama named Michael Taylor, the longtime Monsanto attorney who shepherded transgenic modification into the world, as his food czar. Taylor will be officially interpreting what the Food Modernization Act's demand for "science-based" food requirements means. This phrase, brand-new in history, is used eleven times in the final law. Whose science will it be?

Look at what the food police and their fraternal agencies have already promoted for the last several decades: The unilateral chemicalizing of America's farmlands and lawns. The indiscriminate use of DDT, Roundup, and a host of other deadly chemicals. Chemical fertilizer. Feeding dead cows to cows. Subtherapeutic and indiscriminate antibiotic feeding to livestock. Fumigated vegetable fields. Gassing citrus. Concentrated animal feeding operations. Mandatory irradiation (if they could get it). Transgenic modification. High-fructose corn syrup.

This is a frightening list that represents the overriding science from the government food policy and food police for yea these several decades. Folks, not only is this not normal, it is deadly. Do we really expect these people, operating with this mentality, to actually protect our food from pathogenicity?

The antidote to the pathogen recalls of today is the same as it was in 1906. Withdraw government penetration and the specter of cronyism, let the food system stand on its own two feet. Yes, there will be dirty players. There always have been and always will be. Just because you put a backwards collar on a man doesn't mean he won't chase the church secretary.

At this point, the people who think the government knows best throw up their hands and say, "Well, what do you suggest, just letting everyone sell anything they want, like one big free-for-all, buyer beware and who cares?"

In short, yes. But wait. I'm too much a realist to think that would happen. So here are some ideas that would get us off this dilemma of non-scalable regulations and a factory efficiency mentality prejudiced against small producers.

1. **We should go to empirical benchmarks.** Right now, if you want to sell wheat to Pillsbury for human consumption, it can only contain so many rat turds per ton. The FDA prescribes tolerance levels for all sorts of things in granola and breakfast cereals. If your material is clean enough, it doesn't matter whether you have a hundred pounds or a hundred tons, if it's clean, it's clean. Isn't that what we're after?

   Why do we have to prescribe infrastructure in processing? The fact is, the smaller the operation, the easier it is to keep clean. At our T&E Meats, we process one animal at a time. We spray down the floor between each one. We aren't stacking them up and killing multiples at a time. It's much cleaner than a big operation. Just establish so many parts per million of pathogen, or whatever, and let that be it.

   I proposed this to our area federal meat inspector several years ago and he said, "That would absolutely work, but I wouldn't be needed. No, I'd oppose that." You see, in the final analysis, the sniff and glance is really about job security. If industry can't hide behind inspectors anymore, it will force the industry to be cleaner because now it's their own responsibility instead of someone else's. We can take swab tests, pass them through an R2D2 machine that scans infrared transmissions from bacteria. The technology is here. Remember, the government is always the last to embrace new technologies. The whole point of government is to maintain the status quo. That's why the government technology systems are always behind the industry.

In the ecological agriculture movement, government bulletins are always about ten years behind the industry innovators. It can't go in a government publication until it's gone through double-blind testing and half a dozen committees. By that time, it's already behind the times. I always tell farmers who want the latest information, "Stay away from government offices. They will only give you first-generation stuff."

If the goal is clean food, who cares how many pounds of stainless steel wraps around it? Who cares how many lumens are bearing down? When we had our chickens empirically tested for bacteria culture at the lab, ours were twenty-five times cleaner than the ones in the supermarket. If I can gut chickens in the kitchen sink to a given standard, who cares as long as they are clean? Are we really after clean, or are we after something called denial of market access to upstart innovators? Hmmmmmm?

2. **We could do a periodic test to make sure internal controls are working.** This is a step down from the above, or maybe it's done in conjunction with it. The sticky point here is, who pays for the test? This is a roundabout way the big boys have figured out how to eliminate the competition — expensive testing.

A $500 test once a week is nothing if you're running a $500 million processing plant. But if it's a $1 million mom-and-pop like T&E Meats, that's the entire week's profit. This is a part of food safety that the sincere-minded consumer advocates don't understand. The reason America has lost half of its community-based processing capacities each of the three times the FSIS has been overhauled is because each time, the increasingly onerous regulations have run the little guys out of business.

Now that the local food scene is gaining momentum, start-ups are having to run through a gauntlet that didn't exist for their predecessors and it's exponentially harder to get the business launched in an embryonic form. In order to pay for the regulatory overhead, the start-up must be too big to be birthed. I meet thousands of farmers a year who are ready and willing to bring their local, ecologically friendly food to their community, but they are denied by the capital-intensive and paperwork requirements to birth their dream. Embryos too big do not get birthed, and that is the tragedy of this anti-small prejudiced food police climate. The big guys are desperate to make sure they are protected from entrepreneurial savvy.

Sincere-minded consumer advocates play right into their hands. During the debates over the Food Safety Modernization Act in late 2010, the industry lined right up behind this legislation. Why? Because they were between a rock and a hard place. What if you were the CEO of an industrial food conglomerate? How would you explain to America that you were opposed to increased food safety regulations?

This is where I part company with all my friends who point their fingers at big business and yell, "Conspiracy!" I point my finger at consumer advocates and yell, "Gullibility!" Make no mistake about it, industry does not push for regulations unless and until it feels threatened in the marketplace. As soon as the industry can quantify that threat, it starts the spin rolling to get government intervention that will once again restore confidence in the product. Unfortunately, the naïve and well-meaning consumer advocacy organizations play right into the big boys' hands and actually do much of the dirty work so the industry doesn't have to waste time crafting the legislation.

When this legislation gave the FDA the right to inspect farms without a warrant to ascertain if any procedures violate what is considered "science-based," whose science do you think will be followed? The science that says irradiation changes enzymes and is carcinogenic, or the science that says, like it usually does, "We've tested these procedures and found no credible evidence that there's a problem." Of course, they call irradiation "cold pasteurization" to mask its insidious reality. Talk about cleverspeak.

For the life of me I can't understand why the consumer advocates think it's a good thing when the food manufacturing associations and the industrial food trade organizations join them in the friends circle. Wouldn't you think if the ugly, untrustworthy industry joined up, they must know something you don't? But no, these do-gooders whistle along their way, totally oblivious to the fact that they've been taken in by the industry and that the smart industry has used them to further lock out upstart entrepreneurs.

3. **We could simply have a constitutional amendment that guarantees Americans the right to choose and procure their own food.** Essentially, this would be a freedom of food choice amendment. The only reason we don't have one in this country is because the writers of the Constitution and the Bill of Rights could not have envisioned a day when a neighbor could not sell a gallon of milk from their milk cow to another neighbor across the fence. Even a neighbor who helped milk the cow. Trust me, Thomas Jefferson would roll over in his grave.

Patrick Henry would call what we have now slavery. We could call this amendment a Food Emancipation Proclamation because it would free all the food currently enslaved by bureaucrats. Lest you think you have a lot of choice, consider how hard it is to get raw milk. Homemade pickles. Homemade soups or stew. This list could go on and on and on, but the fact is that our choices are extremely limited.

If a person wants to patronize the government system and eat only government-sanctioned food, then that's fine. Let them do it. But if someone wants food that is not government-sanctioned, she has a right — an inalienable right — as owner of her own body, to acquire what she sees fit. When a bureaucrat gets between my lips and my throat, I call that an invasion of privacy.

For those who fear that such a policy would fill our hospitals with cases of food poisoning, I simply say: Let's try it. If it does, we can deal with the problem. If instead it empties our hospitals, well, that would be a good thing. That brings me to number four.

4. **Pass federal legislation allowing community-based prototypes for intrajurisdictional commerce.** In other words, if my

county wants to try a local food commerce prototype, allowing anyone to buy anything from anyone within the confines of our county, it should be free to do so without jeopardizing federal education funds, highway funds, and other interjursdictional food commerce.

We're back to the prototyping again. The unregulated local commerce folks are at a significant disadvantage in asking for freer local food networking because we don't have a track record of food safety. The only thing we have is that the country operated very well for 150 years without food police and it wasn't until long-distance industrial conglomerates entered the picture that the food police were requested.

With historical precedent, therefore, I would say that prior to industrialization there was no compelling interest for food police. By inference, I would suggest that those kinds of food systems don't require policing. But that's conjecture. It may just be, I admit, that an inspection-free intrajurisdictional food commerce would land everybody in the mortuary. But I would argue that it is just as plausible that it would empty the hospitals because people would eat healthier food.

It would stimulate jobs in local canneries and the cottage industry. It would keep dollars at home, making the local economy boom. Local farmers would quit selling out to development because they would be able to value-add. Indeed, their sons and daughters would return to thriving family businesses. What if all this happened? Then another locality could duplicate. And another. And another.

Right now, with these overburdensome top-down federal food safety laws, a locality can't legally do something innovative like this. The federal agents will swarm in and shut the freedom down — all in the name of protecting safety, of course. That's just wrong. A community that wants to opt out should have the freedom to do so. How a culture treats its lunatic fringe, the ones who want to do something different, says a lot about whether it is a free society or a tyranny. Ours is close to becoming a tyranny, if it's not already there. My friends in China say the food system there is much, much more free than it is here in America.

We've become too sophisticated for our own good. We've analyzed and studied and data-processed until we've lost sight of the big picture. The big picture is about leaving the door open to new ideas and out-of-the box solutions. Federal food policy currently does not allow innovative localized prototyping, and that is plain wrong.

5. **We could let people waive their governmental ownership and cast themselves on their own recognizance.** The reason our culture doesn't want to allow food freedom of choice is because the government runs health care. I can assure you, after having talked to many food police, they sincerely believe that the hospitals will fill up if we start eating from our gardens and cooking things from scratch. I have documents from food police saying that people are simply too ignorant to make food choices. Again, for a more in-depth discussion of this issue, read my book *Everything I Want to Do Is Illegal.*

Government agents truly believe they must protect us from our own ignorance. One of our farm's customers testified at a hearing in Richmond a few years ago that he believes most of what's in the supermarket is hazardous to his health. And it's all government-sanctioned. The cloud of fear that hovers over people when I mention food freedom of choice is palpable. I understand the fear if you're ignorant, but ignorance can be overcome. You can actually learn about food, farming, cooking, preserving, and processing. Your grandmother knew about all these things and she didn't have the gadgetry or the Internet — or this book — to help her.

Invariably, somebody is going to choose something harmful. It might be from a dirty farmer. It might be something injurious, like a poisonous mushroom. But look, people, with childhood leukemia at epidemic proportions, unprecedented obesity, Type II diabetes, and more than half the population on drugs, don't you think it might be worth testing another option besides government-sanctioned industrial sterility? Could it be that government-approved food is killing us? I guess as long as it's slowly enough to give us time to buy pharmaceuticals, that's a good thing.

I propose that anyone who wants to waive their rights of societal ownership should be able to do so. Sign a paper like a living will that I absolve society of ownership over my body. I do not expect society — taxpayers — to pick up the tab for my illness. I will be fully responsible for my health and my food. If I get sick from drinking raw milk, my neighbors aren't liable and if I go to the emergency room, they don't have to treat me and pass the costs on to anybody. I'm completely on my own.

In order for this to work, of course, we would have to allow a totally independent health care system. A totally private, nongovernmental system. Not licensed in any way. These hospitals can play Beethoven into my subcutaneous tissue, and stick acupuncture needles in my ears. The government has no control over this medical care network. If this totally private medical facility can't help me, I can't go to the government. I've already waived any access to public funding and public charity.

You see, when we start down this path, the ugly head of tyranny raises its head, doesn't it? Suddenly we see how we've been duped. Those of you who want to deny me ownership of my own body, the right to choose my own medical care, the right to inform my own destiny — by what authority do you deny me these basic rights of human dignity and individuality? What right have you to demand my pound of flesh?

I hope as we conclude this discussion, you can begin to see just how duped we've been. Here we thought all along that food safety was about me protecting me. Actually, it's about somebody else owning me. Americans voluntarily, eagerly, giving up ownership and autonomy over their own bodies just ain't normal.

Until the last few years, our culture was content to let the local, transparent, traditional, normal food system coexist with the radicalized, industrial, abnormal system. You could shop where you wanted and it was okay. That is fast becoming a thing of the past. Today, this rise of the Church of Industrial Food, with its codification of orthodoxy, threatens to put us heretics on the rack. It is, in fact, beginning to round us up. I think the normal side now could consider itself natives. The

U.S. Cavalry, under the guise of the food police, want us on the reservation where they can keep a good eye on us.

What's wrong with living in a teepee? What's wrong with taking herbal remedies instead of bleeding with leeches? What's wrong with learning how to survive in the wilderness over learning how to recite poetry and figure algebra? What's wrong with different?

Historical normalcy, I argue, is labeled different today. It's even considered heresy by many. Here is what I think. Long after we've experimented with the final bizarre thing to feed cows, they will still do best eating grass. After we've exhausted the drugs, vaccines, and transgenic modification, our animals will still want to express their distinctives, live in historically normal habitats, and fill their traditional role.

Long after the final i-gadget has been discovered, we'll still yearn for hugs, kisses, and personal conversations. When we've traveled to the last exotic place and finished participating in the last recreational or entertainment venue on our list, we will want a haven and we will call it home.

Last fall I went to New Zealand and Australia for a one-month speaking tour. I haven't been gone from this farm or from my family for that long since college. I'm a much more anchored person now. As Teresa and I drove out the lane that morning to go to the airport, I broke down, sobbing uncontrollably. She gently held me and we sat there in the car for several minutes, at the lane entrance, as the depth of these emotions flooded over me.

I finally managed a tearful, "I just love this place." She knew what I meant. It wasn't just this farm, the land — it was everything. It was my grandkids, my kids, my mother, the cows, the chickens, the trees, the grass, the interns, the apprentices. It was my nest, my pantry full of home-canned food, my freezers full of homegrown meat. It was being able to be home and not drive anywhere. It was being completely satisfied in my surroundings, acquainted with the creeks, the hillsides, the terrain, the buildings.

It was my normal. It was historical normal. Today I fear that none of us gets that well acquainted with our place to be this intimate with it. I knew I would miss the earthworm castings and the ducks on the ponds. I started this book with the idea that I've become an anachronism. As the rest of the culture runs helter-skelter, always seeking something outside, demanding care from others, I have found contentment and satisfaction in this place.

I'm surrounded by loving family — multiple generations. I'm surrounded by enthusiastic young people. I'm surrounded by land that I've watched heal over these last fifty years, from a worn-out, gullied mess to verdant pastures supporting poultry, cows, pigs, and rabbits. The intensity of my feelings springs from the intimacy of my knowledge of this place, its surroundings, the weather patterns, the seasons. I believe this is historically normal, and I covet that for others. Now go be a normal person.

Acknowledgments

This book has grown out of a lifetime of different thinking. I do not view that as a curse, but a real blessing. For that I thank my parents, William and Lucille. Although Dad passed away in 1988, his spirit lives here at Polyface still, inspiring and encouraging us to blaze our own trail. Mom, your speaking and theatrical bent have shaped me in profound ways that I am just beginning to fully appreciate.

Teresa, love of my life, wife, partner, and sufferer through all my differentness — thank you. Especially, I appreciate your traditional homemaking and spiritual values that anchor our family in historical normalcy. Our children, Daniel and Rachel, have now passed through the "shake your head and roll your eyes" stage — thank you for being your own individuals and carrying on these traditional values. Daughter-in-law Sheri is a coconspirator in these abnormal times.

Thank you to our winter apprentices and staff who picked up slack especially for me so I could write this winter: Ethan Kelly, Eric Barth, Kristen Long, Brie Aronson, and Wendy Gray.

A special thanks to Lisa DiMona, literary agent extraordinaire, who believed in me several years ago and patiently groomed this project to fruition. This never would have happened without you. Although I've written and self-published seven books, I've never had an editor. What a privilege it's been to work with Center Street editor Kate Hartson, who has shepherded this project from the beginning. Everyone who ends up buying and enjoying this book needs to understand that Lisa and Kate have pushed me beyond anything I would have dreamed on my own — you both are special gifts in my life.

Beyond these named individuals, a whole host of people, both living and deceased, have shaped my thinking with their lives, their examples, and their legacy. Each of us is a composite of our life experiences and awareness. Mine has been especially rich, and I thank you all.

Index